55 Cases in Neurology

55 Cases in Neurology

Case Histories and Patient Perspectives

Mark McCarron
Ulster University

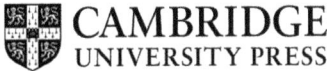

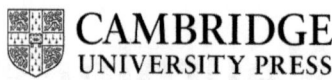

CAMBRIDGE
UNIVERSITY PRESS

Shaftesbury Road, Cambridge CB2 8EA, United Kingdom

One Liberty Plaza, 20th Floor, New York, NY 10006, USA

477 Williamstown Road, Port Melbourne, VIC 3207, Australia

314–321, 3rd Floor, Plot 3, Splendor Forum, Jasola District Centre, New Delhi – 110025, India

103 Penang Road, #05–06/07, Visioncrest Commercial, Singapore 238467

Cambridge University Press is part of Cambridge University Press & Assessment, a department of the University of Cambridge.

We share the University's mission to contribute to society through the pursuit of education, learning and research at the highest international levels of excellence.

www.cambridge.org
Information on this title: www.cambridge.org/9781009214117
DOI: 10.1017/9781009214131

First published 2023

A catalogue record for this publication is available from the British Library.

ISBN 978-1-009-21411-7 Paperback

Contents

*Colour plates can be found between
pages 214 and 215*

Preface

Case reports remain the cornerstone of learning clinical neurology. Although they are less frequently reported in medical and neurological journals, conferences and neurology departments continue to employ case reports as a teaching tool, reflecting the daily experience of neurologists. So why another neurology case report textbook?

Advances in neuroimaging, evolving diagnostic criteria and differential diagnoses, patient access to neurologists in district general hospitals, increasing evidence-based management of neurological disorders and better recognition of patient experience and contribution to management all prompted this collection of case reports aligned with patient perspectives.

While some of the case reports of rare and uncommon neurological disorders have been presented locally (Altnagelvin Area Hospital) and at a regional neuroscience centre (Royal Victoria Hospital, Belfast), common presentations are deliberately included to reflect the daily experience of patients and neurologists. With that in mind, the book is aimed at junior doctors, medical research fellows considering a career in neurology and early neurology trainees.

The 55 case reports are not meant to be a comprehensive neurology collection but rather a glimpse at current neurology practice, including clinical clues, neuroradiology findings and test characteristics of diagnostic investigations. The layout of the history, examination and preliminary investigations allows the reader to think about the potential diagnosis or differential diagnosis before reading about the neurological condition and what happened to the patient.

The author is responsible for any errors. Any learning is to the credit of the patient and reader.

Acknowledgements

55 Cases in Neurology came to print thanks to the generous support, encouragement and reviews from a wide range of colleagues. I am indebted to Dr Peter Flynn (neuroradiology), Dr Gavin McCluskey (neurologist), Dr Ferghal McVerry (neurologist) and Dr Peter McCarron (epidemiologist and psychiatrist) for their timely and critical reviews.

Other colleagues who made important contributions include Stephen Payne (medical photographer), Carrie Wade (personal assistant), Dr Ali Benmusa (pathologist), Dr Brian Herron (neuropathologist) and Rory Durnin (graphic artist). I offer special thanks to the staff of Cambridge University Press for their guidance through the project and their editorial work.

Finally, and most importantly, I thank the patients and relatives who took the time to contribute the patient perspectives in order to educate all of us about the experience of living with a neurological illness.

Weight Loss Effects on Vision and Limbs

History

A 46-year-old right-handed housewife presented with progressive visual disturbance and sensory impairment of her feet and hands. She complained of a six-month history of progressive painful paraesthesiae and numbness in her hands and feet. She had then developed increasingly blurred vision for six to seven weeks prior to presentation. She was a non-smoker and drank a glass of wine once a week.

In her medical history, she had been obese with a weight of 86 kg and body mass index (BMI) of 32.8 kg/m². She had had an 18-month history of nausea, vomiting, anorexia and weight loss. Her weight had dropped by 25 kg (22% of her body weight), and her dress size had dropped from size 20 to size 10–12. Investigations by a gastroenterologist revealed an obstructive liver function pattern with raised alkaline phosphatase and gamma glutamyl transferase. She had a macrocytosis. Serum folate levels were persistently low, between 0.8 and 2 µg/L (normal range >2.2 µg/L) in the eight months prior to a neurology assessment (Figure 1.1). An upper gastrointestinal endoscopy showed only a hiatus hernia. Liver biopsy showed non-alcoholic steato-hepatitis (NASH). Two months prior to presentation to neurology she had been prescribed a one-week course of folic acid replacement; folate levels subsequently improved.

Examination

She had angular stomatitis. She had reduced visual acuity to 6/36 bilaterally. Colour vision tested using Ishihara plates was reduced at 2/14 on the right and 1/14 on the left. There were bilateral central scotomas and mild temporal disc pallor on funduscopy, all consistent with a bilateral optic neuropathy. The remaining cranial nerves were intact. Power was 5/5 in all limbs. There was a sensory neuropathy with reduced fine touch and pinprick sensation in a stocking distribution to her knees. There was reduced proprioception and vibration sensation at both great toes. There was no limb ataxia but her tandem walk was mildly unsteady.

Investigations

A nutritional profile showed normal B12, folate, thiamine, vitamin E, beta carotene and zinc levels. Vitamins A, C and D as well as selenium levels were all deficient (Table 1.1). Other investigations including anti-neuronal antibodies, autoimmune serology (neuromyelitis optica IgG aquaporin 4 and myelin oligodendrocyte glycoprotein antibodies) and immunoglobulin profile were normal.

MRI of brain and spine and cerebrospinal fluid analysis were normal.

Nerve conduction studies demonstrated a severe length-dependent axonal sensory neuropathy.

Visual evoked responses showed no consistent response from either eye. Somatosensory evoked potentials and electroretinogram were normal.

Table 1.1 Micronutrient levels at baseline, 12 and 84 months

Vitamin or mineral	Baseline values	12 months	84 months	Normal ranges
B12 (ng/L)	240	430	1121	175–750
Folate (µg/L)	**<0.8**	>20	>20	>2.2
Vitamin A (µmol/L)	**0.9**	3.4	1.7	1.1–3.5
Vitamin C (µmol/L)	**11.6**	54.2	**12.5**	40–100
Vitamin D (nmol/L)	**31**	72	**37**	50–75
Vitamin E (µmol/L)	–	42.9	32.5	16–35
Vitamin B1 (ngTDP/gHb)	–	537	375	275–675
Selenium (µmol/L)	**0.39**	1.44	0.73	0.6–1.3
Zinc (µmol/L)	10.4	10.6	13.4	8–15
Copper (µmol/L)	16.9	22.0	20.4	12.6–26.7

Low values in bold.

En rules represent no data.

Diagnosis: Nutritional Optic and Sensory Neuropathy (Also Known as Strachan Syndrome)

Management

Dietary supplementation including multivitamins, thiamine, folic acid and an oral selenium supplement were prescribed. On discharge, her weight had increased to 68.9 kg with a BMI of 26 kg/m². At review three months after presentation, her weight was 76 kg with a BMI of 28.9 kg/m². Although there had been an interruption in folic acid supplements, her mean corpuscular volume subsequently normalised to less than 100 fL (Figure 1.1). Visual acuity had improved to 6/24 bilaterally and Ishihara plate colour vision to 5/14 on the right and 6/14 on the left. There was no change in her sensory symptoms. Repeat blood investigations showed that her vitamin A, C, D and selenium deficiencies had resolved. Folate levels remained normal, however B12 levels were found to be low and she started regular hydroxycobalamin injections. Long-term follow-up of her micronutrient status was satisfactory except that vitamin D and C supplements were required (Table 1.2). She was followed up in the longer term by a gastroenterologist with a special interest in functional gut disorders and diagnosed with achalasia.

Comment

A syndrome of optic and peripheral neuropathy, corticospinal tract dysfunction, sensorineural deafness and ataxia was initially described by Henry Strachan, a British medical officer working in the West Indies, in 1897. He noticed that the syndrome was prevalent amongst Jamaican sugarcane workers, and felt at the time that it occurred as a consequence of malaria infection.

A year later in 1898, Domingo Madán reported a similar syndrome of painful sensory neuropathy and amblyopia, which developed during the trade embargo of the Cuban-Spanish-American war (1895–8) [1]. This epidemic was named the 'Amblyopia of the Blockade'. Madán theorised that alcohol was an aetiological factor, but noticed that there was a social gradient of the disease, with the majority of patients being working-class females. He raised the possibility of a nutritional basis for the disease.

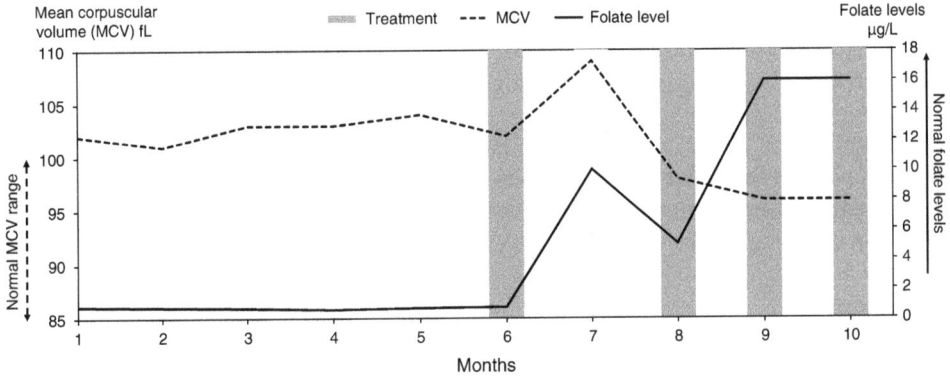

Figure 1.1 Effect of folic acid supplements on serum folate levels and mean corpuscular volume.

Table 1.2 Micronutrient levels 10 years after diagnosis

Vitamin or mineral	10 years+	Normal ranges
B12 (ng/L)	767	191–663
Folate (µg/L)	19.8	3.9–26.8
Vitamin A (µmol/L)	2.3	1.1–3.5
Vitamin C (µmol/L)	34.8	>32.0
Vitamin D (nmol/L)	71	50–75
Vitamin E (µmol/L)	34.6	16.0–35.0
Vitamin B1 (ngTDP/gHb)	548	275–675
Selenium (µmol/L)	0.95	0.75–1.46
Zinc (µmol/L)	11.2	9.6–20.5
Copper (µmol/L)	27.9	11.0–25.0

Similar syndromes were then reported in prisoners of war in camps in Japan and the Far East during the Second World War [2]. A further epidemic occurred in Cuba during the US embargo, which resulted in a collapse of Cuban trade. Over 50,000 cases of optic and peripheral neuropathy were documented in a population of 10.8 million between 1991 and 1994. Records suggested that 52% of patients had an optic form, with progressive bilateral symmetrical loss of central visual function, reduced visual acuity, reduced colour vision and central fields, whilst 48% had a peripheral neuropathy, or mixed form, with a predominantly length-dependent sensory neuropathy, but also motor, dorsal column and auditory nerve involvement. Studies of sural nerve biopsies showed predominantly a large fibre axonal neuropathy.

Epidemiological studies found that most of the affected individuals were men between the ages of 25 and 64 years. The population who had been targeted for nutritional supplementation before the epidemic (pregnant women, children and the elderly) were minimally affected [3]. Tobacco use, low animal product and vitamin B intake, irregular meals, poor food availability, and cassava, sugar and alcohol consumption were identified as risk factors for development of the condition [1]. Following the introduction of polynutritional supplements for the entire population, it was observed that the incidence of new cases declined [3]. Treatment with high-dose parenteral vitamin B complex, oral vitamins A and E, folic acid and a high protein diet was associated with a significant improvement in many patients [1].

Nutritional neuropathies have also been reported in anorexia nervosa patients. Similar syndromes of tropical ataxic neuropathy have been described in Africa and have been attributed to cyanide intoxication due to chronic cassava ingestion. Reports of outcomes vary. In Cuba there have been very few reported long-term sequelae. However, in 1955, Charles Miller Fisher published the results of postmortem studies of 11 Canadian prisoners of war. During captivity they had complained of a combination of numbness, tingling, pain and weakness of the hands and feet, poor vision, deafness and mucocutaneous changes. Despite adequate nutritional supplementation, these patients had residual symptoms and signs of neuropathy and neuropathological changes up to 10 years after disease onset. Miller Fisher was the first to propose that until an aetiological factor could be identified, the syndrome should be named after Strachan.

Strachan syndrome is a rare disorder due to polynutritional deficiency. As there are many causes of optic neuropathy, consideration of Strachan syndrome may not always be on a differential list. However, the macrocytosis, low folate level and optic and peripheral neuropathy were diagnostic clues in our patient (after excluding transverse myelitis, as can occur in neuromyelitis optica spectrum disorder/myelin oligodendrocyte glycoprotein antibody-associated disease).

Strachan syndrome has been reported in association with marked malnutrition and socioeconomic deprivation. The Strachan syndrome patient described here was a 46-year-old Caucasian woman who was not clinically underweight but had had a dramatic weight loss due to achalasia. This report emphasises the importance of prompt nutritional supplementation if considering a diagnosis of Strachan syndrome in a patient who has lost weight and has an optic and peripheral neuropathy.

References

1   Ordunez-Garcia PO, Nieto FJ, Espinosa-Brito AD, Caballero B. Cuban epidemic neuropathy, 1991 to 1994: history repeats itself a century after the 'amblyopia of the blockade'. *Am J Public Health*. 1996 May;86(5):738–43.

2   Denny-Brown D. Neurological conditions resulting from prolonged and severe dietary restriction; case reports in prisoners-of-war, and general review. *Medicine (Baltimore)*. 1947 Feb.;26(1):41–113.

3   Thomas PK, Plant GT, Baxter P, Bates C, Santiago Luis R. An epidemic of optic neuropathy and painful sensory neuropathy in Cuba: clinical aspects. *J Neurol*. 1995 Oct.;242(10):629–38.

Learning Points

- Low serum folate with macrocytosis can be a clue to nutritional deficiency.
- Nutritional deficiencies may cause an optic and/or peripheral neuropathy known as Strachan syndrome.
- Food embargoes have been implicated in large outbreaks of Strachan syndrome.
- Functional gastrointestinal problems can cause nutritional deficiencies.

Patient's Perspective

1. **What was the impact of the condition?**
   a. **Physical (e.g. job, driving, practical support)**
   Loss of power or muscle control in my legs and arms and poor vision.
   b. **Psychological (e.g. mood, future, emotional well-being)**
   Depression – lack of social engagement, loss of friends to socialise with, poor appetite, feeling lost and alone.
   c. **Social (e.g. meeting friends, home)**
   No socialising due to fear of falling has meant disconnection with friends.

2. **What could you no longer do after developing Strachan syndrome?**
   I find it difficult to do a lot of housework, such as making beds or hoovering – due to lack of power.

3. **Was there any change for you because of the diagnosis?**
   Lack of socialising has been the biggest change. However, everyday activities also require more effort. In addition, I have had to give up wearing heels and I have had to give up driving due to my poor eyesight.

4. **What is/was the most difficult aspect of the condition?**
   The feeling of helplessness and having to rely on others for things I previously could do for myself, such as dressing/hair washing.

5. **Was any aspect of the experience good or useful? What was that?**
   Not applicable. It has all been a negative experience.

6. **What do you hope for in the future for your condition (Strachan syndrome)?**
   More understanding of the condition (Strachan syndrome) and hopefully earlier diagnosis.

Adult-Onset Visual Loss

History

A 54-year-old man and taxi driver developed progressive loss of vision over four months. Initially it was thought that he had toxic amblyopia as he drank 14–25 pints of beer per week. He did not smoke cigarettes. However, the diagnosis was revised as a family history of a neurological condition emerged.

Examination

Visual acuity in each eye was reduced to hand movements, with no improvement from pinhole testing. His right optic disc was swollen with haemorrhage. The left optic disc margin was indistinct. Otherwise, his neurological examination was normal.

Investigations

Vitamin B12 and folate were normal. Micronutrients (copper, selenium and zinc) levels were normal. Anti-myelin oligodendrocyte glycoprotein and anti-neuromyelitis optica IgG aquaporin 4 antibodies were negative. MRI of brain, orbits and spine revealed no focal abnormal lesion.

Management

He received supportive measures for visual loss. He stopped drinking all alcohol. He had compensated liver cirrhosis, IgA nephropathy and hypertension.

A diagnostic test was performed.

Diagnosis: Leber Hereditary Optic Neuropathy

A mitochondrial mutation m.11778G>A, one of the three common causes of Leber hereditary optic neuropathy, was identified. Charles Bonnet syndrome developed. He was registered
blind. Optic atrophy ensued.

Comment

Measuring Visual Acuity

Herman Snellen, a Dutch ophthalmologist, devised the Snellen chart in 1862. The usual
Snellen chart has 11 lines of block letters – C, D, E, F, L, O, P, T and Z – with specific geometry
(the thickness of the lines equals the thickness of the white spaces between the lines and the
thickness of the gap in the letter 'C.' The height and width of the letter is five times the thickness of the line.

According to BS 4274–1:2003, only the letters C, D, E, F, H, K, N, P, R, U, V and Z should
be used for the testing of vision as these letters have equal legibility.

At 6 metres distant from the patient, the letters of the 6/6 (or 20/20 in the USA) line sub-
tend five minutes of arc. The minimum standard of vision for driving in the UK is between 6/9
and 6/12, equivalent to reading a number plate from a distance of 20 metres on a car registered
since 2001 (Figure 2.1).

A logarithm (base 10) of the minimum angle of resolution (LogMAR) chart is designed for
a more accurate estimate of visual acuity. An individual who can resolve details as small as one
minute of visual angle scores LogMAR 0 (as base 10 logarithm 1 is 0). Figure 2.1 provides Snellen and LogMAR equivalent acuity readings. Clinical research trials tend to use the LogMAR
chart because of its better accuracy.

Letters	Snellen acuity	LogMAR acuity
H	6/60	1.00
N E	6/36	0.80
V C R	6/24	0.60
R Z N P	6/18	0.50
F H K N P	6/12	0.30
U C D E K N	6/9	0.20
P R U V Z C	6/6	0.00
D E F H K N P	6/5	−0.10

Figure 2.1 Schematic representation of a Snellen chart with Snellen and LogMAR acuities.

Criteria to Be Certified Blind

To be certified severely sight impaired (blind), one of the following criteria is required:

- visual acuity of less than 3/60 with a full visual field;
- visual acuity of between 3/60 and 6/60 with a severe reduction of field of vision, such as tunnel vision;
- or visual acuity 6/60 or better but with a very reduced field of vision.

Differential Diagnosis of Bilateral Optic Neuropathy

There is a large differential diagnosis for optic neuropathy, which can be mistakenly attributed to demyelinating optic neuritis. Some common causes of optic neuropathy are listed in Table 2.1.

Pathophysiology and Epidemiology of Leber Hereditary Optic Neuropathy

Leber hereditary optic neuropathy (LHON) is a mitochondrial genetic disease that causes progressive loss of vision, usually in the second and third decades of life. Although first described in 1848 by Albrecht von Graefe, LHON was subsequently reported by Theodore Leber in

Table 2.1 Differential diagnosis of an optic neuropathy (broad mechanisms of disease)

Glaucoma

Raised intracranial pressure (papilloedema)

Inflammatory
- Idiopathic inflammatory optic neuritis (associated with multiple sclerosis)
- Neuromyelitis optica
- Systemic inflammatory and autoimmune diseases
- Infectious diseases

Vascular
- Anterior or posterior
- Arteritic or non-arteritic
- Post-radiation therapy

Compressive or infiltrative
- Neoplastic
- Non-neopalstic

Paraneoplastic

Toxic

Nutritional

Hereditary

Traumatic

Optic nerve head drusen

Congenitally anomalous optic nerve

Glaucoma is by far the most common cause of optic neuropathy and a leading cause of blindness; inflammatory optic neuritis is the most common subacute optic neuropathy in young people; non-arteritic anterior ischaemic optic neuropathy is the most common acute optic neuropathy in patients older than 50 years.

Adapted from Biousse and Newman [1] with permission from Elsevier.

1871. Three common mutations in the mitochondrial genome (m.3460G>A, m.11778G>A and m.14484T>C) affect complex I of the mitochondrial respiratory chain. These mutations account for over 90% of patients with LHON in Europe and North America. The m.11778G>A mutation (70% of Northern European and 90% of Asian cases) causes more severe disease. There is a defect in the synthesis of adenosine triphosphate and oxygen-free radicals damage the retinal ganglion cell layer. In Northern Europe prevalence of LHON is at least 1 in 30,000 (3.2–4.4 per 100,000).

A lower heteroplasmy rate correlates with less disease manifestation. In addition, penetrance of LHON varies with sex; 50% of males and just 10% of female carriers develop visual loss. Environmental factors, particularly smoking, have been implicated in visual loss in LHON [2]. Alcohol has a modifying effect, excess consumption being associated with earlier visual loss. Mitochondrial DNA-haplotype background is also thought to influence the occurrence and severity of visual loss in LHON.

In 75% of patients, acute central visual loss is unilateral before the other eye is affected weeks to months later. In the reminder (as in our patient), the acute visual loss begins bilaterally. The visual failure is painless. LHON has associations with multiple systems. Tremor, neuropathy, movement disorders and a leukoencephalopathy mimicking multiple sclerosis have all been described in LHON.

Treatment Research

Idebenone is an antioxidant that inhibits lipid peroxidation. It is a short chain benzoquinone with mitochondrial effects that activate viable but inactive retinal ganglion cells. An openlabelled study and a randomised controlled trial (the RHODOS trial) assessed idebenone. The primary outcome in the RHODOS trial was not met (change from baseline to 24 weeks in best visual acuity). However, a sub-group analysis in patients with discordant visual acuity found improvements in visual acuity. In the RHODOS trial, 12 out of 61 patients taking idebenone (300 mg tid) who could read no letters on the chart at baseline were able to read at least five letters by week 24 compared to 0 out of 29 in the placebo group (p = 0.008). The trial demonstrated that patients with m.11778G>A and m.3460G>A mutations had the largest treatment effect. The m.14484T>C mutation has a high spontaneous recovery rate. Idebenone had minimal side effects [3].

An expanded access programme has suggested idebenone 900 mg/day was associated with clinically relevant recovery in nearly half of patients (46%).

The Scottish Medicines Consortium (SMC No. 1226/17) indication for idebenone restricts use of idebenone to patients with LHON who are not yet blind. In 2019, NHS England deemed that idebenone did not have sufficient evidence for the treatment of patients with LHON.

However, genetic treatment of LHON is emerging, which may be less controversial. Lenadogene nolparvovec (rAAV2/2-ND4) is an adeno-associated viral vector that has the modified cDNA encoding human wild-type mitochondrial ND4 protein, the defect in m.11778G>A LHON. Patients with LHON due to an m.11778G>A mutation were enrolled if visual loss was 12 months or less. A single intravitreal injection of lenadogene nolparvovec has shown sustained improvement in best corrected visual acuity in both eyes and improvement in quality of life in two phase 3 trials [4]. Gene therapy may become an important treatment for LHON if efficacy and safety can be maintained.

References

1.   Biousse V, Newman NJ. Diagnosis and clinical features of common optic neuropathies. *Lancet Neurol.* 2016;15(13):1355–67.

2.   Kirkman MA, Yu-Wai-Man P, Korsten A et al. Gene-environment interactions in Leber hereditary optic neuropathy. *Brain.* 2009;132(9):2317–26.

3.   Catarino CB, von Livonius B, Priglinger C et al. Real-world clinical experience with idebenone in the treatment of Leber hereditary optic neuropathy. *J Neuro-Ophthalmology.* 2020;40(4):558–65.

4.   Biousse V, Newman NJ, Yu-Wai-Man P et al. Long-term follow-up after unilateral intravitreal gene therapy for Leber hereditary optic neuropathy: the RESTORE study. *J Neuro-Ophthalmology.* 2021;41(3):309–15.

Learning Points

- Leber hereditary optic neuropathy (LHON) is a mitochondrial genetic disorder that can cause progressive, painless visual loss more often in males than females.
- In LHON, environmental factors such as alcohol and smoking play a role in visual loss.
- Genetic treatment has shown early promise in improving vision in patients with recent (<12 months) visual loss due to LHON.

Patient's Perspective

1.   **What was the impact of the condition on you?**

   a. **Physical (e.g. job, driving, practical support)**
   Shock, fear and how I will I be able to cope with loss of my sight.

   b. **Psychological (e.g. mood, future, emotional well-being)**
   I became very depressed. I did not want to leave the house and I had a fear of losing my cane.

   c. **Social (e.g. meeting friends, home)**
   I was nervous about meeting people and embarrassed eating out in restaurants etc.

2.   **What can you no longer do?**
   I had to stop driving. I can no longer watch television, read newspapers or go to Gaelic matches, which I loved to attend.

3.   **Was there any other change for you due to your medical condition?**
   Yes, I developed Charles Bonnet syndrome. This had a major impact and was very disturbing as I had visual hallucinations of machinery, animals, people from period times, both at home and when I was outside.

4.   **What is/was the most difficult aspect of the condition for you?**
   Learning to adapt to living my life in a new way.

5.   **Was any aspect of the experience good or useful? What was that?**
   Yes, eventually after a few years I became more confident dealing with all the above-mentioned changes.

6.   **What do you hope for in the future for your condition?**
   It would be good if medicine improved to maybe be able to enhance people's lives with sight loss.

History

A 44-year-old right-handed female driver developed a new onset moderately severe headache with vomiting. She attended hospital and had a CT scan of her brain and a lumbar puncture; both were reported as normal. She was discharged from hospital but over the next week the headaches became more severe and vomiting recurred. Then, 11 days after the onset of headache, she developed slurred speech and impaired concentration. She giggled inappropriately and became confused. Her condition fluctuated but did not return to normal. She had no oral or genital ulcers but had noticed decreased hearing on her right side. She was re-admitted to hospital and a neurological opinion was sought.

She had two children. She did not smoke cigarettes but drank one bottle of wine at weekends.

Examination

She had no rash and no mouth ulcers. She was dysphasic and encephalopathic, smiling out of context. She knew the month but not the day. She recognised that she was in hospital. She could not explain a doctor's role. She had decreased hearing on the right. Clinical examination of her eyes was normal. The remaining cranial nerves were normal. Neurological examination of her limbs was normal. Her cardiovascular examination was normal.

Clinical differential diagnosis from the neurological consultation included:

1. an immune-mediated brain, ear and eye (BEE) syndrome such as Susac syndrome
2. autoimmune encephalitis
3. infective encephalitis, Lyme disease or tuberculosis
4. nutritional encephalopathy
5. a demyelinating condition such as multiple sclerosis
6. vasculitis
7. a connective tissue disorder
8. a mitochondrial disorder

Investigations

An MRI scan of the brain demonstrated callosal lesions, left thalamic (pulvinar) and bilateral cerebellar lesions (Figure 3.1A–3.1D). There were also lesions in the posterior pons at the level of the medial longitudinal fasciculus and rostral midbrain. Following contrast, there was no abnormal enhancement. An MRI of the spine revealed no definite lesions.

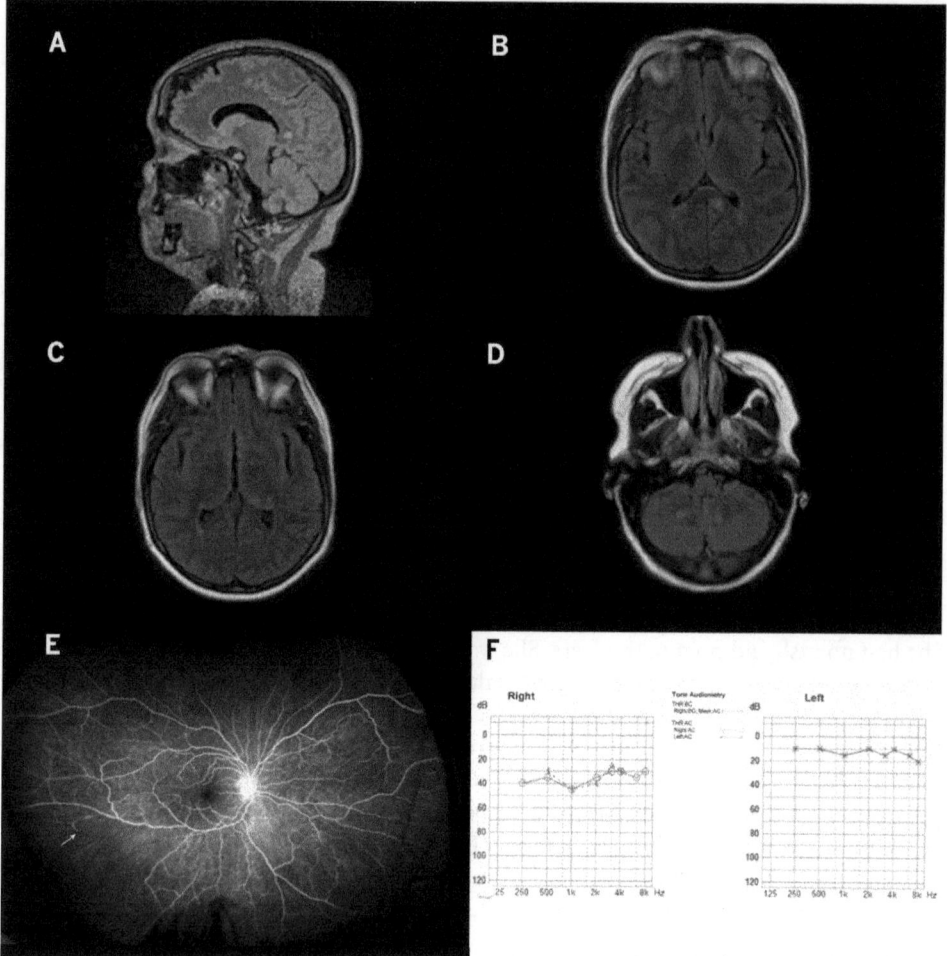

Figure 3.1 A (A) sagittal and (B) axial T2 FLAIR MRI scan of the brain, showing corpus callosal lesions. An axial MRI brain showing pulvinar lesion in (C) the left thalamus and (D) bilateral cerebellar lesions. Fluorescein angiography (E) shows a BRAO (arrow). (F) Audiometry demonstrates a right hearing deficit more prominent at lower frequencies.

She had two lumbar punctures. The cerebrospinal fluid (CSF) findings are shown in Table 3.1.

An EEG showed a marked excess of slow waves, most notably over the temporal regions but affecting both hemispheres in keeping with an encephalopathy.

Tests for antibodies to N-methyl-D-aspartate receptor (NMDAR), myelin oligodendrocyte glycoprotein (MOG), neuromyelitis optica (NMO) aquaporin 4 and voltage-gated potassium channel (leucine-rich, glioma-inactivated 1 (or LGI1) and contactin-associated protein-like 2 (or CASPR2)) in blood and CSF were all negative. A nuclear autoantibody screen was negative. The thyroid profile, ammonia, B12 and folate levels were normal. Fluoroscein angiography showed a branch retinal artery occlusion (BRAO) (Figure 3.1E). Audiometry revealed right hearing loss, worse at lower frequencies (Figure 3.1F).

Table 3.1 CSF findings

Measurement (normal range)	LP 1	LP 2 (two weeks later)
Opening pressure (6–25 cmCSF)	18 cmCSF	29 cmCSF
CSF white cells (<5/µL)	1	1
CSF red cells	107	65
CSF glucose/serum glucose	3.4 mmol/L/5.5 mmol/L	3.0 mmol/L/9.0 mmol/l
CSF protein (<0.4g/L)	0.53 g/L	1.55 g/L
Oligoclonal bands	Not done	Not detected
Enterovirus PCR	Negative	Negative
Herpes simplex virus 1 and 2 and varicella zoster virus PCR	Negative	Negative
Neisseria meningitidis/Streptococcus pneumoniae/Haemophilus influenza	Negative	Negative
Parechovirus PCR	Negative	Negative
NMDAR antibody	Not done	Negative
Voltage-gated potassium channel antibodies (LGI-1 and CASPR2)	Not done	Negative

Diagnosis: Susac Syndrome

Comment

Susac syndrome is an immune-mediated, pauci-inflammatory, occlusive microvascular endotheliopathy or basement membranopathy that affects the brain, retina and inner ear [1]. Brain manifestations include cognitive, psychiatric, headache and focal neurological deficits. There have been very few epidemiological studies; one study from Austria reported an incidence of 0.024 per 100,000 per year (95% CI 0.010–0.047).

Differential Diagnosis

There is a wide range of differential diagnoses for Susac syndrome, but the triad of clinical features of encephalopathy, deafness and BRAO suggests Susac syndrome. There is a need for fluorescein angiography to confirm BRAO because BRAO can be asymptomatic. The condition may be radiologically and clinically diagnosed as multiple sclerosis because multiple sclerosis is a much more common neurological disorder in young adults. Clinicians, however, should think of other causes, particularly if the brain, ear and eye are involved. Recognised immune-mediated BEE syndromes include multiple sclerosis, antiphospholipid syndrome, neurosarcoidosis, systemic lupus erythematosus, neuromyelitis optica spectrum disorder, Behçet disease, Vogt–Koyanagi–Harada disease (systemic granulomatous autoimmune disease against melanocyte-containing tissues – uvea, retina, leptomeninges, inner ear and skin), Cogan syndrome (an autoimmune disease affecting eye, audio and vestibular apparatus with antibodies to connexion 26, which can also cause meningitis, encephalitis, psychosis, seizures and cerebral infarction) and Susac syndrome.

History of Susac Syndrome

Susac syndrome was named after John Susac (1956–2012) following his report of the condition in 1979. The condition had previously been described as small infarction of cochlear, retinal and encephalic tissue (SICRET) syndrome or retinocochleocerebral vasculopathy.

Susac was criticised when he argued that this neurological disorder was not multiple sclerosis. Involvement of the retina, cochlea and brain explains the clinical triad of visual loss due to BRAOs, sensorineural hearing loss (in the low to moderate range frequencies) and encephalopathy. The encephalopathy includes cognitive impairment, psychiatric disturbance, headache, seizures and focal neurological deficits. More than 300 cases had been described by 2013, but most patients do not present with the full clinical triad. Partial presentations may have a role in delaying diagnosis. In addition, vestibular abnormalities are very common in Susac syndrome. The mechanism of the immune-mediated endotheliopathy is not clear.

Pathophysiology of Susac Syndrome

Anti-endothelial cell antibodies in serum of patients with Susac syndrome have been identified, although their exact role is unclear. However, in 2019, a CD8+ T cell-mediated endotheliopathy was identified as a mechanism in the neuro-inflammation of Susac syndrome [2]. The authors of this paper revealed that blocking T-cell adhesion (with anti-α4 integrin – a transmembrane heterodimer that acts as an adhesion receptor for extracellular ligands) not only improved the disease in a preclinical mouse model, but also resulted in less severe disease in four patients when treated with natalizumab, albeit along with other therapy. Clinical trial data are awaited.

Diagnostic Confirmation

Retinal fluorescein angiography can confirm arterial occlusion in the region of suspected BRAOs. Asymptomatic BRAOs and vessel-wall hyperfluorescence remote from bifurcations where emboli may lodge can confirm diffuse endothelial-cell damage.

Pathognomonic MRI Findings in Susac Syndrome

The central corpus callosum is supplied by small-calibre blood vessels. MRI lesions in the centre of the corpus callosum are referred to as 'snowball' lesions. Central callosal 'icicle' and 'spoke' lesions in contact with the roof of the corpus callosum support a diagnosis of Susac syndrome; these are said to differ in location from other inflammatory conditions including multiple sclerosis. A 'string of pearls' appearance from microinfarcts in the internal capsule has also been described. Common areas of MRI brain abnormalities include periventricular regions, centrum semiovale, cerebellum, brainstem and middle cerebellar peduncles. Many of these lesions were identified in our patient (Figure 3.1). Grey and white matter lesions often enhance. Widespread axonal damage has been recognised.

Suggested diagnostic criteria are based on the recognised triad of features in Susac syndrome [3]. The European Consortium classification for a definite diagnosis of Susac syndrome requires a full triad of brain, ear and eye involvement. Brain symptoms include new cognitive impairment and/or behavioural changes and/or new focal neurological symptoms and/or headache with hyperintense, multifocal small round lesions on a T2 FLAIR MRI of the brain, at least one of which must be in the corpus callosum 'snowball.' Retinal findings include BRAOs or arterial wall hyperfluorescence, while vestibulocochlear symptoms include tinnitus and/or hearing loss and/or vertigo in the presence of hearing loss documented on an audiogram [3]. A probable diagnosis of Susac syndrome exists if any two of the three features are present.

Management of Susac Syndrome

Clinical experience suggests that therapy targeting both B cells and T cells has efficacy but there is a lack of randomised controlled trials and prospective treatment studies [1]. The first aim of therapy is to induce remission with intravenous methylprednisolone followed by a slow taper of oral glucocorticoid therapy over several months. For severe disease, rituximab has also been used. Next, glucocorticoid-sparing maintenance immunotherapy involves rituximab, mycophenolate or azathioprine. Expert recommendations suggest acute treatment for several months to 2.5 years. A gradual withdrawal of therapy may be considered if the disease has been inactive for 24 months. Lack of long-term data necessitates long-term follow-up. A group in Cleveland, US has extensive experience and has recommended treatment based on a qualitative severity scale [1].

Follow-up management involves serial audiometry, fluorescein angiography and MRIs of the head.

References

1. Rennebohm RM, Asdaghi N, Srivastava S, Gertner E. Guidelines for treatment of Susac syndrome: An update. *Int J Stroke Off J Int Stroke Soc.* 2020;15(5):484–94.
2. Gross CC, Meyer C, Bhatia U et al. CD8+ T cell-mediated endotheliopathy is a targetable mechanism of neuro-inflammation in Susac syndrome. *Nat Commun.* 2019;10(1):5779.

3. Kleffner I, Dörr J, Ringelstein M et al. Diagnostic criteria for Susac syndrome. *J Neurol Neurosurg Psychiatry*. 2016;87(12):1287–95.

Learning Points

- Susac syndrome causes deafness, branch retinal artery occlusions and an encephalopathy.
- Susac syndrome is an immune-mediated BEE syndrome.
- Corpus callosal snowball lesions on MRI brain scanning are found in Susac syndrome.
- Pathophysiology of Susac syndrome may be a T-cell mediated endotheliopathy.
- Empirical aggressive initial immunosuppressant treatment with high-dose corticosteroids is often used.

Patient's Perspective

1. **What was the impact of the condition?**

   a. Physical (e.g. job, driving, practical support)
   Susac syndrome took away my independence as I was totally confused in all aspects of life. I could not do the following tasks:
   drive or work;
   care for my home or my teenage daughter;
   make financial decisions as I didn't comprehend what was required for me; and
   initially, read or write.
   I needed full-time care, which I received from my family, as I was not able to bathe, make food, eat/feed myself or shop for basic groceries. I suffered continuous exhaustion and headache.

   b. Psychological (mood, future, emotional well-being)
   I found myself in a very dark place, often having suicidal thoughts. I suffered a continual low mood, having many tearful episodes. I have been short-tempered with many mood swings. Overall, I would say depressed with PTSD. I have anxiety attacks daily.

   c. Social (e.g. meeting friends, home)
   I have felt very unsure of myself, losing all confidence in going anywhere alone. I feel isolated and paranoid as I didn't want anyone to see me like 'this'. 'This' meaning – a few stone heavier. I felt people were talking about me, as they may not have recognised me. I also was not fit for visitors coming to me.

2. **What can or could you not do because of the condition?**
   Initially I didn't recognise my closest family and friends. I could not make any decisions, financial or for daily tasks. I couldn't read or understand the content of letters or process any information. Managing appointments was left to others, as was cooking, laundry and shopping.

3. **Was there any other change for you due to your medical condition?**
   Yes, I developed vertigo and tinnitus. I found my eyesight impaired and lost my hearing on the right. I also suffer from joint pain and generalised body pains daily. My sleeping pattern is also disturbed and, due to my medication my toileting habits are also unpredictable.

4. **What is/was the most difficult aspect of the condition for you?**
   Trying to adjust to the new me. I struggle daily with the effects of Susac syndrome. I feel like I have lost myself to this condition. My life has changed dramatically as I still cannot function anywhere near the way I did pre-Susac's.

5. **Was any aspect of the experience of the condition good or useful? What was that?**
   In a word – no. I can't find anything positive about this condition other than the care I have received.

6. **What do you hope for in the future for people with this condition?**
   My hope is that there may be a treatment available that doesn't impact daily life or even a cure in the near future. Maybe more awareness and research would be good too.

CASE 4 Multiple Problems

History

A 23-year-old right-handed student presented with a one-year history of unsteadiness and a six-month history of urinary and bowel urgency with incontinence. Four weeks before hospital admission, she also had a change in the vision from her right eye, only seeing the periphery of the visual field. Three weeks prior to hospital admission, she had right-hand numbness and weakness and was admitted to hospital when she developed left-leg weakness and numbness.

Past medical history included depression, breast augmentation and mastoplexy. She also had B12 deficiency. She had no history of miscarriage, oral or genital ulcers, deep venous thrombosis or pulmonary emboli.

Medication was sertraline 100 mg/day and B12 replacement.

Examination

She was alert, orientated and systemically stable. She had marked truncal ataxia. Visual acuity on a Snellen chart was $6/6^{-2}$ on the right and $6/6$ on the left, both unaided. She had normal upper limb tone and strength. Tone was normal in the legs but there was a pyramidal distribution of weakness in her left leg (hip flexion, knee flexion and ankle dorsiflexion grade 4/5). She had brisk reflexes and bilateral ankle clonus, more sustained on the left. Joint position sense, pinprick and cold sensation were intact.

Investigations

Full blood count, electrolytes, liver function tests, thyroid profile, B12 and folate levels and nuclear autoantibody screen were all normal. HIV, syphilis, Lyme serology, HTLV-1, anticardiolipin antibodies, lupus anticoagulant and angiotensin converting enzyme tests were negative or normal.

An MRI of the brain showed multiple periventricular lesions. An MRI of the spine showed a medulla lesion and multiple spinal lesions (Figure 4.1).

Lumbar puncture results are shown in Table 4.1.

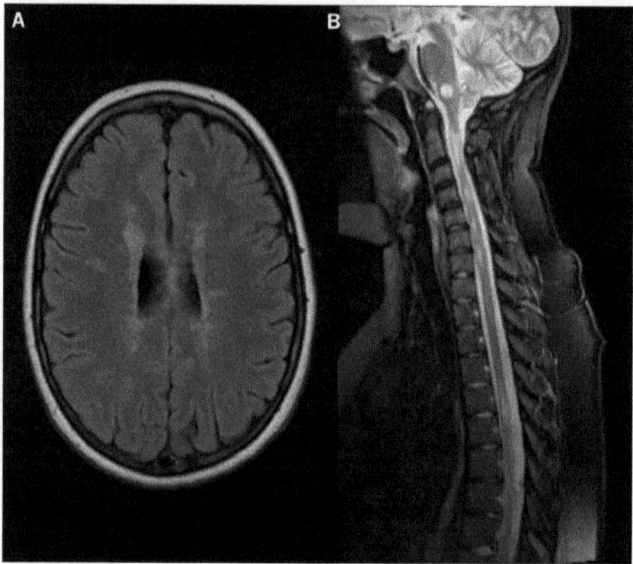

Figure 4.1 (A) Non-contrast axial T2 FLAIR MRI scan of brain shows multiple bilateral periventricular and some subcortical lesions. (B) A T2 sagittal MRI scan of the spine demonstrates a round medullary lesion and at least five 'droplet-like' lesions in the spinal cord.

Table 4.1 Blood and cerebrospinal fluid investigation results

Measurement (normal range)	Value
Opening pressure (6–25 cmCSF)	20 cmCSF
White cell count (<5/μL)	3/μL
Red cell count	4/μL
Cerebrospinal fluid protein (<0.4g/L)	0.44 g/L
Cerebrospinal fluid glucose	3.2 mmol/L
Serum glucose	5.5 mmol/L
Oligoclonal bands restricted to cerebrospinal fluid	Positive
Lupus anticoagulant/anti-beta-2-glycoprotein antibody/ anticardiolipin antibody	Negative
Neuromyelitis optica IgG aquaporin 4 antibody	Negative
Myelin oligodendrocyte glycoprotein antibody	Negative
Anti-gastric parietal cell antibody	Negative
Anti-intrinsic factor antibody	Negative
John Cunningham (JC) virus	Negative

Diagnosis: Relapsing-Remitting Multiple Sclerosis

Management

A five-day course of intravenous methylprednisolone (500 mg/day) was given, which was associated with a good improvement in her left leg strength. Subsequently, monthly natalizumab was started and well tolerated.

Over the next four years, she remained clinically and radiologically stable, with no evidence of new demyelinating lesions or progressive multifocal leucoencephalopathy. However, in the fourth year after her diagnosis, she had three episodes of generalised seizure activity. A repeat MRI brain scan had shown no new lesions. An EEG demonstrated fairly frequent slow activity over the left temporal region. She was treated with lamotrigine. Three years on, she has been seizure-free and continues on natalizumab and lamotrigine.

Comment

The Epidemiology of Multiple Sclerosis

Multiple sclerosis is an immune-mediated disease of the central nervous system that affects mostly young individuals and, increasingly, females. Epidemiological studies have demonstrated a north-south gradient in the incidence rate of the disease. Lack of vitamin D, particularly from sunlight, may play an aetiological role in multiple sclerosis but evidence of benefit from supplementary oral vitamin D (prevention of relapse) has not been consistently identified. Infection with Epstein Barr virus has been associated with a markedly increased risk of developing multiple sclerosis. There is now better evidence for a causal role of Epstein-Barr virus in multiple sclerosis.

The Clinical Presentation and Pathology of Multiple Sclerosis

Classically, multiple sclerosis has been classified into relapsing-remitting multiple sclerosis, clinically isolated syndrome, radiologically isolated syndrome, primary progressive multiple sclerosis and secondary progressive multiple sclerosis. Fred Lublin then added the presence of active and non-active descriptions to each of the subtypes [1]. Activity is determined by clinical relapse and/or MRI activity. Progression is measured by an annual clinical evaluation.

Four stages of pathology have been recognised in multiple sclerosis [2].

Although multiple sclerosis has been classified as an inflammatory disorder of white matter, acute demyelinating lesions can occur with neuronal loss and meningeal inflammation.

Recognised Pathological Stages of Multiple Sclerosis

Pattern 1 (15%)

   Active demyelination and remyelination. Oligodendrocyte precursor cells

   Variable loss of oligodendrocytes at lesion edge

   Lymphocytes, activated microglia/macrophages

Pattern 2 (60%)

   Active demyelination and remyelination. Oligodendrocyte precursor cells

   Variable loss of oligodendrocytes at lesion edge

   Immunoglobulin and complement deposition on myelin and on myelin debris within macrophages

   Inflammatory cells

Pattern 3 (24%)

    Active demyelination (preferential loss of myelin-associated glycoprotein); no remyelination

    Extensive oligodendrocyte apoptosis throughout lesion and beyond

    Initial damage to parts of the oligodendrocyte most distal from its cell body

    Inflammatory cells

Pattern 4 (1%)

    Profound oligodendrocyte loss in periplaque white matter

Bladder Symptoms in Multiple Sclerosis

Bladder symptoms are frequent in multiple sclerosis. Bladder storage symptoms include urinary frequency, urgency with or without incontinence. Voiding problems manifest with hesitancy, poor or interrupted urinary stream, sensation of incomplete emptying and double voiding. Both types of bladder symptoms can develop in multiple sclerosis. Lesions above the pons can cause storage symptoms due to loss of inhibition on the detrusor muscle. Spinal lesions (often present in multiple sclerosis) can cause a mixture of storage and voiding symptoms. Lesions in the conus medullaris may cause voiding symptoms. A post-void residual over 100 ml may require clean intermittent self-catheterisation. Otherwise, an anti-cholinergic drug is indicated, ideally with more muscarinic M3 specificity for the bladder and less central muscarinic effects on cognition.

Epilepsy and Multiple Sclerosis

There is a positive association between multiple sclerosis and epilepsy (as observed in our patient). The pooled prevalence of epilepsy among patients with multiple sclerosis is 3% compared to 0.4–1.2% in the general population.

Criteria for Diagnosing Multiple Sclerosis (a Will Rogers Phenomenon)

Allowing a disease to be diagnosed at an earlier stage can seem to improve outcome when measured as disability or survival. The 2017 revised McDonald criteria for multiple sclerosis [3] lead to diagnosis of more patients with less active multiple sclerosis compared to previous iterations of the McDonald criteria. The 2017 McDonald criteria are best used in populations in which multiple sclerosis is relatively common and in patients in whom there is a typical presentation.

    MRI evidence of dissemination in space requires two of the following:

- one or more periventricular lesions
- cortical or juxtacortical lesion
- infratentorial lesion
- spinal cord lesion.

    Dissemination in time requires one of the following criteria:

- a second attack/relapse
- new lesions on a follow-up MRI scan
- simultaneous enhancing and non-enhancing lesions on an MRI scan
- restricted oligoclonal bands in the cerebrospinal fluid.

Table 4.2 The 2017 McDonald criteria for diagnosing relapsing-remitting multiple sclerosis

Number of clinical attacks (separated by 30 days)	Number of lesions with objective clinical evidence	Additional data needed for a diagnosis of multiple sclerosis
≥2	≥2	None
≥2	1 (as well as clear-cut historical evidence of a previous attack involving a lesion in a distinct anatomical location†)	None
≥2	1	DIS – clinical episode at another site or MRI
1	≥2	DIT by clinical episode, MRI or restricted oligoclonal bands
1	1	DIS by further clinical episode at another site or by MRI *and* DIT by further clinical episode, by MRI or restricted oligoclonal bands

DIS= disseminated in space; DIT = disseminated in time

Adapted from Thompson et al. [3] permission from Elsevier.

Table 4.2 highlights different scenarios in which multiple sclerosis can be diagnosed. The original 1965 Schumacher criteria were purely clinical (patients 10–50 years old, attacks lasting at least 24 hours, separated by at least a month, or for progressive multiple sclerosis a slow or stepwise progression over at least six months, and evidence of white matter disease in two or more distinct sites) and were more restrictive than current criteria. Earlier and therefore milder disease is now recognised as multiple sclerosis. Aware of the shortcomings of the revision, the authors stated that neurologists should 'recognise that the McDonald criteria were not developed to differentiate multiple sclerosis from other conditions but to identify multiple sclerosis or a high likelihood of the disease in patients with a typical clinically isolated syndrome once other diagnoses have been deemed unlikely' [3].

Accurate Diagnosis of Multiple Sclerosis

Accurate diagnosis of multiple sclerosis relies on both an appropriate history and examination findings suggestive of demyelination with correct interpretation of neuroimaging. The National Academy of Medicine (previously known as the Institute of Medicine) has emphasised the 'moral, professional and public health imperative' to improve the diagnostic process [4]. An incorrect diagnosis of multiple sclerosis can lead to harmful consequences as some of the disease-modifying therapies licensed for multiple sclerosis can exacerbate another demyelinating disease – neuromyelitis optica. Academic centres suggest that misdiagnosis of multiple sclerosis can include conditions such as fibromyalgia, non-specific or non-localising neurological symptoms with an abnormal MRI and neuromyelitis optica spectrum disorder. There is a large differential diagnosis for multiple sclerosis, but there are a number of conditions to be considered from migraine to sarcoidosis, anti-myelin oligodendrocyte glycoprotein antibody-associated disease, neuromyelitis optica spectrum disorder, lymphoma, autoimmune glial fibrillary acidic protein astrocytopathy (a rare disorder associated with steroid-responsive encephalitis, meningitis, myelitis or meningoencephalitis first described in 2016) and Fabry disease.

While neuromyelitis optica is a recognised cause of longitudinal extensive myelitis (defined on a spinal MRI scan as a lesion extending over three or more vertebral segments), such spinal lesions can occur in 3% of patients with multiple sclerosis; 0.7% of multiple sclerosis patients can present with longitudinally extensive myelitis. Other causes of longitudinally extensive myelitis include myelitis associated with systemic autoimmunity such as systemic lupus erythematosus, infectious (HIV, syphilis, tuberculosis) or paraneoplastic myelitis, metabolic (B12 or copper deficiency) and vascular causes (spinal cord infarction).

History of Disease-Modifying Treatments in Multiple Sclerosis

Over 20 drugs have been approved and are currently used as disease-modifying treatments for relapsing-remitting, primary progressive and secondary progressive multiple sclerosis (Table 4.3). Primary progressive multiple sclerosis and secondary progressive multiple sclerosis have fewer disease-modifying treatments, possibly reflecting a different pathological process. Ocrelizumab may be effective in reducing progression in primary progressive multiple sclerosis. For relapsing-remitting multiple sclerosis, the less effective and earlier-licensed drugs (glatiramer acetate, interferon beta-1b and interferon beta-1a) appear to have safer profiles and require less monitoring than subsequent oral and infusion therapies. Siponimod is used to treat active (relapses or MRI showing new or growing lesions) secondary progressive multiple sclerosis. Autologous haemopoietic stem cell transplantation (aHSCT) is a relatively new treatment for patients with highly active relapsing-remitting multiple sclerosis that has not responded to disease-modifying treatment. As treatment-related mortality from aHSCT has declined to less than 1%, future robust evidence of efficacy may result in more use of aHSCT.

Table 4.3. Some disease-modifying treatments in multiple sclerosis

Name of drug	Year of license	Mode of administration	Mode of action
Interferon beta-1b	1995	Subcutaneous	Alters pro- and anti-inflammatory agents in the brain, decreasing inflammatory cell access across the blood–brain barrier
Interferon beta-1a	1997	Intramuscular	Alters pro- and anti-inflammatory agents in the brain, decreasing inflammatory cell access across the blood–brain barrier
Mitoxantrone	2001	Intravenous	Intercalation of DNA, preventing repair and inhibiting B and T cell proliferation
Glatiramer acetate	2001	Subcutaneous	Induction of anti-inflammatory antigen-presenting cells
Natalizumab	2006	Intravenous or subcutaneous	Inhibition of α4β1 integrin, a selective adhesion molecule blocking VCAM-1 and leukocyte migration across the blood–brain barrier
Fingolimod	2011	Oral	Sphingosine 1-phosphate receptor modulator – prevents lymphocytes entering the central nervous system

Table 4.3. (cont.)

Name of drug	Year of license	Mode of administration	Mode of action
Teriflunomide	2013	Oral	Dihydro-orotate dehydrogenase inhibitor, a key mitochondrial enzyme in pyrimidine synthesis, leading to a reduction in proliferation of activated T and B lymphocytes
Alemtuzumab	2013	Intravenous infusion	Monoclonal antibody-depleting CD52-expressing T and B cells
Dimethyl fumarate	2014	Oral	Enhances nuclear factor erythroid 2 related factor 2 transcriptional pathway and inhibits nuclear factor kappa B
Cladribine	2017	Oral	Inhibits DNA polymerase and ribonucleotide reductase, depleting T and B lymphocytes
Ocrelizumab	2018	Intravenous infusion	Selectively targets CD20-expressing B cells
Autologous haemopoietic stem cell transplant	2019–first RCT	Intravenous	Re-diversification of the T cell repertoire
Siponimod	2020	Oral	Sphingosine 1-phosphate receptor modulator – prevents lymphocytes entering the central nervous system
Ofatumumab	2021	Subcutaneous injection	Selectively targets CD20-expressing B cells

An MRI scanning surveillance system allows confirmation of escalating disease burden with or without clinical relapses. Such scanning may be facilitated by artificial intelligence or computer-aided design in order to identify patients in need of escalation of disease-modifying therapy. The ultimate goal of therapy is safety and no evidence of disease activity (NEDA). Earlier treatment with more efficacious drugs appears to lessen long-term disability. Rates of NEDA for aHSCT between 61 and 92% at two years have been recorded.

The history of two disease-modifying drugs in multiple sclerosis is summarised in the next section.

Natalizumab and Progressive Multifocal Leucoencephalopathy

Natalizumab is a humanised anti-α4 integrin monoclonal antibody blocking the binding of α4β1 and α4β7 integrins to their endothelial receptors in order to reduce inflammation. Natalizumab also inhibits the interaction of α4-positive leucocytes, fibronectin and osteopontin. Following interim data analysis of two phase three trials (AFFIRM and SENTINEL), natalizumab was approved by the US Food and Drug Association in 2004 for relapsing-remitting multiple sclerosis. However, in 2005, it was taken off the market because three patients developed progressive multifocal leucoencephalopathy, two with multiple sclerosis and one with Crohn's disease. Further use, including European Union approval, followed in 2006, with restricted distribution focussed on safety. The status of John Cunningham virus (JC virus) is checked and monitored in treated patients, who are then repeatedly consented for treatment with natalizumab.

Progressive multifocal leucoencephalopathy is due to activation of the polyomavirus. Infection with the JC virus is usually asymptomatic in immunocompetent individuals. However, latent infection means that it can reactivate under appropriate conditions. Other disease-modifying drugs for multiple sclerosis have been implicated in progressive multifocal leucoencephalopathy, but the risk with natalizumab has been more frequent.

Alemtuzumab

Alemtuzumab, initially called Campath 1H (to reflect Cambridge pathology) is a monoclonal antibody against CD52, which depletes B cells. Hermann Waldmann at the University of Cambridge had suggested that the Cambridge academic neurology team consider using this drug in multiple sclerosis. It had already gained a license in 1991 for childhood chronic lymphocytic lymphoma. Alemtuzumab had a chequered path to licensing for treatment of relapsing-remitting multiple sclerosis. Multiple drug companies, regulations, large investments of time and money as well as individual interventions eventually yielded the MS CARE 1, 2 and extension studies, revealing an effective licensed product, albeit with recognised adverse effects (Grave's disease 30%, idiopathic thrombocytopenic purpura 1–3%, Goodpasture's syndrome 0.1%). Intriguingly, a lymphocyte-depleting drug is associated with autoimmune adverse effects. Alemtuzumab was launched in 2013 and recommended by NICE for its full indication in May 2014.

This annual treatment for two years (infusion ×5 days in year 1 and infusion ×3 days in year 2) became well established as one of the more effective disease-modifying treatments for multiple sclerosis. Like some other drugs (natalizumab and fingolimod), alemtuzumab also had demonstrated sustained disability improvement, although the mechanism for this has not been clearly elucidated. In the studies (MS CARE 1, 2 and extension studies), early treatment was initiated, hinting at the need for prompt initiation for maximum benefit. However, in 2019, a safety alert was raised. The European Medicines Agency reported rare serious disorders within one to three days of the alemtuzumab infusion, including myocardial infarction, intracerebral haemorrhage, cervical arterial dissection, pulmonary alveolar haemorrhage and thrombocytopenia. Delayed autoimmune complications were also a concern, including autoimmune hepatitis, haemophilia A, idiopathic thrombocytopenic purpura, thyroid disorders and rarely, nephropathies or haemophagocytic lymphohistiocytosis. There was also increased risk of serious infections and reactivation of Epstein–Barr virus. Restricted used of alemtuzumab ensued.

References

1. Lublin FD, Reingold SC, Cohen JA et al. Defining the clinical course of multiple sclerosis. *Neurology* 2014;83(3):278–86.

2. Lucchinetti C, Bruck W, Parisi J, Scheithauer B, Rodriguez M, Lassmann H. Heterogeneity of multiple sclerosis lesions: implications for the pathogenesis of demyelination. *Ann Neurol.* 2000;47(6):707–17.

3. Thompson AJ, Banwell BL, Barkhof F et al. Diagnosis of multiple sclerosis: 2017 revisions of the McDonald criteria. *Lancet Neurol.* 2018;17(2):162–73.

4. Institute of Medicine. *Improving Diagnosis in Health Care.* Washington, DC: National Academies of Sciences, Engineering, and Medicine, 2015 (http://iom.nationalacadmies.org/Reports/2015/Improving-Diagnosis-in-Healthcare.aspx), page 2.

Learning Points

- Multiple sclerosis is a common cause of neurological disability, which shows latitudinal variation in incidence.
- Since 1995, an increasing number of disease-modifying drugs have emerged that reduce the relapse rate of patients with relapsing-remitting multiple sclerosis. Different blood-monitoring strategies are required for disease-modifying drugs.
- Individuals with multiple sclerosis are at increased risk of epilepsy.
- The ultimate goal of a disease-modifying drug in multiple sclerosis is NEDA.
- Risks of complications from disease-modifying therapy have emerged from phase 4 or post-marketing surveillance data from larger numbers of patients.

Patient's Perspective

1. **What was the impact of the condition on you?**

   a. Physical (e.g. job, driving, practical support)
   Loss of feeling in my right hand, my right leg was a dead weight and my left leg gave way. I had poor balance and poor co-ordination. I had memory loss, I could not retain information. I could not control my bladder and bowels, in that at times I did not get a warning.

   b. Psychological (e.g. mood, future, emotional well-being)
   Depression and anxiety due to constant fatigue, frustration, confusion, loss of vision from my left eye, and later diagnosed with epilepsy.

   c. Social (e.g. meeting friends, home)
   Social meetings were minimal. Family events were not attended due to my poor walking ability.

2. **What can or could you not do because of the condition?**
   I had difficulty remembering or planning things, writing or signing, holding my bladder and control of bowel movements. I could not walk very well and I could not concentrate. Now my memory and concentration have improved.

3. **Was there any other change for you due to your medical condition?**
   I dropped out of college due to depression, fatigue, lack of memory and poor concentration.

4. **What is/was the most difficult aspect of the condition for you?**
   Carrying the weight of my right leg and numbness in my right hand was most frustrating. My bladder and bowel problems caused me to fear of going out. Optic neuritis and seizures were by far the scariest experience!

5. **Was any aspect of the experience good or useful? What was that?**
   Overcoming obstacles. Exercise slightly helped my mobility. Reminders helped my memory. I learned to write and do tasks with my left hand. The OT [occupational therapist] helped my balance and movement a lot. The monthly infusions have helped a lot, especially with the fatigue.

6. **What do you hope for in the future for your condition?**
   In the future, I hope that patients with MS [multiple sclerosis] do not lose hope. I hope they know to help themselves alongside the treatment. Lifestyle changes worked for me. I hope that one day there will be a cure.

History

A 65-year-old man developed a swelling of his left medial canthus. He was referred from out-patient Ear, Nose and Throat to Ophthalmology. However, prior to an Ophthalmology assess-ment, he developed horizontal diplopia. A neurologist confirmed a left VI cranial nerve palsy. He had visual acuity of 6/6 bilaterally. A non-contrast MRI scan of the brain was reported as normal. The diplopia resolved within two months, as confirmed by an ophthalmologist and a neurologist.

He was a non-smoker and drank one or two glasses of wine per day. His mother had a melanoma at the age of 70 years.

Five months after the onset of diplopia, the medial canthus lesion was excised; it was noted that the lesion was adherent to underlying bone. Clinically, there was a patch of numbness in the distribution of the left inferotrochlear nerve (a branch of the nasociliary nerve supplying medial upper and lower eyelids, lateral part of nose above the medial canthus and medial con-junctiva). Histology showed a squamous cell carcinoma with immunohistochemistry stain-ing for cytokeratin 5/6 and epithelial membrane antigen (Figure 5.1). Further clearance was performed but identified no further evidence of tumour.

Seven months later, a mild left-sided headache developed. Double vision recurred. He was neurologically re-assessed.

Examination

He had a fair skin complexion. Visual acuity was 6/6 and there was a normal pupillary light reaction. There was left proptosis and failure of left eye abduction and impaired left eye upgaze. There was no optic nerve head swelling and no other neurological deficit. He was re-investigated.

Investigations

An MRI of the brain and orbits with contrast revealed a left intraorbital abnormality, suspi-cious for malignant infiltration (Figure).

A further left orbital biopsy was performed, confirming a poorly differentiated squamous cell carcinoma (strong staining with cytokeratin 5/6 and epithelial membrane antigen).

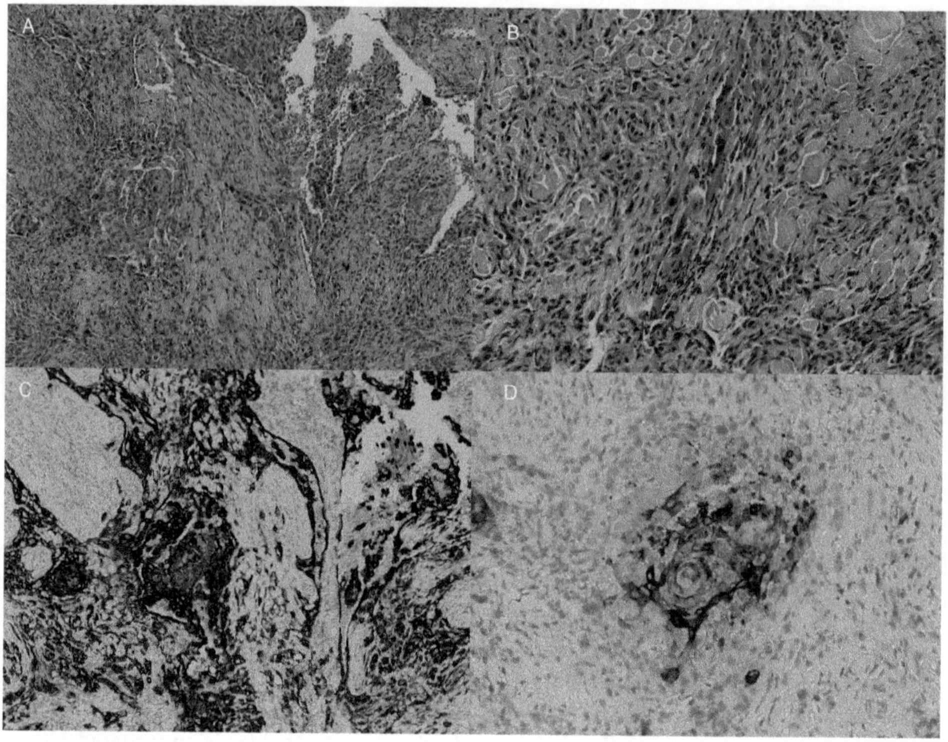

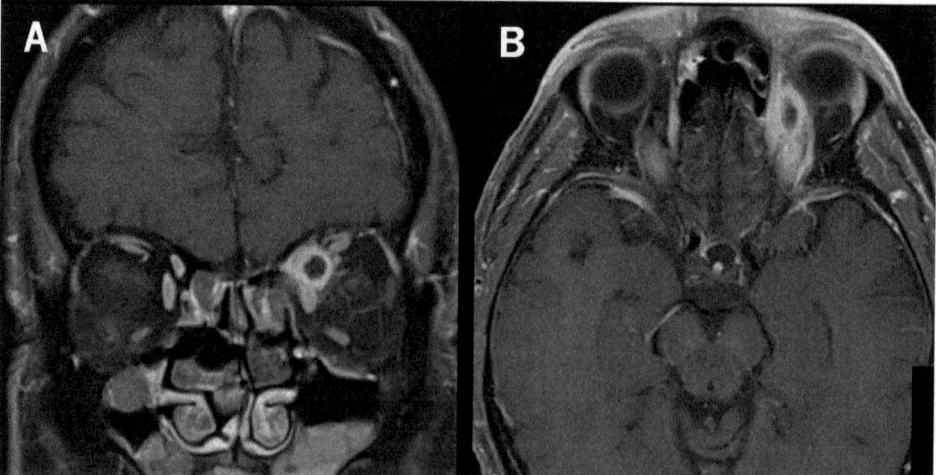

Figure 5.1 (A) Histology of the canthal tissue biopsy shows granulation tissue that is infiltrated by pleomorphic squamoid cells exhibiting dense eosinophilic cytoplasm, intercellular bridges and some keratinisation is seen focally. These atypical cells form nests and large groups with irregular contours as well as trabeculae and single cell forms. (B) Focally, sarcomatoid morphology with elongated spindle cell-like appearances and conspicuous mitotic figures are seen. There are also entrapped skeletal muscle bundles. (C) Cytokeratin 5/6 immunohistochemistry confirms the squamous phenotype of the lesional cells and highlights the tumour silhouette. (D) Epithelial membrane antigen immunohistochemistry shows patchy focal positivity that is consistent with squamous cell carcinoma.

Figure 5.2 (A) Coronal and (B) axial fat suppressed T1 MRI of the orbit with contrast showing thickened and enhancing soft tissue with central necrosis in the superomedial left orbit.

Diagnosis: Superior Orbital Fissure Syndrome or Rochon-Duvigneaud Syndrome (from Perineural Infiltration of Squamous Cell Carcinoma of the Orbit)

Management

A specialist multidisciplinary management plan was developed. The patient underwent a left orbital exenteration with clear margins followed by radiotherapy (66 Gray in 33 fractions) in order to reduce the risk of relapse. He developed a naso-orbital fistula. The weeping discharge severely restricted outdoor and social activities as frequent dressings were required. A prosthesis was fitted. The fistula was subsequently treated with three osseo-integrated implants. However, the fistula persisted with ongoing discharge. A paramedian forehead flap hampered the fitting of the prosthesis.

Comment

Differential Diagnosis of VI Cranial Nerve Palsy

The VI cranial nerve emerges anteriorly at the pontomedullary junction and then ascends in front of the brainstem. It makes a sharp angle over the tip of the petrous bone into Dorello's canal (under the petroclinoid ligament) before entering the back of the cavernous sinus. It next enters the orbit through the superior orbital fissure to pass laterally to the lateral rectus muscle.

Six syndromes of the VI cranial nerve (abducens) are recognised, defined by the anatomical location of the nerve injury (Figure 5.3), which can provide clinical clues.

1 Brainstem syndrome – The VI cranial nerve nucleus supplies the lateral rectus muscle and abducens internuclear neurones, which project via the medial longitudinal fasciculus to the contralateral oculomotor nerve for medial rectus innervation. A nuclear VI cranial nerve palsy therefore causes ipsilateral conjugate horizontal gaze palsy. Involvement of other pontine structures may cause Millard–Gubler syndrome (VI cranial nerve palsy, ipsilateral VII cranial nerve palsy and contralateral hemiparesis), Raymond's syndrome (VI cranial nerve palsy and contralateral hemiparesis) and Foville's syndrome (horizontal conjugate gaze palsy due to ipsilateral VI cranial nerve palsy and involvement of the parapontine reticular formation, ipsilateral V, VII and VIII cranial nerve palsies with ipsilateral Horner syndrome).

2 Subarachnoid space (prepontine cistern) syndrome– Downward displacement of the brainstem may displace the VI cranial nerve. This is the explanation for a VI cranial nerve lesion in patients with idiopathic intracranial hypertension; one third of patients with idiopathic intracranial hypertension have a VI cranial nerve lesion.

3 Petrous apex syndrome – The VI cranial nerve can be damaged at the tip of the petrous pyramid in Dorello's canal. Gradenigo syndrome (as can occur with infection of the petrous temporal bone from otitis media) consists of VI cranial nerve palsy, ipsilateral decreased hearing, ipsilateral facial pain from V cranial nerve involvement and ipsilateral facial weakness.

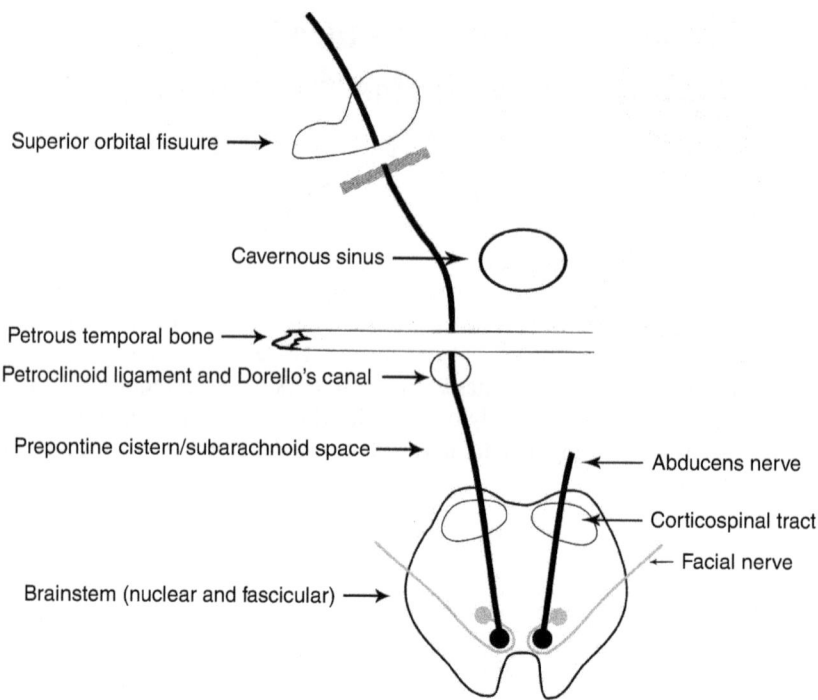

Superior orbital fisuure →

Cavernous sinus →

Petrous temporal bone →

Petroclinoid ligament and Dorello's canal →

Prepontine cistern/subarachnoid space →

← Abducens nerve

← Corticospinal tract

← Facial nerve

Brainstem (nuclear and fascicular) →

Figure 5.3 Schematic diagram of the course of the left VI cranial nerve and potential sites of injury.

4   Cavernous sinus syndrome – Lesions in the cavernous sinus cause VI cranial nerve palsy in association with III, IV and Va–b cranial nerve lesions, Horner syndrome, optic nerve or optic chiasm lesion and pituitary involvement.

5   Orbital apex syndrome-visual loss (optic nerve involved)/superior orbital fissure syndrome-vision spared (optic nerve not involved) – Early proptosis can suggest an orbital cause for VI cranial nerve lesion. It is difficult to distinguish between III, IV and VI cranial nerve palsies and mechanical restriction of the globe. Cranial nerve Va is also affected.

6   Isolated VI cranial nerve palsy – This syndrome has none of the signs in the other VI cranial nerve syndromes. Isolated VI cranial nerve palsy is usually an ischaemic mononeuropathy in adults. This was the presumed aetiology in our patient's initial presentation, particularly because of the recovery. Presumed microvascular VI cranial nerve palsy may mimic early perineural cutaneous squamous cell carcinoma invasion [1].

Cutaneous Periorbital Squamous Cell Carcinoma

Malignant tumour spread can occur via direct invasion, or by lymphatic and vascular routes, but perineural spread can also occur via layers of the perineurium and the endoneurial compartment guided by neurotrophins, growth factors and axonal guidance receptors dependent on the expression of neural cell adhesion molecules.

Squamous cell carcinoma accounts for 5–10% of periocular tumours. Increasing age, prolonged sun exposure, male sex, fair complexion, some skin disorders (e.g. albinism) and immunosuppression (particularly for renal transplant) all increase the risk of cutaneous squamous cell carcinoma. Between 2 and 6% of patients with cutaneous basal and squamous cell carcinomas have evidence of perineural invasion [2]. Mid-face location, male sex, high histological grade and increasing tumour size are risk factors for perineural invasion. Cranial nerves V and VII are most commonly involved due to their extensive subcutaneous distribution.

Management of Periocular Cutaneous Squamous Cell Carcinoma

Management of periocular cutaneous squamous cell carcinoma is challenging, requiring a specialist oculo-facial plastic surgeon to co-ordinate interdisciplinary management, surgical reconstruction and post-operative surveillance.

Delay in Diagnosis

A delayed, missed or incorrect diagnosis is defined as a misdiagnosis. Cognitive or heuristic errors (faulty clinical reasoning) [3], system-related errors and an incorrect interpretation of diagnostic tests constitute the important domains or themes underlying many misdiagnoses.

Should perineural invasion have been suspected when this patient initially presented with VI cranial nerve palsy? The resolved lateral rectus weakness with initial normal neuroimaging (albeit without contrast) pointed towards the initial VI cranial nerve palsy being due to microvascular ischaemic disease. The medial canthus lesion was not biopsied at that stage. A partial resolution of a VI cranial nerve palsy has been reported in periorbital squamous cell carcinoma [1], but a spontaneous and full resolution of a VI cranial nerve would be unusual in the presence of a tumour.

Nomenclature and Definitions

There are a number of terms used to describe the anatomical location of pathological processes affecting cranial nerves in and around the orbit.

The **orbital apex syndrome** involves the optic nerve, the oculomotor nerve, the trochlear nerve, the abducens nerve and the ophthalmic division of the trigeminal nerve. Clinically, there is loss of vision plus painful and limited eye movements. The term orbital apex syndrome is now reserved for such patients with loss of vision. There may also be proptosis, altered corneal reflex, a relative afferent pupillary defect, optic disc oedema or atrophy and choroidal folds.

The **superior orbital fissure syndrome** (also known as Rochon-Duvigneaud syndrome) is caused by lesions anterior to the orbital apex and in close proximity to the annulus of Zinn (ring of fibrous tissue that is the common origin for four rectus muscles and surrounds the optic nerve). There is impaired function of cranial nerves III, IV, Va and VI. As in our patient, the optic nerve is generally spared.

The **cavernous sinus syndrome** and the superior orbital fissure contain the same structures, making it clinically difficult to state whether a lesion is in the cavernous sinus or the superior orbital fissure. The maxillary division of the trigeminal nerve may occasionally be involved in the cavernous sinus syndrome but not in the superior orbital fissure syndrome. Sympathetic carotid plexus involvement also occurs in the cavernous sinus syndrome.

References

1. Koukkoulli A, Koutroumanos N, Kidd D. Perineural spread of cutaneous squamous cell carcinoma manifesting as ophthalmoplegia. *Neuro-Ophthalmology.* 2015;39(3):144–6.

2. Mendenhall WM, Amdur RJ, Hinerman RW et al. Skin cancer of the head and neck with perineural invasion. *Am J Clin Oncol Cancer Clin Trials.* 2007;30(1):93–6.

3. Vickrey BG, Samuels MA, Ropper AH. How neurologists think a cognitive psychology perspective on missed diagnoses. *Ann Neurol.* 2010;67(4):425–33.

Learning Points

- Accompanying features of a VI cranial nerve palsy may provide clues to the anatomical location of the pathology.

- Superior orbital fissure syndrome is caused by lesions anterior to the orbital apex and annulus of Zinn. Cranial nerves III, IV, Va and VI are impaired but the optic nerve is generally spared in the superior orbital fissure syndrome.

- Squamous cell carcinoma can invade perineurally, particularly cranial nerves V and VII due to their extensive subcutaneous distribution.

Patient's Perspective

1. **What was the impact of the condition on you?**

   a. Physical (e.g. job, driving, practical support)
   The initial symptom was sudden onset of double vision, which was attributed to a VI nerve palsy possibly due to a TIA. This was alleviated by the use of corrective spectacles. An MRI was also arranged. This was believed to show nothing suspicious. Later examination of scan indicated growth behind the eye, which biopsy confirmed to be a squamous cell carcinoma. Treatment involved orbital exenteration followed by six weeks of radiotherapy. Also, the hospital dental surgeon advised that a particular tooth should be removed prior to treatment to avoid this at a later date. I was told that I would need to use a high fluoride toothpaste for life.

   b. Psychological (e.g. mood, future, emotional well-being)
   Depression at disfiguration due to loss of eye (with no easy cosmetic solution due to an empty socket). Fear of further spread of condition. Decrease in weight due to loss of taste and appetite due to side-effects of radiotherapy. Disinclination to mix with people.

   c. Social (e.g. meeting friends, home)
   Reluctant to meet people and having to explain what had happened and that it would not improve.

2. **What could you not do because of the condition?**
   Due to the need to have the wound dressed every couple of days, holidays became impossible for several years. Having no binocular vision meant loss of depth perception. This meant that any intricate tasks became very difficult. Due to my restricted field of vision, I became reluctant to drive even though permitted by DVLA [the Driver and Vehicle Licensing Agency].

3. **Was there any other change for you due to your medical condition?**
   Protein drinks were provided for several months to help compensate for loss of appetite and consequent weight loss. Several sessions of antibiotic due to infection of the wound.

4. **What is/was the most difficult aspect of the condition for you?**
   The surgery resulted in a fistula between [my] nasal cavity and eye socket. The ongoing issue with this is an inability to blow my nose without air and mucus being expelled into the eye socket. Discharge from the nose into the eye socket seems to be the principal cause of the requirement to dress the wound every few days (four years after the surgery). The surgery caused permanent numbness down the left side of my face.

5. **Was any aspect of the experience of the condition good or useful? What was that?**

I was accommodated at the City Hospital in Belfast during the weeks of my radiotherapy. A volunteer from Derry drove several patients to and from Belfast for treatments. Also, the Macmillan centre in Belfast offered a number of helpful activities including reflexology. One positive period was when I was given appointments with a maxillofacial prosthetist. He spent a lot of time producing a prosthesis that required glue to hold it in place. Later an operation was performed to fit magnetic screws. This enabled a magnetic prosthesis to be fitted a few months later. This is a much more convenient cosmetic solution. Excellent support was provided by district nurses and later nurses in my doctor's treatment room. They recommended and applied dressings (initially maggots) until recently when my wife has taken on the task. Further scans have helped reduce the worry of a recurrence.

6. **What do you hope for in the future for people with this condition?**

The biggest improvement in treatment would be much earlier closure of the fistula. This could obviate the necessity of the years of dressing the wound. That operation was planned for this summer, only to be delayed due to the COVID-19 crisis.

High Pressure

History

A 17-year-old woman presented with six weeks of moderately severe headache, and intermittent double and blurred vision. She had visual obscurations (darkening or black-out of vision) triggered by postural change. She denied any pulsatile tinnitus.

Examination

Her weight was 90.1 kg and body mass index was 40.5 kg/m². She had marked optic disc swelling (Figure 6.1A). Visual acuity was 6/12 on the right and 6/6 on the left. She had weakness of right eye abduction. Face and corneal sensation were intact. Visual fields were peripherally constricted to confrontation. She had no other focal neurological deficits.

Investigations

An MRI scan of the brain showed no abnormality. A CT venogram was normal. At lumbar puncture, there was an opening pressure of 41 cm cerebrospinal fluid (CSF), 2 white cells/µL, 55 red blood cells/µL, CSF glucose of 3.5 mmol/L, serum glucose of 5.4 mmol/L and CSF protein of 0.14 g/L.

Visual perimetry showed bitemporal constriction (Figure 6.1B).

Management

A ventriculoperitoneal shunt was inserted. Headaches, visual fields and optic disc swelling all improved (Figure 6.1C and 6.1D).

Some years later, the shunt was converted to a ventriculo-atrial shunt due to a peritoneal infection. This also became infected and she subsequently had two 8 mm stents placed in the right transverse sinus.

At follow-up she had ongoing headaches and optic atrophy.

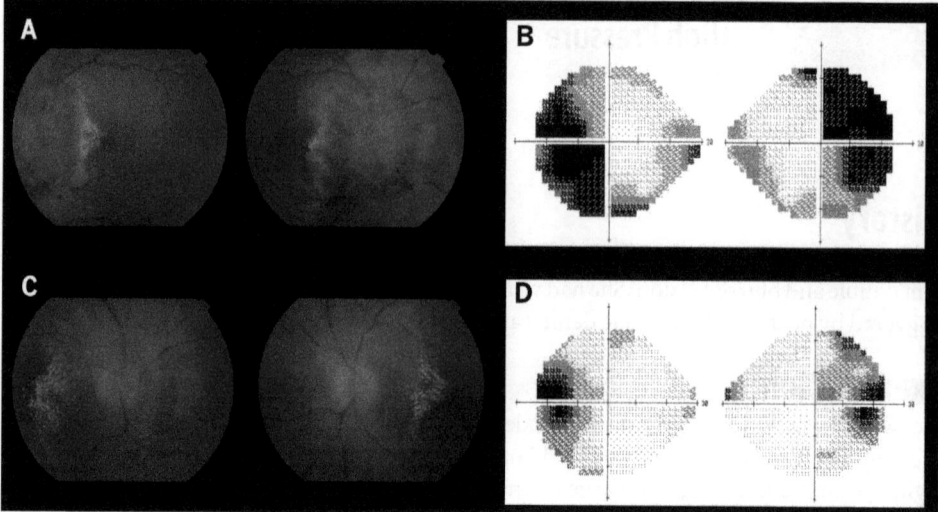

Figure 6.1 (A) Funduscopic photographs showing marked optic disc swelling alongside (B) perimetry showing predominantly bitemporal visual field constriction. Following shunt insertion, the (C) optic discs and (D) visual field appearances improved.

Diagnosis: Idiopathic Intracranial Hypertension

Comment

History

The diagnostic criteria of idiopathic intracranial hypertension first described by Walter Dandy in 1937 required the presence of papilloedema with an opening pressure of ≥ 25 cm CSF. The criteria have evolved, putting increasing emphasis on neuroimaging, and neuroimaging exclusion of cerebral venous sinus thrombosis is now required.

The 2013 Friedman criteria for idiopathic intracranial hypertension (also called pseudotumour cerebri syndrome) are listed in Box 6.1 [1].

Criteria A–E make the diagnosis of idiopathic intracranial hypertension definite. The diagnosis is considered probable if criteria A–D are met but the measured CSF pressure is lower than specified for a definite diagnosis [1].

Epidemiology and Secular Trends

Idiopathic intracranial hypertension occurs predominantly in young, obese women. The UK has recorded a particularly high incidence of idiopathic intracranial hypertension. The obesity prevalence in a country correlates positively with the incidence of idiopathic intracranial hypertension [2]. The increase in the incidence of idiopathic intracranial hypertension since 2002 in England has been over-represented among socially deprived populations. A Welsh study has confirmed increasing incidence (as high as 7.8 per 100,000 per year) associated with increasing BMI and increasing socio-economic deprivation.

Box 6.1 Diagnostic criteria for idiopathic intracranial hypertension (pseudotumour cerebri syndrome)

The following are required for diagnosis of idiopathic intracranial hypertension

A. Papilloedema
B. Normal neurological examination except for cranial nerve abnormalities
C. Neuroimaging: Normal brain parenchyma without evidence of hydrocephalus, mass, or structural lesion and no abnormal meningeal enhancement on MRI, with and without gadolinium, for typical patients (female and obese), and MRI, with and without gadolinium, and magnetic resonance venography for others; if MRI is unavailable or contraindicated, contrast-enhanced CT may be used
D. Normal CSF composition
E. Elevated lumbar puncture opening pressure (≥ 25 cm CSF in adults and ≥ 28 cm CSF in children (25 cm CSF if the child is not sedated and not obese) in a properly performed lumbar puncture

Diagnosis of idiopathic intracranial hypertension (pseudotumour cerebri syndrome) without papilloedema can be made in the following circumstances

In the absence of papilloedema, a diagnosis of idiopathic intracranial hypertension (pseudotumour cerebri syndrome) can be made if B–E are satisfied, and in addition the patient has a unilateral or bilateral abducens nerve palsy

In the absence of papilloedema or VI cranial nerve palsy, a diagnosis of idiopathic intracranial hypertension (pseudotumour cerebri syndrome) can be suggested but not made if B–E are satisfied, and in addition, at least three of the following neuroimaging criteria are satisfied:

i.   Empty sella
ii. Fattening of the posterior aspect of the globe
iii. Distention of the perioptic subarachnoid space with or without a tortuous optic nerve
iv. Transverse venous sinus stenosis

Adapted from Friedman et al. [1] with permission from Wolters Kluwer.

Putative Pathology

Idiopathic intracranial hypertension appears to be a systemic metabolic condition in which there is an insulin- and leptin-resistant phenotype. Metabolic interventions are undergoing active research.

Differential Diagnosis of Papilloedema

There are multiple causes of papilloedema (optic disc oedema due to intracranial hypertension) and optic disc oedema without elevated intracranial pressure (Table 6.1).

Clinical Features of Idiopathic Intracranial Hypertension

Headache, transient visual obscurations and diplopia in a young and overweight or obese woman are typical features of idiopathic intracranial hypertension. Pulsatile tinnitus may also occur. More non-specific symptoms include dizziness, neck and back pain and blurred vision. Some patients may, however, be asymptomatic and optic nerve swelling may only be detected by an optician during a routine vision test.

In addition to optic disc oedema, there may be exudates, retinal haemorrhages and an obliterated central cup, as present in our patient. Venous pulsations are usually absent. The presence of venous pulsation suggests that the CSF pressure is probably < 20 cm CSF.

Visual field loss in idiopathic intracranial hypertension begins with enlarged blind spots. Further visual field loss usually begins nasally and leads to generalized constriction. Our patient was unusual, having mostly bitemporal field loss.

Management Evidence for Idiopathic Intracranial Hypertension

Guidelines to manage idiopathic intracranial hypertension have been produced in the UK based on accumulating evidence [3]. These include a diagnostic workup (blood pressure to exclude malignant hypertension, visual acuity, dilated funduscopy, formal visual fields, brain imaging and venography prior to lumbar puncture).

Repeated lumbar punctures can improve headache but an exacerbation of headache may occur, suggesting little overall benefit from this type of management. Migraine is a common type of headache in idiopathic intracranial hypertension for which migraine treatments appear effective. Indeed, migraine is over-represented in idiopathic intracranial hypertension cohorts prior to clinical presentation. Further emphasis on headache (and migraine) management in idiopathic intracranial hypertension could improve quality of life.

Acute management is required if there is evidence of declining visual function. A temporising lumbar drain may be used but CSF diversion in the form of shunting is the preferred procedure for declining visual function and was employed in our patient. Optic nerve

Table 6.1 Some causes of optic nerve oedema with and without intracranial hypertension

Causes of papilloedema – swollen optic disc with intracranial hypertension	Causes of optic nerve disc oedema without intracranial hypertension
Idiopathic intracranial hypertension	Inflammatory – papillitis
Cerebral venous sinus thrombosis	Ocular disease – uveitis, vein occlusion
Mass lesion	Infiltrative – lymphoma
Infection	Vascular – ischaemic optic neuropathy, arteritis
Infiltrative process	Metabolic – dysthyroidism
	Optic disc tumour – glioma
	Drusen

fenestration and CSF diversion work well in the short term but may fail over time, emphasising the need for weight reduction to avoid recurrence of idiopathic intracranial hypertension. A precise threshold for employing CSF diversion therapies has not been established, but it is estimated that 1% of patients with idiopathic intracranial hypertension go blind. In the UK, all patients who drive and have a ventriculo-peritoneal shunt should inform the Driver and Vehicle Licensing Agency. Shunt complications can ensue (blocked shunt, infection, migration of catheter and even visual deterioration). Although venous sinus stenting has a good early safety profile and has been shown to improve headaches, pulsatile tinnitus and papilloedema, the UK guidelines recommend more research as the role of this procedures is not yet established.

Weight reduction was first shown to decrease symptoms when Barbara Newborg reported a decrease in symptoms and weight with a low-calorie rice-based diet in 1974. A strict weight reduction regime of 425 kcal per day for three months led to decreased weight, reduced intracranial pressure, reduced headache and papilloedema in a cohort of 25 UK women with idiopathic intracranial hypertension.

The first randomised placebo-controlled clinical trial for idiopathic intracranial hypertension (the Idiopathic Intracranial Hypertension Treatment Trial) enrolled newly diagnosed patients with mild visual field loss to assess the effect of acetazolamide therapy. The acetazolamide group experienced moderate improvements in visual field assessments, papilloedema grade and quality-of-life measures compared with the placebo group.

A randomised controlled trial of bariatric surgery in 66 patients with idiopathic intracranial hypertension and a BMI of ≥ 35 kg/m^2 achieved lower opening pressures of CSF (beginning as early as two weeks after surgery), more weight reduction and better quality of life for the bariatric surgery group at 12 and 24 months. However, neither of these trials addressed management of early visual loss in idiopathic intracranial hypertension.

In the longer term, public health interventions aimed at reducing childhood and young adult obesity will be required to reduce the increasing incidence of idiopathic intracranial hypertension.

References

1. Friedman DI, Liu GT, Digre KB. Revised diagnostic criteria for the pseudotumor cerebri syndrome in adults and children. *Neurology*. 2013;81(13):1159–65.

2. McCluskey G, Doherty-Allan R, McCarron P et al. Meta-analysis and systematic review of population-based epidemiological studies in idiopathic intracranial hypertension. *Eur J Neurol*. 2018;25(10):1218–27.

3. Mollan SP, Davies B, Silver NC et al. Idiopathic intracranial hypertension: consensus guidelines on management. *J Neurol Neurosurg Psychiatry*. 2018;89:1088–100.

Learning Points

- Idiopathic intracranial hypertension, a disease predominantly affecting young women, has increased in incidence with increases in national obesity prevalence.

- Visual constriction is the main neurological risk of idiopathic intracranial hypertension, with a 1% risk of blindness. Urgent CSF diversion, mainly with ventriculoperitoneal shunt, is indicated for progressive visual loss.

- Weight reduction is the mainstay of management of idiopathic intracranial hypertension.

- Migraine headaches are frequent in idiopathic intracranial hypertension and may respond to migraine therapies.

Patient's Perspective

1. **What is/was the impact of the condition?**
    Cooking was a struggle as the heat set off headaches. There are days when I cannot get out of bed at all.
    IIH [idiopathic intracranial hypertension] left me very low. It still does 13 years later. I feel useless, tired and get upset that I can't do things.
    Because of the headaches I have to miss out on quite a lot of social events including my grandmother's wedding.

2. **What can you no longer do?**
    It varies day to day. Some days I can't walk far as I fall, some days I can't get out of bed. Doing my hair is a massive struggle.

3. **Was there any other change for you due to your medical condition?**
    Yes, my arms and legs have become so weak. One side of my face doesn't move like the other side, which leaves me paranoid about it.

4. **What was/is the most difficult aspect of the condition?**
    The amount of time I missed and still miss with my children from either being sick with a headache or being in hospital.

5. **Was any aspect of the experience good or useful? What was that?**
    Learning a lot about the brain and body and starting me on a healthier lifestyle to lose weight.

6. **What do you hope for in the future for your condition?**
    That the headaches stay away for at least a month at a time instead of having them everyday with different intensity.

History

A 49-year-old man developed blurred vision from his left eye two days after the onset of a moderately severe global headache. His left eye vision deteriorated further over one week. He had an unremarkable past medical history. He was on no medication. He did not smoke cigarettes. He drank three cans of beer and two whiskeys at the weekend.

Examination

Visual acuity in the left eye was reduced to hand movements, colour vision in the left eye was reduced to 0/14 Ishihara plates. He had a left relative afferent pupillary defect, full range of eye movements in both eyes but had pain in his left eye when gazing superiorly and medially. Ophthalmological examination revealed that the cornea was clear in the left eye and the anterior chamber was deep and quiet. Normal optic disc and macula were visualised. Examination of the right eye was normal.

Investigations

MRI of the brain showed non-specific white matter changes. All of these were subcortical and not periventricular. The left optic nerve had high signal in the intracanalicular and intracranial segment (Figure 7.1).

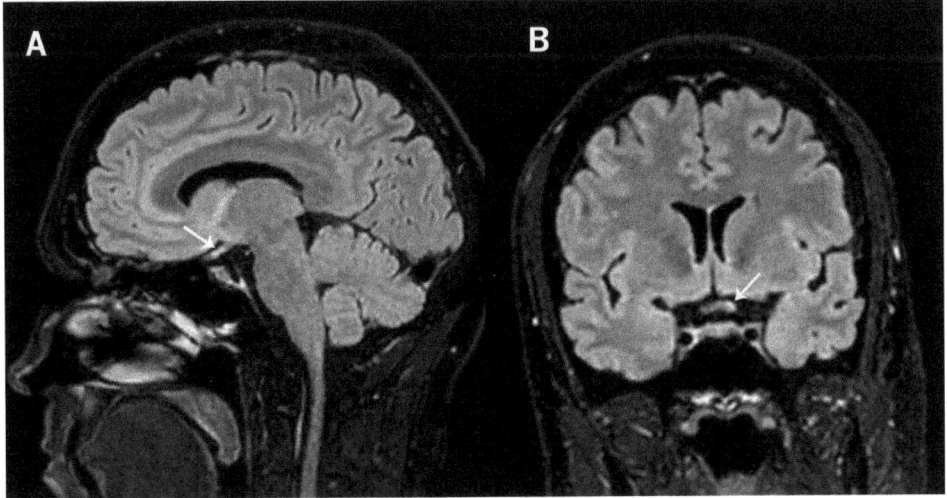

Figure 7.1 A (A) sagittal and (B) coronal T2 FLAIR MRI scan showing high signal in the intracranial left optic nerve (arrow) at the junction with the optic chiasm.

Blood investigations yielded negative neuromyelitis optica (NMO) aquaporin 4 immunoglobulin G (AQP4-IgG) from a fixed commercial assay and myelin oligodendrocyte glycoprotein (MOG) antibody.

At lumbar puncture, opening pressure was 12.5 cm of cerebrospinal fluid (CSF). There were no white cells/μL and 44 red cells/μL. CSF glucose was 3.6 mmol/L (serum glucose 4.5 mmol/L) and CSF protein was 0.69 g/L (normal range 0.15–0.4 g/L). CSF was negative for oligoclonal bands.

A diagnostic test was performed.

Working Diagnosis: Left Optic Neuritis

Management and Follow-up Investigations

He was diagnosed with left eye optic neuritis and admitted to hospital for three days of intravenous methylprednisolone. At two months follow-up, vision improved to 6/9–2 on the left.

A live cell-based NMO AQP4-IgG assay was requested. A positive NMO AQP4-IgG was then identified.

Optical coherence tomography (OCT) confirmed left retinal nerve fibre layer (RNFL) thinning (67 μm on the left versus 103 μm on the right; Figure 7.2).

Diagnosis: Neuromyelitis Optica Spectrum Disorder (NMOSD) with AQP4-IgG

He was referred to a national NMO centre. Prior to assessment, he started mycophenolate and prednisolone 20 mg/day. The prednisolone was then gradually reduced over months to 10 mg/day.

Comment

The Optic Nerve

The optic disc (5 degrees across) sits 15 degrees to the nasal side of the optical axis. The optic nerve has four components:

1. the intraocular optic nerve (1–2 mm in length);
2. the intraorbital optic nerve (20–30 mm), which is longer than the distance from the globe to the optical canal to allow for rotation and stretching;
3. the intracanalicular optic nerve (10 mm), which is attached to the dura of the lesser wing of the sphenoid bone;
4. and the intracranial optic nerve, which is 10–15 mm in length before joining the optic chiasm.

In multiple sclerosis, optic neuritis is usually unilateral and covers a short segment of the optic nerve. Longitudinally extensive optic neuritis is found in NMO and MOG antibody-associated disease, both of which may also cause bilateral optic neuritis. NMO is a demyelinating condition of the central nervous system distinct from multiple sclerosis. Since 1894, bilateral visual and spinal disease was known as Devic's NMO [1]. However, since 2004, the condition has been associated with a pathogenic serum AQP4-IgG, which may or may not be found in CSF [2]. Since the discovery of the AQP4-IgG, different clinical features of AQP4-IgG-positive patients have been described: recurrent optic neuritis and myelitis, posterior reversible encephalopathy, acute demyelinating encephalomyelitis, and brainstem and area postrema syndromes. The combination of positive AQP4-IgG and these conditions constitute NMO.

In 2015, criteria were updated to include NMO spectrum disorders (NMOSDs) to account for more restricted disorders (i.e. patients who may not have both optic neuritis and acute myelitis) but also to account for more extensive central nervous system disease phenotypes [3].

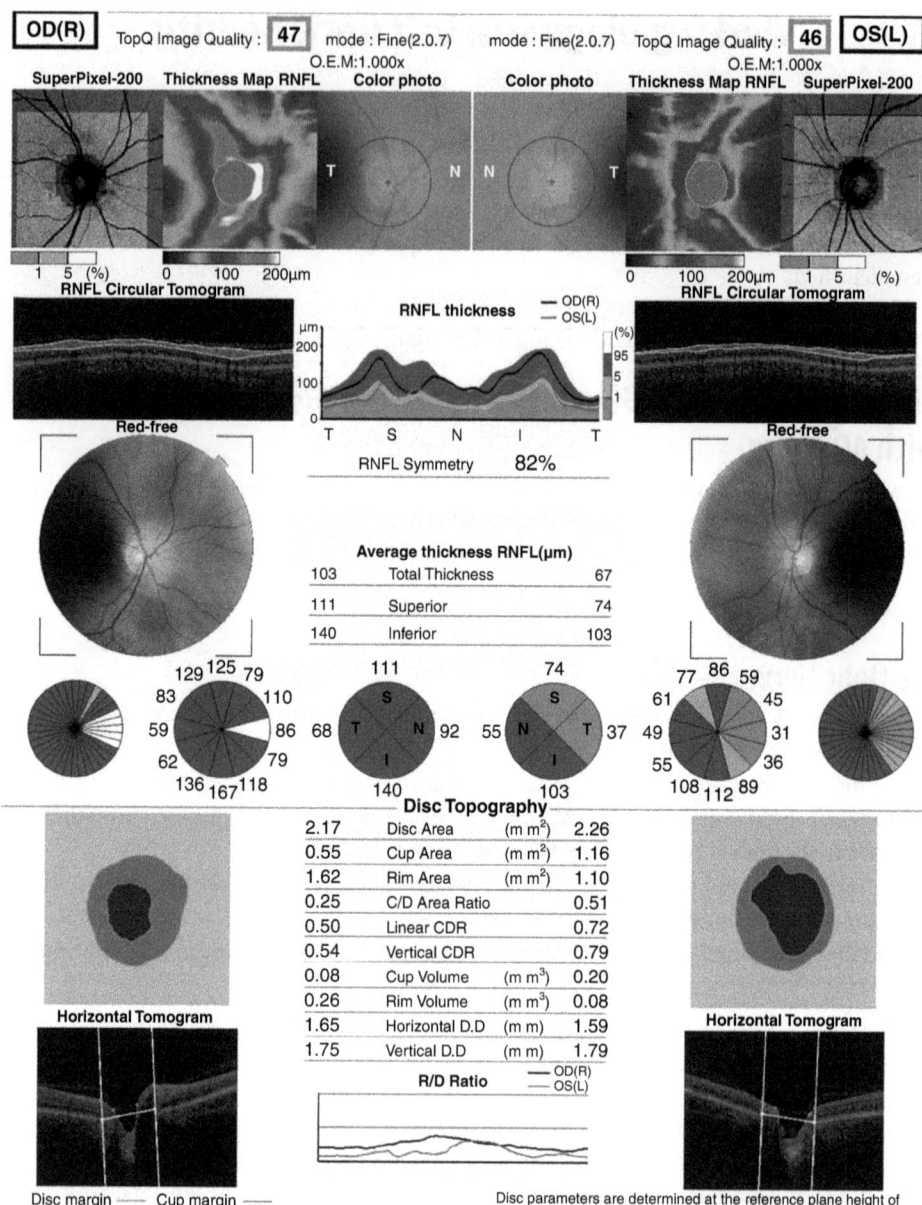

Figure 7.2 OCT demonstrating left retinal fibre layer thinning.

Box 7.1 Diagnostic criteria for NMOSDs

Diagnostic criteria for NMOSD with AQP4-IgG

1. At least one core clinical characteristic (optic neuritis, acute myelitis, area postrema syndrome, acute brainstem syndrome, symptomatic narcolepsy or acute diencephalic clinical syndrome with NMOSD-typical diencephalic MRI lesions or symptomatic cerebral syndrome with NMOSD-typical brain lesions)
2. Positive test for AQP4-IgG using best available detection method (live cell-based assay)
3. Exclusion of alternative diagnoses

Diagnostic criteria for NMOSD without or unknown AQP4-IgG

1. At least two core clinical characteristics occurring as a result of one or more clinical attacks and meeting the following criteria:
   a. At least one core clinical criteria must be optic neuritis, longitudinally extensive transverse myelitis or area postrema syndrome
   b. Dissemination in space of two or more clinical characteristics
   c. Fulfilment of additional MRI requirements
2. Negative tests for AQP4-IgG using best available detection method or test unavailable
3. Exclusion of alternative diagnoses

Core clinical characteristics

1. Optic neuritis
2. Acute myelitis
3. Area postrema syndrome: episode of otherwise unexplained hiccups or nausea and vomiting
4. Acute brainstem syndrome
5. Symptomatic narcolepsy or acute diencephalic clinical syndrome with NMOSD-typical diencephalic MRI lesions
6. Symptomatic cerebral syndrome with NMOSD-typical brain lesions

Additional MRI requirements for NMOSD without AQP4-IgG and NMOSD with unknown AQP4-IgG status

1. Acute optic neuritis, which requires a brain MRI showing:
   a. normal findings or only non-specific white matter lesions
   OR
   b. optic nerve MRI T2-hyperintense lesion or T1-weighted gadolinium-enhancing lesion extending over more than half of the optic nerve length or involving optic chiasm
2. Acute myelitis, which requires
   a. associated intramedullary MRI lesion extending over ≥ 3 contiguous segments (longitudinal extensive transverse myelitis)
   OR
   b. ≥ 3 contiguous segments of focal spinal cord atrophy in patients with history compatible with acute myelitis
3. Area postrema syndrome, which requires associated dorsal medulla/area postrema lesions
4. Acute brainstem syndrome, which requires associated periependymal brainstem lesions

Adapted from Wingerchuk et al. [3] with permission from Wolters Kluwer.

The 2015 NMO criteria [3] are itemised in Box 7.1, which includes the core clinical characteristics and the additional MRI requirements for NMOSD without AQP4-IgG and NMOSD with unknown status of AQP4-IgG.

The classification is not straightforward and has been further complicated in that another entity, MOG-antibody disease can overlap with NMOSD.

However, the classification has been important in managing patients. Some treatments for multiple sclerosis can be deleterious in NMOSD. New drugs have emerged with proven efficacy in NMOSD. Some of these emerging drugs are listed in Table 7.1. It makes sense to target B lymphocytes and complement, which have been recognised to play a pathological role. The broader immunosuppressing regimes of azathioprine and mycophenolate continue to be used.

Table 7.1 Emerging evidence-based therapies for NMOSD

Drug	Target
Rituximab	Anti-CD20 lymphocytes
Inebilizumab	Anti-CD19 lymphocytes
Eculizumab	Complement C5 blockade
Satralizumab	Interleukin 6 receptor signalling

Test Characteristic

The initial negative fixed commercial assay for NMO AQP4-IgG was less sensitive than the live cell-based assay. A test with a low sensitivity is misleading. The pre-test probability in our patient was high because of the phenotype (optic neuritis) and the location plus extent of the optic neuritis.

The prevalence of a disease in the population being tested is crucial in determining both the positive predictive value (presence of the target disease among patients with a positive result; PPV) and the negative predictive value (NPV) of an investigative test. The prevalence of multiple sclerosis is about 230 per 100,000 in Northern Ireland, whereas the prevalence of NMOSD has been estimated to be 1–2 per 100,000 (i.e. 115–230 times less prevalent than multiple sclerosis). If the prevalence of a disease in a population is very low, then testing that population yields a low PPV. This can be demonstrated graphically because PPV can be plotted against prevalence of disease, as shown in Figure 7.3.

PPV is calculated from the following equation:

$$\frac{(\text{sensitivity} \times \text{prevalence})}{(\text{sensitivity} \times \text{prevalence}) + ((1\text{-specificity}) \times (1\text{-prevalence}))}$$

Widespread testing in populations with low prevalence of NMOSD is problematic as without a specificity of 100% (the proportion of those who do not have the disease who test negative), false positive results can occur. Increasing test sensitivity has little impact on the

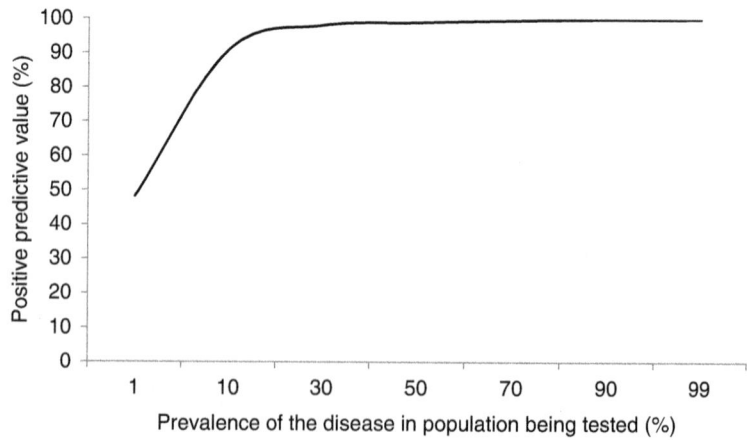

Figure 7.3 Effect of prevalence on PPVs for NMO AQP4-IgG testing (specificity 99% and sensitivity 92%).

PPV–prevalence curve. Testing all patients suspected of multiple sclerosis and/or NMOSD for AQP4-IgG means a low PPV, with the prevalence of NMOSD being at most 2% of the tested population.

This theme of the influence of prevalence on the PPV of a test has been demonstrated in many publications. In summary, diagnostic test characteristics and prevalence of disease are important.

Optical Coherence Tomography

Optical coherence tomography uses low coherence near-infrared light to produce structural cross-images. This non-invasive technique, first used as a clinical tool in 1996, can produce high-resolution, three-dimensional images of retinal structures. For ophthalmologists, OCT has developed a particular role in the diagnosis and long-term monitoring of glaucoma. It can also aid diagnosis of optic neuritis and can be used for monitoring. Retinal nerve fibre thinning has an increasing severity spectrum from patients with multiple sclerosis to MOG-antibody disease to NMO.

Other neurological applications of OCT in diagnosis, monitoring and prognostication are summarised in Table 7.2. Optical coherence tomography imaging of the optic disc and macula are of neurological interest. A circle scan of the optic disc measures peripapillary retinal nerve fibre thickness. Red, yellow and green bands represent population cut-offs for 1%, 5% and 95%. Atrophy and ganglion cell loss can be measured via a composite of the ganglion cell layer and inner plexiform layer.

The total RNFL is 110–120 μm at the age of 15 years and then declines to 90 μm by the age of 70 years. Our patient's left RNFL at his left optic disc was 67 μm compared to 103 μm in his right optic disc (Figure 7.2). This interocular asymmetry of the RNFL thickness is the OCT evidence of previous optic neuritis.

Table 7.2 Optical coherence tomography in neurological disorders

Neurological issue	Use of OCT
Idiopathic intracranial hypertension	Diagnosis and monitoring of the swollen optic nerve. Optic nerve head volume correlates with intracranial pressure. Identifies Patton's (retinal lines) and choroidal folds – other changes in papilloedema
Optic disc drusen	Diagnosis of drusen can be distinguished from papilloedema
Optic neuritis	In the chronic phase, thinning of the RNFL to < 75–80 μm is associated with clinically significant visual impairment (our patient). RNFL thinning at the macula can be seen within weeks. In secondary progressive multiple sclerosis, an unaffected eye may exhibit faster thinning of the RNFL than in relapsing-remitting multiple sclerosis. RNFL thinning in multiple sclerosis is associated with MRI lesion load and atrophy. NMOSD has more severe RNFL thinning than multiple sclerosis
Leber's hereditary optic neuropathy	Asymptomatic carriers thickening of the RNFL. When symptomatic thickening of the superior and inferior RNFL occurs before normalisation and thinning
Cystoid macular oedema	Patients taking fingolimod or siponimod can develop macular oedema

Relative Afferent Pupillary Defect

The afferent pupillary defect is an important clinical sign that can confirm pathology in the afferent visual system from the optic nerve to the lateral geniculate ganglion or the pretectal fibres in the dorsal midbrain (at the Edinger Westphal nucleus). Dr Lee provides an excellent tutorial on YouTube on the anatomy of this sign (www.youtube.com/watch?v=AFYY1qxF0T0).

In a unilateral optic neuropathy (as in our patient), the consensual light reflex from shining light on the unaffected eye is a stronger pupillary constrictor than the direct light reflex in the affected eye. This results in the Marcus Gunn pupil, in which a swinging torchlight shining on the unaffected eye causes consensual pupillary constriction but on swinging the torchlight on the affected eye, there is relative pupillary dilatation (i.e. a relative afferent pupillary defect).

References

1. Jarius S, Wildemann B. The history of neuromyelitis optica. *J Neuroinflammation*. 2013;10(8):1–12.
2. Lennon VA, Wingerchuk DM, Kryzer TJ et al. A serum autoantibody marker of neuromyelitis optica: distinction from multiple sclerosis. *Lancet*. 2004;364(9451):2106–12.
3. Wingerchuk DM, Banwell B, Bennett JL et al. International consensus diagnostic criteria for neuromyelitis optica spectrum disorders. *Neurology*. 2015;85(2):177–89.

Learning Points

- Neuromyelitis optica spectrum disorder (NMOSD) is an inflammatory demyelinating disorder with a predilection for optic nerves and spinal cord.
- NMOSD can recur with debilitating consequences, requiring early immune therapy.
- Think carefully when requesting a diagnostic test. Ensure the test can explain the phenotype and consider the prevalence of the disease in the tested population.

Patient's Perspective

1. **What is/was the impact of the condition?**

    a. Physical (e.g. everyday life, practical support, work, hobbies)
    As the condition only affects my left eye, the blurriness particularly when I am tired, would make working at the computer or reading a bit difficult. Reading small print sometimes would be a problem and I would close my left eye and only use my right eye. Otherwise, the condition doesn't really impact on day-to-day life.

    b. Psychological (e.g. mood, emotional well-being)
    Apart from the initial shock when I was told that I possibly had a neurological condition, when I felt very fit and well, the condition doesn't really affect my mood or emotional well-being. I just hope that I will not be unlucky enough to have another attack, although when I am taking daily medication, the reminder is always there that there is something wrong with me.

    c. Social (e.g. meeting friends and family, home life)
    My home, social life and meeting friends haven't really changed apart from myself being more aware in not being excessive with either food or alcohol. I do not make anyone aware even close family that I have this condition as I do not want to be thought of or made feel any different than before.

2. **What can or could you not do because of the condition?**
    I cannot do anything that I couldn't do before my diagnosis, but I am more aware that I just can't take everything I do physically for granted anymore.

3. **Was there any other change for you due to your medical condition?**
Making sure that I have my medicines in stock and being aware that I will now have doctors' appointments to attend in the future is the only real change due to my condition.

4. **What is/was the most difficult aspect of the condition for you?**
The most difficult part is the unknown. Whilst I tell myself I am fine and I will not have any more attacks, there is always a doubt. Before the diagnosis, I would have no problem making decisions or taking risks in relation to the financial future, whereas now I must consider, will I still be able to work in the future?

5. **Was any aspect of the experience of the condition good or useful? What was that?**
The experience has made me humbler. When I think of other people getting a very different or a terminal diagnosis, I appreciate that I am quite lucky and again hope that I will have no further attacks.

6. **What do you hope for in the future for people with your condition?**
In the future I hope that people with my condition can be told with certainty that with proper medication and lifestyle, they will live a normal life with the same life expectancy as a normal healthy person.

8 Temporary Visual Failure

History

A 45-year-old woman from Thailand was admitted to hospital with visual loss. Her optician had told her that she had 'papilloedema'.

Two months earlier, she had had an admission to another hospital with headache and weakness in her left arm and left leg, which resolved spontaneously after one day. A CT scan of brain was reported as normal. She was diagnosed with migraine with aura. Two days later, she was found unconscious. She was readmitted to the same hospital. Her husband described generalised shaking for a few minutes without incontinence or tongue-biting. She had an MRI scan of the brain, which was reported as showing no abnormality. A lumbar puncture had normal cerebrospinal fluid (CSF) constituents except for the presence of 6 white cells/µL. An infective screen of CSF (herpes simplex virus types 1 and 2, varicella zoster virus and meningeal sepsis screen) was negative. Human immunodeficiency virus and syphilis immunoassay tests were negative. She was discharged but further headache ensued and she was admitted a third time to the same hospital. Another CT brain scan was performed and reported as normal. A contraceptive pill was stopped.

Two weeks later, her vision deteriorated. After her optician had reported papilloedema, she was admitted to this hospital. At that time, she had no headache.

Past medical history was unremarkable. She had one grown-up son. Her mother was alive and well. Her father had had an epileptic fit and died at 62 years of age. She ate a balanced diet including meat. She was a non-smoker and drank little alcohol. She was on no medication. She denied any illicit drug use.

Examination

She was alert and orientated. Visual acuity was $6/18^{-1}$ on the right and $6/18$ on the left (not improved with pinhole). No relative afferent pupillary defect. Ishihara plates were reduced to $6/17$ bilaterally. There was bilateral optic nerve swelling. Neurological examination of the remaining cranial nerves and limbs was normal.

Investigations

Full blood count, ESR, electrolytes, thyroid profile, B12 and folate levels were all normal. Hepatitis screen was negative. Nuclear autoantibody and vasculitic screens were negative. Zinc, selenium and copper levels were normal. Complement C3 and C4 were normal.

An MRI scan of the brain showed a left juxtacortical high signal in the posterior cingulate gyrus that enhanced with contrast (Figures 8.1A and 8.1B). There was FLAIR, DWI and T2 hyperintensity in the optic nerves, which also enhanced with contrast (Figures 8.1C and 8.1D)

A diagnostic test was performed.

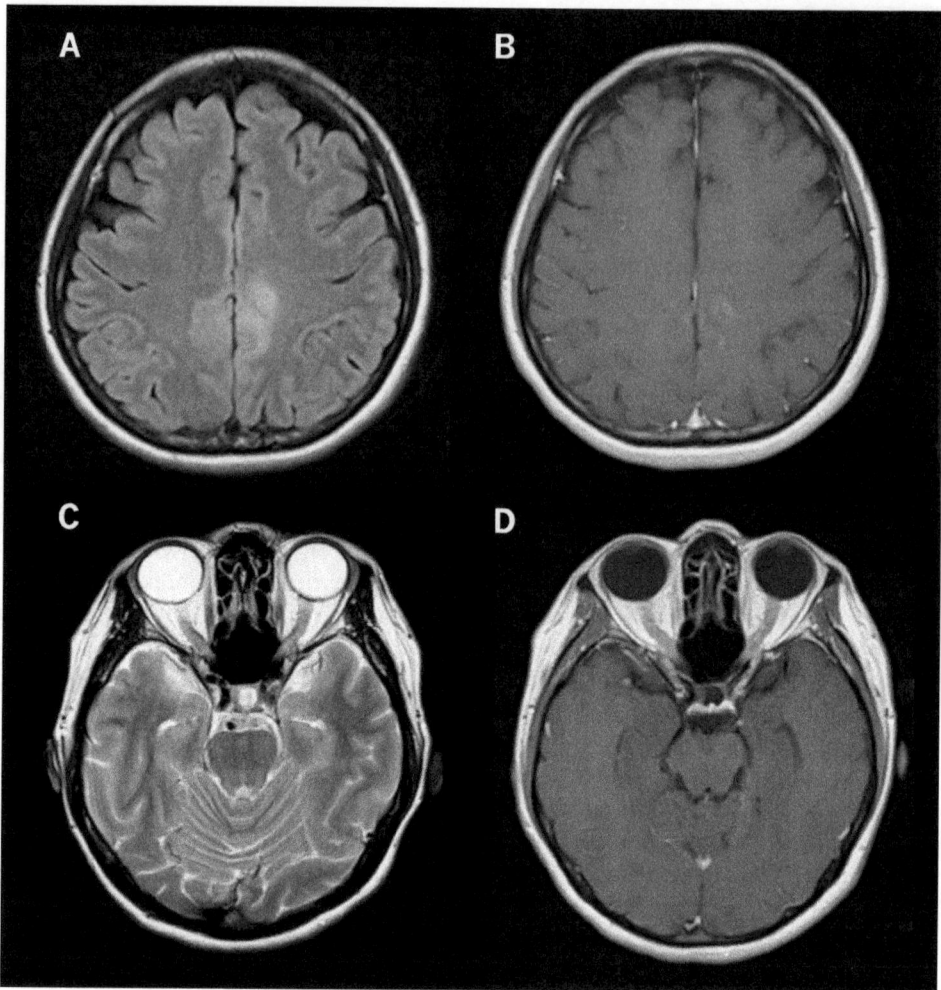

Figure 8.1 (A) Axial T2 FLAIR MRI brain scan showing cortical and subcortical high signal in the posterior cingulate area. (B) Axial T1 MRI with contrast demonstrates faint enhancement of the same lesion. (C) Axial T2 MRI brain scan showing bilateral hyperintense optic nerves and (D) axial T1 MRI scan showing contrast enhancement of the optic nerves.

Other Investigations

A repeat lumbar puncture had an opening pressure of 17 cm of CSF. No organisms were seen. Cerebrospinal fluid revealed 1 white cell/μL, 30 red cells/μL, protein 0.33 g/L, glucose 2.9 mmol/L (plasma glucose 5.0 mmol/L). Oligoclonal bands were detected.

Plasma myelin oligodendrocyte glycoprotein (MOG) antibody was positive. Plasma neuromyelitis optica (NMO) aquaporin 4 immunoglobulin G (AQP4-IgG) was negative. Live cell-based assays were used for these tests.

Diagnosis: Myelin Oligodendrocyte Glycoprotein (MOG) Antibody-Associated Disease

Management

She was treated with intravenous methylprednisolone before switching to oral steroid therapy. Because of her poor vision, plasma exchange treatment was started but she could only tolerate three sessions.

Her right eye vision deteriorated to 6/60 and epileptic seizures recurred within six months. She declined further steroid treatment. She was treated with levetiracetam, reaching 500 mg twice daily and, after appropriate counselling, aziothioprine at 100 mg/day (weight 48 kg). Her visual acuity in the right eye improved to 6/9, as was the left eye visual acuity.

After 30 months, her MOG antibody assay was negative. Azathioprine was reduced and stopped. As she was seizure-free, levetiracetam was also withdrawn.

Comment

Epidemiology and MOG Antibody

Recognition of antibody-associated neurological disorders has increased, and none more so than demyelinating disorders of the central nervous system. AQP4-IgG causes an autoimmune astrocyopathy known as NMO. Although not all patients with a disease phenotype suggestive of NMO have AQP4-IgG, they can still be categorised as NMO spectrum disorder (NMOSD). A sub-group of AQP4 antibody-negative NMOSD patients produce an antibody response against MOG, which is expressed on the outer lamella of the myelin sheath. This protein is only expressed in mammals and has up to 15 isoforms in humans. It is expressed in late embryogenesis but its function is not clear.

MOG antibody can fix complement, suggesting potential pathogenicity, but it is acknowledged that the antibody may in fact just be a biomarker of tissue damage [1]. Cell-based assays have shown that an MOG antibody humoral response is extremely rare in adult multiple sclerosis and virtually absent in AQP4 antibody-positive NMO. It has therefore been suggested that MOG antibody-associated demyelination of the central nervous system is a distinct novel disease, known as MOG antibody (-associated) disease. Live MOG-IgG cell-based assays are preferred as they are reproducible for strong positive and clearly negative samples.

Clinical Features and Natural History of MOG Antibody Disease

MOG antibody disease has been studied particularly in Oxford, England. In a landmark publication on 252 UK patients with MOG antibody disease, patients presented with isolated optic neuritis (ON; 55%, bilateral in almost half, as in our patient), transverse myelitis (TM; 18%) or acute disseminated encephalomyelitis (ADEM)-like illness (18%) [2]. Cortical encephalitis and isolated brainstem attacks have also been reported in MOG antibody disease. Just over half of MOG antibody disease patients are female without an ethnic bias. The disease occurs in adults and children and can be monophasic or relapsing.

Currently less than 25% of MOG antibody disease patients fulfil the diagnostic criteria for NMOSD (Figure 8.2A), while others with MOG antibody can have single site or limited disease (Figure 8.2B). Dual positive AQP4 and MOG antibodies is very rare [1].

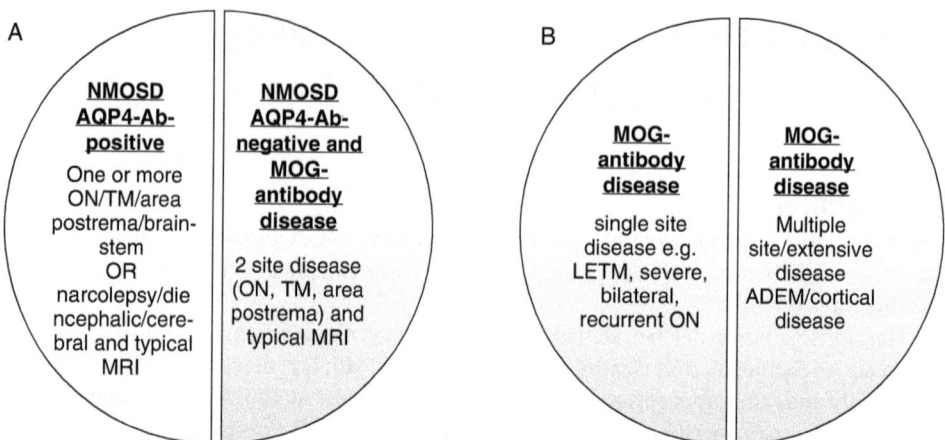

Figure 8.2 (A) Overlap of NMOSD and MOG-antibody disease. (B) MOG antibody disease that is not part of the NMOSD. LETM = longitudinal extensive TM.

The ON in MOG antibody disease frequently is associated with papillitis (anterior or optic nerve head inflammation). Extensive intraorbital optic nerve involvement is recognised. Despite poor vision in the acute phase, most patients recover, such that 80–90% return to normal vision. Posterior optic nerve and chiasm involvement occurs in AQP4 antibody-positive NMOSD.

In MOG antibody disease, TM often but not always involves more than three vertebral segments (longitudinal extensive TM or LETM) and affects the lower thoracic and conus areas, which can cause sphincter (and in men, erectile) dysfunction. Persistent urogenital (bladder and sexual) and bowel dysfunction are recognised despite good motor recovery. However, overall permanent disability is less frequent in MOG antibody disease than in AQP4 antibody NMOSD.

Acute disseminated encephalomyelitis is a typical presentation of MOG antibody disease in children. Large bilateral white matter lesions are not typical of the ovoid periventricular lesions found in multiple sclerosis. Persistent MOG antibody in children increases the risk of relapses.

Cortical encephalitis can present with seizures (demonstrated in our patient), behavioural change or focal symptoms. The prognosis is good as the seizures and MRI lesions often resolve.

Elevated white cell counts (5–10%) and elevated protein (50%) can be present in the CSF during the acute attack. Oligoclonal bands restricted to the central nervous system are found in 15% of MOG antibody disease patients compared to 90% in multiple sclerosis patients. Another distinguishing feature from multiple sclerosis is the absence of accumulating clinically silent lesions in MOG antibody disease.

Neuroimaging in MOG Antibody Disease

MRI findings may be suggestive of MOG antibody disease [3]. Optic neuritis often shows bilateral, anterior and longitudinal extensive involvement (more than half of the optic nerve). Optic nerve head swelling can occur [3]. Optic perineuritis occurs with circumferential optic nerve sheath and orbital fat enhancement.

Transverse myelitis may cause longitudinally extensive or short lesions (pseudo-dilatation of the ependymal canal) on sagittal T2 MR imaging, which may involve grey and white matter. They are characteristically central lesions, which are often swollen in the acute phase similar to AQP4 antibody-positive NMOSD, but unlike multiple sclerosis. The brain lesions are similar in MOG antibody disease and AQP4 antibody-positive NMOSD. Brainstem lesions may be fluff-like in the pons, medulla and cerebellar peduncles.

Relapses and Treatment of MOG Antibody Disease

MOG antibody disease can be monophasic or relapsing in nature. Half of patients may relapse within two or three years, and most relapses occur in the early months after the onset of the attack [1]. The disappearance of MOG antibodies (18–25% within one year) is associated with relapse cessation [2]. There is a suggestion in the literature that patients treated with prednisolone for three to six months may have a lower relapse rate than patients treated with steroids for a shorter period of time [2]. Maintenance intravenous immunoglobulin therapy has also been associated with a decreased relapse rate.

The evidence base for treating MOG antibody disease is not as well established as that for NMO treatment. Acute relapses are treated with intravenous or oral methylprednisolone followed by oral prednisolone. A poor response can prompt plasma exchange or intravenous immunoglobulin therapy.

As noted, relapses seem to occur only in patients with persistent MOG antibody, but not all patients with persistent MOG antibody will relapse. A steroid-sparing immunosuppressant such as azathioprine (as used in our patient), methotrexate or mycophenolate mofetil is recommended for patients who relapse. Maintenance intravenous immunoglobulin therapy and rituximab have also been used. The duration of immunosuppression, as with many autoimmune (neurological) disorders, is uncertain. Our patient was weaned off azathioprine when she became seronegative.

Investigation Guidance for MOG Antibody

Because of the MOG antibody IgG1 assay limitation (i.e. false positives can occur), the prevalence of disease impacts on the positive predictive value of this test. It is therefore suggested that testing is restricted to the phenotypes suggestive of MOG antibody disease such as: ADEM, multiphasic disseminated encephalomyelitis, ON and TM co-presenting, bilateral optic neuropathy, ON with papillitis, recurrent ON, LETM and brainstem/cerebral cortical encephalitis.

References

1. Juryńczyk M, Jacob A, Fujihara K, Palace J. Myelin oligodendrocyte glycoprotein (MOG) antibody-associated disease: practical considerations. *Pract Neurol*. 2019;19(3):187–95.

2. Jurynczyk M, Messina S, Woodhall MR et al. Clinical presentation and prognosis in MOG-antibody disease: a UK study. *Brain*. 2017;140(12):3128–38.

3. Denève M, Biotti D, Patsoura S et al. MRI features of demyelinating disease associated with anti-MOG antibodies in adults. *J Neuroradiol*. 2019;46(5):312–8.

Learning Points

- MOG antibody disease is a demyelinating disorder of the central nervous system.
- MOG antibody disease presents with optic neuropathy (including papillitis), TM, ADEM, and less frequently with cortical encephalitis and brainstem attacks.

- Some forms of MOG antibody disease fall into the NMOSD classification.
- Monophasic and relapsing disease can occur in MOG antibody disease. While vision usually recovers in MOG-associated disease, sphincter disturbance can persist following immunotherapy.
- Severe or frequent relapses of MOG antibody disease are treated with long-term immunosuppression.

Patient's Perspective

1. **What was the impact of the condition on you?**

   a. Physical (e.g. practical support at home)
   I could not cook with the fear of taking unwell and not being able to turn off the gas. I was frightened in case I caused a fire.

   b. Psychological (e.g. mood, emotional well-being)
   My condition drained me mentally, not being able to get out and about to socialise or work. It made me feel very lonely and isolated.

   c. Social (e.g. meeting friends, home)
   My condition meant that I could not socialise with the fear of taking unwell anywhere and not being able to work to be with my work-friends.

2. **What could you not do because of the condition?**
   Unfortunately, I was unfit to drive. Not being able to drive meant that I could not make it to and from work or to meet up with friends.

3. **Was there any other change for you due to the medical condition?**
   Change in my vision – my eyesight went downhill.
   Change in my fitness – I had a lot of pain in muscles.

4. **What is/was the most difficult aspect of the condition?**
   The most difficult part would be the tiredness, constantly feeling physically drained. Also, the visual loss was a scary thing and frustrating. It took a lot from me including my independence.

5. **Was any aspect of the experience good or useful? What was that?**
   No.

6. **What do you hope for in the future for people with this condition?**
   A lot more research and treatment for the condition
   More mental health support.

Chasing the Clot

History

A 44-year-old self-employed male driver had been to Alicante on holiday. There he had been SCUBA driving down to 30 m. One week after returning from holiday, he developed a moderately severe headache. On the following day, the headache was still present. He broke out in a sweat. He felt unwell and so left work. That evening, he had a loose stool and vomited once at home. The headache persisted and three days into the headache he noticed blurred vision from his left eye. He went to an optician who told him there was swelling behind his eyes and advised him to attend an emergency department.

Past medical history was unremarkable. He had no history of diabetes mellitus, heart disease, deep venous thrombosis or stroke.

He was on no medication.

Examination

He was alert and orientated. He was apyrexic with a BMI of 27 kg/m^2. Visual acuity was 6/6 unaided bilaterally. Visual fields assessed to confrontation and monocularly were normal. There was bilateral optic nerve head swelling, on the right more prominent than the left. The remaining cranial nerves and neurological limb examination were normal. He had a normal general examination including normal cardiovascular assessment.

Investigations

A CT of the brain was reported as normal. A lumbar puncture demonstrated an opening pressure of 45 cm of cerebrospinal fluid (CSF). The CSF contained no white cells/μL, 250 red cells/μL, protein of 0.69 g/L and glucose of 3.4 mmol/L (with plasma glucose 5.7 mmol/L).

A diagnostic test was performed.

A CT venogram showed extensive cerebral venous sinus thrombosis involving the jugular bulb extending into the torcula and superior sagittal sinus (Figures 9.1A and 9.1B). Deep veins enhanced normally.

Diagnosis: Cerebral Venous Sinus Thrombosis Secondary to Dehydration

Cerebral Venous Sinus Thrombosis Investigations

An MRI scan of the brain and MR venogram confirmed the CT venogram findings. A CT of the chest abdomen and pelvis identified no evidence of malignant disease. Full blood count and coagulation screen were normal. A thrombophilia screen was performed (lupus anticoagulant negative, nuclear autoantibody screen negative, anticardiolipin immunoglobulin G (IgG) and immunoglobulin M (IgM) antibodies and anti-β2 glycoprotein IgG and IgM antibodies negative, prothrombin 20210A mutation negative, factor V Leiden negative). Homocysteine was normal.

Management

He was treated initially with subcutaneous enoxaparin and then warfarin. Formal visual perimetry was normal. Haematology advice was sought on duration of anticoagulation. The European Stroke Organisation guidelines suggested that in the presence of a single episode and no identified thrombophilic tendency, then anticoagulation could stop after 3–12 months. A follow-up CT venogram 10 months later revealed chronic thrombus in the left transverse sinus and left sigmoid sinus. Warfarin was stopped.

One month after stopping warfarin, the patient re-presented to hospital. He had developed new episodes of pins and needles in his left hand for a couple of minutes. His left hand then felt weak for another couple of minutes. He had drunk a half bottle of vodka. His left-hand sensory disturbance recurred on the following day with a contiguous spreading phenomenon before he had a third episode on the next day, after which he woke up in an ambulance. His wife had witnessed his left arm and hand turning in before he went stiff and then started jerking with grunting noises. Another family member witnessed rolling of his eyes, dilated pupils and foaming at the mouth.

A non-contrast CT brain was reported as normal but at review a right cortical vein signal was suspicious for thrombosis (Figure 9.1C). An MRI scan of the brain (Figure 9.1D) and contrast MR venogram revealed no new parenchymal abnormalities but confirmed right cortical vein thrombus in addition to chronic thrombus in the left transverse sinus and middle third of the superior sagittal sinus.

Management changed to anti-epileptic medication (lamotrigine) and re-anticoagulation. He was advised not to drive until he was one year seizure-free and had informed the Driver and Vehicle Licensing Agency of his seizures. Enoxaparin was switched to long-term rivaroxaban.

Comment

Epidemiology of Cerebral Venous Sinus Thrombosis

Cerebral venous sinus thrombosis mainly occurs in a younger population than arterial stroke, with peaks in childhood and young adulthood. Incidence is estimated at 0.22–1.57 per 100,000 per year and female patients account for two-thirds of cases. Women aged 40–44 years have the highest incidence (2.7 per 100,000 per year). With an almost 100-fold lower

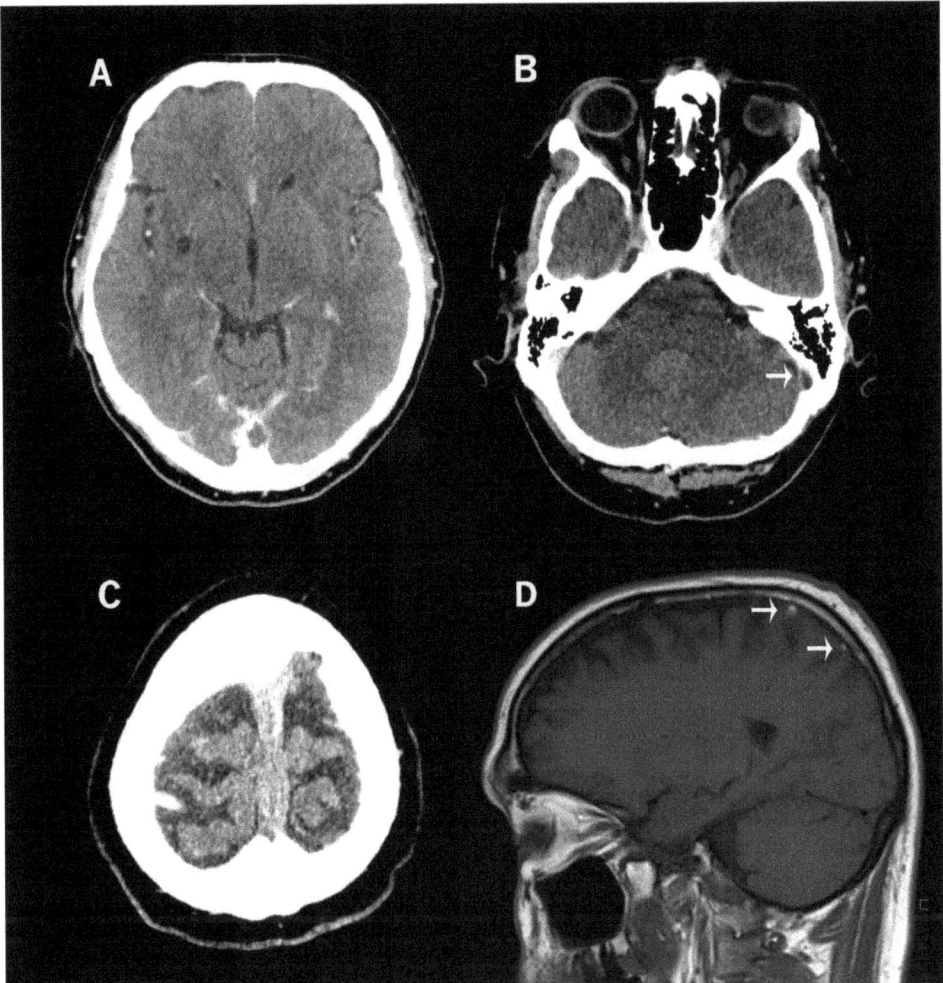

Figure 9.1 A CT venogram at initial presentation showing empty delta sign at (A) the torcula and a filling defect in the left transverse sinus (arrow in B). At second presentation, (C) a CT brain scan showing a prominent and dense right cortical vein suspicious for thrombosis. Parasagittal T1 MRI scan of the brain showing high signal in cortical veins (arrows in D) consistent with cortical vein thrombus.

incidence than arterial stroke, the clinician and radiologist need to carefully consider a diagnosis of cerebral venous sinus thrombosis, particularly in young patients with a stroke-like presentation.

A genome-wide association study has identified that individuals with blood groups A, B or AB have 2.85 times the risk of cerebral venous sinus thrombosis compared with individuals with blood group O.

Pathophysiology and Clinical Presentation
Two pathophysiological mechanisms are recognised in cerebral venous sinus thrombosis. This patient demonstrated both mechanisms.

Dural sinus thrombosis leads to increased venous pressure and impaired absorption of CSF from arachnoid villi, preventing drainage into the superior sagittal sinus, ultimately resulting in raised intracranial pressure. However, there is no pressure gradient between the subarachnoid spaces on the surface of the brain and the ventricles, meaning that hydrocephalus does not usually develop. Headache develops over hours or days and becomes severe in 70–90% of patients with dural sinus thrombosis. Coughing, bending and movement can worsen the headache. Papilloedema is thought to develop over days to weeks following dural sinus thrombosis. Importantly, thunderclap headache occurs in a minority of patients (differential diagnostic symptom for aneurysmal subarachnoid haemorrhage).

Cerebral vein thrombosis causes infarction and focal neurological symptoms from cytotoxic and vasogenic oedema. Focal onset seizures and stroke deficits are presenting features of venous infarction. Paresis may occur from infarction of frontoparietal regions (vein of Trolard) and dysphasia may result from temporal lobe infarction (vein of Labbé). Encephalopathy and coma can occur with multiple sinus and deep cortical venous thrombosis [1].

Clinically important aspects of seizures in cerebral venous sinus thrombosis have emerged [2]. Seizures occur acutely in 34% and chronically in 11% of patients with cerebral venous sinus thrombosis. This compares with a 3% risk of both from arterial ischaemic stroke. Patients with acute seizures in the setting of cerebral venous sinus thrombosis do not usually need long-term anti-epileptic treatment, whereas late seizures carry a high risk of seizure recurrence (mandating anti-epileptic treatment). The extent of cortical damage, particularly haemorrhage, predicts the risk of early and late seizures, but observational evidence does not currently suggest that routine seizure prophylaxis is required [2].

Diagnosis of Cerebral Venous Sinus Thrombosis

A CT and MRI of the brain with contrast-enhanced venography are the ideal investigations for suspected cerebral venous sinus thrombosis. A venous filling defect (increased density on non-contrast CT brain and low density or 'empty delta sign' on CT venography) can confirm superior sagittal sinus thrombosis. An equivalent appearance in the transverse sinus can be seen on sagittal and coronal planes. The empty delta sign reflects dural wall enhancement without intrasinus enhancement. Technical issues are important for a good-quality scan as intracranial hypertension can delay filling of the sinuses.

Venous stroke manifests as an oedematous region with mixed infarction, haemorrhage and contrast enhancement, which does not respect arterial territory boundaries.

Causes of Cerebral Venous Sinus Thrombosis

Table 9.1 highlights some potential causes of cerebral venous sinus thrombosis. Clues for investigation include thrombocythaemia associated with *JAK2* mutation, which increases the risk of venous thrombosis. Genetic prothrombotic predisposition may be present in 22% of patients with cerebral venous sinus thrombosis. Mastoiditis can be associated with transverse sinus thrombosis, particularly in so-called developing countries.

Hypercoagulabe states from heparin-induced thrombocytopenia, autoimmune heparin-induced thrombocytopenia (not triggered by heparin) and vaccine-induced thrombotic thrombocytopenia are associated with thrombosis, a low platelet count and disseminated intravascular coagulation. Platelet-activating antibodies to platelet factor 4 are found in these conditions.

In 2021, SARS-CoV-2 vaccination, particularly with ChAdOx1 nCoV-19, was noted to be associated with a pathogenic platelet factor 4-dependent syndrome that caused thrombosis in

Table 9.1. Potential causes of cerebral venous sinus thrombosis

Risk factors	Examples
Female conditions	Pregnancy and puerperium
Systemic conditions	Iron deficiency anaemia, malignancy, inflammatory bowel disease, systemic lupus erythematosus, Behcet's disease and neurosarcoidosis infections including SARS-CoV-2 and obesity
Blood issues	Myeloproliferative disease (e.g. *JAK2* mutation), dehydration, antithrombin deficiency, factor V Leiden mutation and prothrombin 20210 mutation homocystinaemia, nephrotic syndrome and antiphospholipid syndrome
Local conditions	Infections – otitis media, sinusitis, mastoiditis, meningitis and lumbar puncture Trauma – head injury and neurosurgical procedures
Drugs	Oral contraceptive pill, hormone replacement therapy and SARS-CoV-2 vaccine

unusual sites such as cerebral venous sinuses as well as portal, splanchnic and hepatic veins. Typically, thrombosis and thrombocytopenia syndrome manifested within two weeks of adenovirus vector-based SARS-CoV-2 vaccination. Such patients were mostly female with a mean age of 45 years with no known prothrombotic risk factors. Initial mortality was reported as being as high as 40%; however, early immunoglobulin therapy and anticoagulation with non-heparin-based therapies may improve survival.

Treatment of Cerebral Venous Sinus Thrombosis

The 2017 European Stroke Organisation guideline for the diagnosis and treatment of cerebral venous sinus thrombosis recommends acute treatment with low molecular weight heparin, despite low quality of evidence [3].

Warfarin was historically used in the longer term, but there is evidence that direct oral anticoagulants are equivalent outside of antiphospholipid syndrome. Duration of anticoagulation in the absence of ongoing risk factors varies from 3 to 12 months. However, recurrent thrombosis may need permanent anticoagulation. Our patient continues on rivaroxaban for long-term recurrence prevention.

Endovascular therapy does not have supportive trial evidence, whereas decompressive hemicraniectomy may be beneficial for patients with large venous infarction and clinical or imaging evidence of brain herniation or raised intracranial pressure.

Neurological Complications of SCUBA Diving

Underwater diving exposes the body to elevated ambient pressure (atmospheric pressure plus hydrostatic pressure). Decompression sickness (nitrogen bubbles in the bloodstream after reduction in the ambient pressure) may manifest as fatigue, joint pain or malaise (type 1). The lungs, vestibular system (vertigo and nystagmus) and neurovascular complications of the brain or spinal cord (coma, seizures, monoparesis or paraparesis) occur in type 2 decompression sickness. In pulmonary barotrauma, breath-holding ascent can cause gas expansion, leading to pneumothorax, mediastinal and subcutaneous emphysema or cerebral arterial air embolism if gas bubbles enter the vascular system. Nitrogen narcosis or 'rupture of the deep' can occur when breathing compressed air at a depth of 30 m. Impaired judgement and/or excessive self-confidence can ensue. High pressure neurological syndrome can occur when diving at depths beyond 100 m. Helium has an effect on the lipid membrane at these very high ambient pressures, resulting in headache, nausea, dizziness, a tremor of 8–12 Hz, myoclonus, opsoclonus, impaired co-ordination, cognitive and neuropsychiatric changes and seizures. Middle ear barotrauma during the descent can be exacerbated by eustachian tube obstruction. Paranasal sinus barotrauma can cause pain and paraesthesia in the distribution of the infraorbital nerve. Meningitis and empyema are rare complications of sinus barotrauma. Internal carotid artery dissection has been reported in divers due to neck trauma or cervical spine hyperextension, excessive rotation of the head and the weight of diving gear. Venous thrombosis is not thought to be related to diving, but diving is not recommended if an individual is taking an anticoagulant because of the increased risk of haemorrhage.

References

1. Ropper AH, Klein J. Cerebral venous thrombosis. *N Engl J Med*. 2021;385:59–64.
2. Bentley P, Sharma P. Distinguishing early from late seizures after cerebral venous thrombosis: cinderepilepsy. *Neurology*. 2020;95(12):513–14.
3. Ferro JM, Bousser MG, Canhão P et al. European Stroke Organization guideline for the diagnosis and treatment of cerebral venous thrombosis: endorsed by the European Academy of Neurology. *Eur J Neurol*. 2017;24(10):1203–13.

Learning Points

- Cerebral venous sinus thrombosis should be considered in the differential diagnosis of acute neurological presentations (including seizure, stroke and papilloedema), particularly in the young.
- A thorough investigation for predisposing factors is required for patients presenting with cerebral venous sinus thrombosis.
- Occult malignancy can underlie a new presentation of cerebral venous sinus thrombosis.
- For acute treatment of cerebral venous sinus thrombosis, a balance between thrombosis prevention and haemorrhagic risk favours anticoagulation, even in the presence of haemorrhagic venous infarction.
- Vaccine-induced immune thrombotic thrombocytopenia has been recognised as a cause of cerebral venous sinus thrombosis shortly after exposure to adenovirus vector-based SARS-CoV-2 vaccines.

Patient's Perspective

1. **What was the impact of the condition?**

   a. Physical (e.g. job, practical support)
   After the diagnosis of cerebral venous sinus thrombosis I had a number of seizures including a grand mal seizure. This led to a diagnosis of epilepsy, albeit no seizures in the last eight years. I requested my wife to drive for me for one year.

   b. Psychological (e.g. mood, emotional well-being)
   Uncharacteristically I was emotionally down. However, after the reduction of Lamictal medication, I felt less low. I had a feeling of uneasiness about my mortality due to the unexpected nature of the condition.

   c. Social (e.g. meeting friends, home)
   Little to no impact as I had a great support system. We have a strong faith, which shored us up as a family. I reduced my alcohol consumption.

2. **What could you not do because of the condition?**
   I was not permitted to drive for one year. I am not permitted to dive (SCUBA) although I had enjoyed this regularly.

3. **Was there any other change for you due to your medical condition?**
    At the beginning taking Rivaroxaban, I was concerned about cutting myself or falls. I also had some memory issues (forgot the type of car I driving).

4. **What is/was the most difficult aspect of the condition for you?**
    Day to day the condition has little impact. However, the inability to SCUBA-dive is frustrating as I feel capable of doing it. Also, being on medication for life.

5. **Was any aspect of the experience good or useful? What was that?**
    Learned to work smarter with less stress. Started a second business online. The condition isn't fatal and I can live a relatively normal life.

6. **What do you hope for in the future for your condition?**
    Early diagnosis and with correct medication people can live normal lives.

CASE
10   Losing Volume

History

A 65-year-old man woke up with new onset vertigo, headache and nausea. He vomited later that day. He had a pressure feeling in his ears. The headache improved on lying down. He had no history of trauma. He was admitted to hospital where a CT brain scan was reported as showing bilateral subdural collections including evidence of haemorrhage (Figure 10.1A). After the medical team had sought neurosurgical advice, conservative management was advised and he was discharged.

He continued to lie down at home for relief of his headache. Seven days later, he was re-admitted to hospital. He had developed tingling of his left arm and leg, which persisted for 10 hours. An MRI brain scan confirmed persistent 'small uncomplicated subdural collections' (Figure 10.1B). He was discharged again.

Two days later, he had a third admission to hospital because of ongoing postural headache and vertigo. A neurology opinion was sought.

Past medical history included radiotherapy for prostate carcinoma. He neither smoked cigarettes nor drank alcohol.

Examination

General and neurological examinations were normal. In particular, there was no neck stiffness, visual or hearing abnormality.

Investigations

A review of the neuroimaging confirmed bilateral subdural collections. However, there was obliteration of the third ventricle and blunting of the angle between the pons and midbrain with sagging of the brainstem (Figure 10.1C).

An MRI scan of the spine revealed perineural cysts at C6/7 and C7/T1.

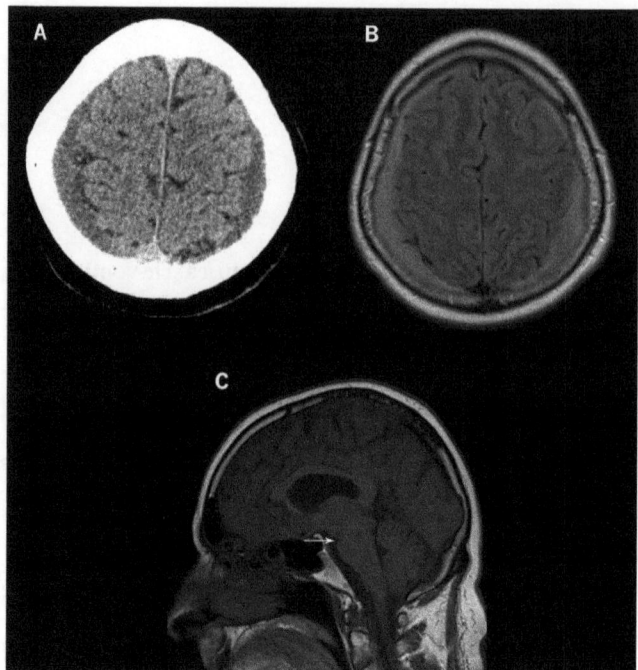

Figure 10.1 (A) CT brain scan showing subdural collections. (B) Axial FLAIR MRI brain scan demonstrating subdural collections. (C) Sagittal T1 MRI brain scan showing blunting of the angle between the midbrain and pons (arrow).

Diagnosis: Spontaneous Intracranial Hypotension

Management
An epidural blood patch was performed, which yielded almost instantaneous relief of the headache.

Comment
Epidemiology of Spontaneous Intracranial Hypotension
Spontaneous intracranial hypotension is an uncommon neurological disorder characterised by spinal cerebrospinal fluid (CSF) leak and resulting in decreased CSF volume, and displacement of cerebral structures, causing headache and other neurological symptoms [1]. Despite the name of spontaneous intracranial hypotension, CSF pressure can in fact be normal. Spontaneous intracranial hypotension manifests acutely with postural or orthostatic headache (worse in the upright posture, as demonstrated by our patient) but also with an increasingly wide phenotype, including coma, dementia and apathy – so-called brain sagging dementia, which can manifest as gradually progressive cognitive and behavioural changes similar to behavioural variant frontotemporal dementia. Spontaneous intracranial hypotension has been frequently under-recognised and misdiagnosed. The incidence of spontaneous intracranial hypotension is 3–4 per 100,000 per year.

The third edition of International Classification of Headache Disorders (ICHD-3) lists the diagnostic criteria for spontaneous intracranial hypotension as a headache related to low CSF pressure or CSF leakage that is not better accounted for by another headache diagnosis from ICHD-3 [2]. The low CSF pressure is established by a measurement of CSF pressure of < 6 cmCSF and/or neuroimaging evidence of a CSF leakage. However, a dural puncture is not necessary in patients who already have MRI evidence of CSF leakage such as dural enhancement on a contrast MRI brain scan. A lumbar puncture in such patients risks worsening symptoms. Another part of the ICHD-3 criteria for headache attributed to spontaneous intracranial hypotension is that the criteria do not apply to a patient who has had a dural puncture within the prior month or trauma causing CSF leakage.

Pathogenesis
Two mechanisms have been proposed for spontaneous intracranial hypotension. In the Munro–Kellie doctrine, the intracranial volumes (of brain, CSF and blood) must remain constant or intracranial pressure will change. Loss of CSF in spontaneous intracranial hypotension lowers intracranial pressure and causes intracranial venous structures to dilate. As some patients apparently have reduced volume without a CSF pressure of < 6 cmCSF, spontaneous intracranial hypotension is really a misnomer and the name should reflect reduced intracranial CSF volume. The second proposed mechanism is a shift in the hydrostatic indifference point. Normally there is zero pressure in the upper cervical spine. Erect posture increases CSF expulsion, with possible venous dilatation causing orthostatic headache.

Sources of CSF Leak

There are three recognised sources of CSF leakage.

Protruding meningeal diverticula (usually thoracic and upper lumbar) are potential sources of CSF leakage but such perineural cysts are a common finding, and by themselves do not necessarily indicate a CSF leak.

Ventral (less often dorsal) tears of the dura from calcified disc herniations and speculated endplate osteophytes are also sources of CSF leakage. Evidence has shown that microspurs may be aetiologically relevant in at least some patients with intractable symptoms of spontaneous intracranial hypotension. Intracranial hypotension may therefore result from a duropathy. These patients may then develop superficial siderosis of the central nervous system. Many of the apparently idiopathic cases of superficial siderosis (approximately one-third) may develop in association with intracranial hypotension. The mechanism of the bleeding in the presence of low CSF pressure has not been comprehensively demonstrated. Direct dural trauma and traction on superior vermian veins are possible sources of bleeding.

A third source of CSF leakage involves CSF-venous fistulas, which represent an aberrant connection between the subarachnoid space and a spinal epidural vein usually along lower thoracic root nerves. This mechanism highlights how a leak may not be identified despite thorough investigation. Specialised spinal imaging (digital subtraction myelography or dynamic CT myelography) may detect CSF-venous fistulas in patients in whom an extradural spinal CSF collection has not been found [1].

Importantly, a skull base CSF leak does not usually cause spontaneous intracranial hypotension symptoms. The intracranial pressure is normally less than atmospheric pressure and, under the influence of gravity, the pressure gradient increases in a caudal spinal axis on standing, disappearing on lying.

Management of Spontaneous Intracranial Hypotension

Based on expert recommendation, management of spontaneous intracranial hypotension consists of treatments including conservative measures, epidural patching and surgery. Conservative management includes bed rest, caffeine and oral hydration, but the impact of conservative management has not been validated with robust outcome measures. This evidence relies solely on case series. Corticosteroids, indomethacin and theophylline have anecdotally helped some patients.

Mechanical interventions include epidural blood patching (introduced in 1960 and regarded as the best treatment), epidural fibrin glue injection and surgical repair performed in decreasing order of frequency. Non-targeted or blind epidural blood patching involves injection of autologous blood into the lower thoracic or lumbar epidural space, which worked very well in our patient. Targeted epidural blood patching involves injecting autologous blood into the area of the suspected leak based on spinal imaging studies. Failures or short-lived responses can occur. Multiple blood patches are sometimes required to achieve success. The volume of blood, the length of the anterior epidural fluid collection on an MRI of the spine and the midbrain-pons angle have emerged as factors that influence initial epidural blood patch response rates.

Patients in whom CSF leakages have been confidently located and epidural blood patching has failed may be surgical candidates. Rebound intracranial hypertension has been recognised after closure of a leak. A new headache, which is now worse when lying down and frontal or periorbital in location, can emerge. Acetazolamide and therapeutic lumbar puncture may be required.

Subdural Collection and Transient Neurology

Our patient had focal sensory disturbances attributed to the subdural collections. Such transient neurological deficits have been recognised in chronic subdural collections. The mechanism is unknown but hypotheses have included mechanical pressure from the collection, parenchymal swelling, repeated haemorrhages in the subdural space, seizure activity and cortical spreading depolorisation (as implicated in transient focal neurological events due to cerebral amyloid angiopathy).

Improvement in recognition of spontaneous intracranial hypotension has been attributed to increasing familiarity with typical findings from MRI brain scans in affected patients. Contrast MRI of the brain is required to demonstrate dural enhancement. Our patient did not have contrast at the time of the MRI brain scan. There were, however, sufficient features from the history and available neuroimaging to secure the diagnosis of spontaneous intracranial hypotension.

MRI features identified in spontaneous intracranial hypotension:
- subdural fluid collection
- dural enhancement
- venous distension
- sagging of the brain
- pituitary enlargement/hyperaemia
- reduction in volume of optic nerve sheath subarachnoid space.

References

1. Schievink WI. Spontaneous intracranial hypotension. *N Engl J Med.* 2021;385(23):2173–8.
2. Headache Classification Committee of the International Headache Society (IHS). The International Classification of Headache Disorders, 3rd edition. *Cephalalgia.* 2018;38(1):1–211.
3. Schievink WI, Maya MM, Jean-Pierre S et al. A classification system of spontaneous spinal CSF leaks. *Neurology.* 2016;87(7):673–9.

Learning Points

- Eliciting a history of postural headache should raise suspicion of intracranial hypotension.
- Features on an MRI of the brain of spontaneous intracranial hypotension include pachymeningeal (dural) enhancement, subdural collections, sagging of the brain, pituitary enlargement/hyperaemia, venous engorgement and reduction in the volume of optic nerve sheath subarachnoid space.
- It is not necessary to perform a lumbar puncture in order to diagnose spontaneous intracranial hypotension.
- Epidural blood patching is regarded as the best treatment for spontaneous intracranial hypotension if conservative measures fail.

Patient's Perspective

1. **What was the physical, psychological and social impact of the condition?**
   a. Physical (e.g. job, driving, practical support)
   I had extreme headaches and felt sick for most of the time I was in hospital on and off for three weeks. They could not work out why I had a bleed on the brain but within 15 minutes of seeing the neurologist, he told me the problem.

b. **Psychological (e.g. mood, future, emotional well-being)**
I was worried about what was happening to me – feeling sick, always wanting to lie down and sleep.

c. **Social (e.g. meeting friends, home)**
I could not go anywhere and I was not interested when people called at home.

2. **What could you no longer do after developing spontaneous intracranial hypotension?**
I was totally floored, stuck at home all of the time; the only ease was lying down.

3. **Was there any change for you because of the diagnosis?**
Since that time, sometimes when I get headaches, I am not sure if the problem is returning. I may not feel too well for about four days and so just lie on the couch until it passes.

4. **What is/was the most difficult aspect of the condition?**
When at home and my condition became so severe that I went to Casualty as I felt that I was close to passing out. There I had to be given oxygen. It was a terrible feeling.

5. **Was any aspect of the experience good or useful? What was that?**
Nothing was good about it but I was glad that the neurologist understood what was happening and the blood patch worked.

6. **What do you hope for in the future for your condition?**
I hope that doctors can understand the condition and diagnose it earlier. Most people on the ward were not aware of the condition.

Where Is the Pus?

History

A 60-year-old man developed low back pain along with flu-like symptoms. He had returned to Northern Ireland from a nine-day trip to Florida one month before his presentation. The pain increased over a few hours. The pain radiated from his right lower back into his groin and right upper leg as far as his right knee. He felt nauseated, faint-like and experienced severe pain. He was admitted to hospital.

In hospital, right low back pain radiating to both groins was worse when lying on his right side. He had no rigors. He was treated empirically with intravenous flucloxacillin and piperacillin with tacobactam.

Past medical history included asthma, gout and diabetes mellitus. He had stopped a statin two months earlier due to myalgia. He had no recent dental work and denied a history of rheumatic fever.

Examination

His temperature was 38°C on the day before a neurology assessment. He walked with an antalgic gait. Straight leg raising was limited to 60° on the left and 45° on the right. Cranial nerve and limb examinations were normal except for pain at right hip flexion and absent ankle jerks.

Investigations

His CRP was elevated and fluctuated (Figure 11.1). Blood cultures grew Gram-positive cocci, confirmed as *Staphylococcus aureus*. A diagnostic test was performed.

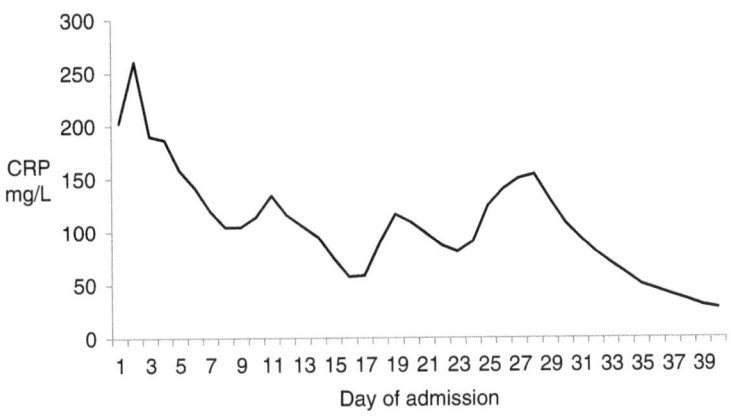

Figure 11.1 Course of CRP during hospital admission.

An MRI of the lumbosacral spine identified an epidural phlegmon (Figure 11.2). Subsequent imaging confirmed a multiloculated spinal epidural abscess.

He was transferred to a spinal orthopaedic ward but was managed medically. At follow-up, he was pain-free and had no neurological deficit.

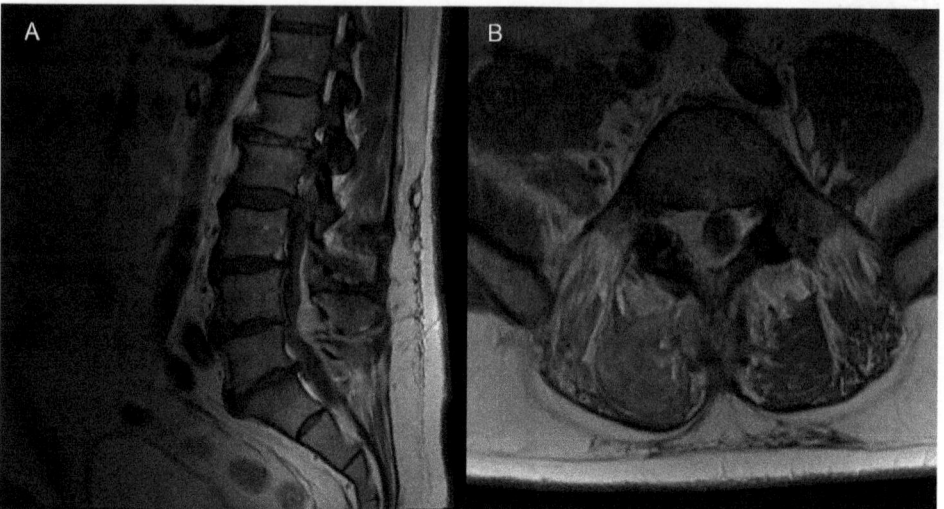

Figure 11.2 T1 MRI scan of the lumbosacral spine with contrast. (A) Sagittal imaging shows extensive abnormal signal in the spinal canal from L3 to S2. (B) Axial imaging shows enhancing paravertebral muscles with inflammatory tissue in the spinal canal extending through a right lumbar neural exit foramen consistent with phlegmon.

Diagnosis: Spinal Epidural Phlegmon/Abscess Due to *S. aureus* Infection

Comment

Abscess versus Phlegmon

An abscess is walled in and is confined to the area of infection. A phlegmon is unbounded and can keep spreading out along connective tissue and muscle. Phlegmonous epidural infection may precede the development of a frank epidural abscess and is less amenable to surgical drainage.

A spinal epidural abscess is rare, and is often initially misdiagnosed or even not diagnosed. Giovanni Morgagni first described a spinal epidural abscess in 1761. Successful operations have been documented since the 1930s. The diagnosis is important for a number of reasons. Firstly, the incidence of spinal epidural abscess is increasing, now estimated at 2–8 cases per 10,000 hospital admissions. Although mortality is decreasing (between 3.7 and 5%), one-third of patients still have a poor neurological outcome [1]. Such abscesses are most frequently due to *S. aureus* (50–93% of cases in which an organism is isolated). The *Streptococcus* species and Gram-negative organisms have also been identified in spinal epidural abscesses. Infection can spread via any of three primary mechanisms – haematogenous spread (e.g. the vertebral venous plexus), extension from adjacent infected tissue and direct external inoculation.

Presentation of an Epidural Abscess

Most patients present with back pain or localised tenderness and fever. This progresses to radicular pain and, if not treated, ultimately to neurological deficits. Although the triad of back pain, fever and neurological deficit has high specificity, it has low sensitivity; our patient lacked a neurological deficit. Up to one-third of patients have thoracic back pain. Infection was suspected in our patient; imaging helped confirm the location of the infection.

Back pain, fever, and raised CRP were all strong clues, and subsequently a cultured organism confirmed the infective cause. A lumbar puncture was not performed as it risks seeding the infection. Prolonged delays in diagnosing spinal epidural abscess are common and yet prompt treatment is required to prevent irreversible neurological sequelae.

Predisposing Factors to Spinal Epidural Abscess

Diabetes mellitus (present in our patient) has been reported in 21–43% of patients with a spinal epidural abscess. Morbid obesity, malignancy, long-term corticosteroid use, pregnancy, trauma, end-stage renal disease, liver disease and cirrhosis are all strongly associated with spinal epidural abscess. Intravenous drug abuse, alcoholism and HIV infection are also risk factors for spinal epidural abscess.

Radiology

Advanced imaging is important for the diagnosis of a spinal epidural abscess. In patients with severe back pain and elevated ESR/CRP, the threshold for urgent imaging is low. Imaging of the entire spine with and without contrast is required. Epidural abscesses are not well recognised on T2 as the abscess displays a similar signal to CSF. The characteristic MRI findings include high signal on T2 and low signal on signal T1. A post-contrast MRI scan can define the anatomical location and extent of an abscess. The radiological differential diagnosis includes vertebral metastasis, epidural haematoma, disc protrusion, vertebral osteomyelitis and osteodiscitis without abscess [1].

Management

Medical versus surgical management decisions are derived from case series, cohort studies and expert opinions. To date, there have been no randomised controlled trials for guidance. Management involves medical treatment (antibiotic) plus or minus surgical intervention (laminectomy). There has been a trend in the last 40 years to manage an increasing minority of patients medically. Standard care may be medical treatment alone if there are no neurological deficits (as in our patient) or patients with very high surgical risk. However, a number of factors may influence the decision regarding medical or surgical management such as age, co-morbidities, CRP level, blood culture, sepsis, anatomical location, spinal instability and decline in neurological function.

Mortality was 34% in 1954–60, 15% in 1990–7 and is now 5% or less. The main issue with a spinal epidural abscess is early diagnosis before neurological deficits ensue.

Cauda Equina Syndrome

Another cause of acute low back pain – cauda equina syndrome – merits consideration in this context. Cauda equina syndrome is a clinical manifestation of compression of lumbosacral roots (below the spinal cord) within the lumbosacral canal which requires prompt diagnosis and surgical treatment in order to prevent irreversible incontinence. Cauda equina syndrome usually involves L4/L5 or L5/S1 central disc prolapse. The incidence of cauda equina syndrome is 7 per 100,000 per year in the working-age adult population whereas low back pain is much more common and can also be associated with urinary symptoms. For the diagnosis of cauda equina syndrome, a finding of reduced anal tone is often quoted but this is not a very sensitive (as low as 22%), specific or reliable sign [2]. Saddle anaesthesia appears more sensitive (~59% of cases with cauda equina syndrome). These test characteristics can make the diagnosis of cauda equina syndrome difficult. However, red flag features should prompt urgent investigation in patients with sciatica and include: 1. onset of bilateral numbness or leg weakness; 2. onset of a sensation of anal numbness ('numb bum') or pins and needles; and 3. any alteration in sensation of a full bladder, desire to pass urine or awareness of passing urine. By the time urinary incontinence has developed, it is usually too late to treat successfully.

Scan-negative cauda equina syndrome is a similarly important diagnosis. It is estimated that 6,000–7,000 patients in the UK alone present to hospitals each year with scan-negative cauda equina syndrome. These patients also require early diagnosis, particularly as triggers appear to be pain, anxiety/panic, medication side effects and features of functional neurological disorder [3].

References

1. Sharfman ZT, Gelfand Y, Shah P et al. Spinal epidural abscess: a review of presentation, management, and medicolegal implications. *Asian Spine J.* 2020;14(5):742–59.

2. Barraclough K. Cauda equina syndrome. *BMJ.* 2021;372:6–10.

3. Hoeritzauer I, Stanton B, Carson A, Stone J. 'Scan-negative' cauda equina syndrome: what to do when there is no neurosurgical cause. *Pract Neurol.* 2022;22(1):6–13.

Learning Points

- New onset back pain with tenderness and fever should raise clinical suspicion of a spinal epidural abscess.
- Mortality from a spinal epidural abscess is decreasing (5% or less) but the incidence is increasing. A delayed diagnosis can result in severe neurological disability.
- An MRI including T1 sequences with contrast can help diagnose a spinal epidural abscess.
- *S. aureus* is responsible for the majority of cases of spinal epidural abscesses.

Patient's Perspective

1. **What was the impact of the condition on you?**

   a. Physical (e.g. job, driving, practical support)
   Massive physical impact. I was unable to walk unaided and needed help for most everyday tasks such as washing and dressing etc.

   b. Psychological (mood, future, emotional well-being)
   Mood was very down; I was depressed due to the pain and limited movement as previously I was very active.

   c. Social (meeting friends, home)
   I was unable to go out to meet with friends. My low energy levels meant very little social interaction.

2. **What could you not do because of the condition?**
   I could not work. I could not do normal, everyday tasks (washing and dressing). I was unable to walk unaided.

3. **Was there any other change for you due to the condition?**
   No.

4. **What is/was the most difficult aspect of the condition for you?**
   The physical limitations, which led to a loss of independence.

5. **Was any aspect of the experience good or useful? What was that?**
   No.

6. **What do you hope for in the future for people with this condition?**
   Prompt diagnosis and early intervention.

History

A 59-year-old woman developed symptoms of a chest infection. She had not taken any medi-cation for this. She woke at midnight and felt that she had to cough as she felt that she had choked. She had a burning chest pain radiating into her arms and head. A severe headache developed but became worse throughout the night, particularly when she repeatedly coughed. She was nauseated. Ten hours after headache onset, she was admitted to hospital. There her headache worsened, with at least three separate thunderclap exacerbations. Attempted def-ecation also worsened the headache. Prior to this episode, she had no history of headache.

Past medical history was unremarkable except for a cholecystectomy and a varicose vein operation. She never smoked cigarettes and did not drink alcohol. She had no history of hypertension.

Examination

She was alert and orientated with stable observations including a pulse of 72 beats per minute and blood pressure of 137/64 mmHg. He neck was slightly stiff on rotation. Her visual acuity was 6/9 unaided with normal fundi. The remaining cranial nerves were normal. Neurological examination of her limbs was normal.

Investigations

A CT brain scan 14 hours after onset revealed a sulcal subarachnoid haemorrhage high up in the left convexity (Figure 12.1A). A lumbar puncture 16 hours after the initial headache onset did not have a recorded opening pressure. There were no white cells/μL, 131 red cells/μL, no organisms, cerebrospinal fluid (CSF) glucose of 3.4 mmol/L, serum glucose of 6.1 mmol/L, CSF protein of 0.35 g/L and spectrophotometry showed no elevation of bilirubin or oxyhaemoglobin.

An MRI scan of the brain on day 3 confirmed the sulcal haemorrhage from the hyper-intense or 'dirty' signal on the FLAIR sequence (Figure 12.1B). There was now, however, evidence of right basal ganglia haemorrhage seen with blooming effect from gradient echo sequence (Figure 12.1C).

A CT angiogram on day 6 showed a change in calibre of the anterior cerebral arteries, the right middle cerebral artery and distal components of both posterior cerebral arteries (Figure 12.1D). There was no evidence of a cerebral aneurysm.

A follow-up MRI scan of the brain showed resolution of the sulcal convexity haemorrhage and partial resolution of the right basal ganglia haemorrhage. A three-month CT angiogram revealed normal calibre intracranial arteries.

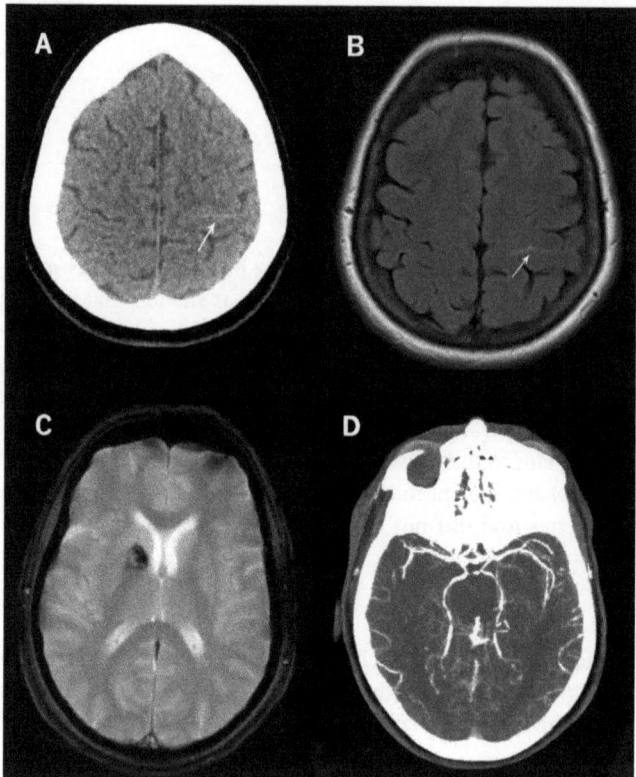

Figure 12.1 (A) A CT scan of the brain showing convexity subarachnoid haemorrhage also present on axial FLAIR MRI scan of brain (B) as a 'dirty CSF signal' (arrow). (C) An axial gradient echo MRI scan of brain showing a low signal consistent with right basal ganglia haemorrhage. (D) A CT angiogram demonstrates multiple narrowings of both distal posterior cerebral arteries.

Diagnosis: Reversible Cerebral Vasoconstriction Syndrome

Comment

Nomenclature for Reversible Cerebral Vasoconstriction Syndrome

In reversible cerebral vasoconstriction syndrome (RCVS), clinical and radiological manifestations are attributed to a transient disturbance of cerebral arterial tone. Sudden and acute, or thunderclap, headache (peaking within seconds) is often the first symptom and can recur for one to two weeks [1]. The condition has had many previous names (e.g. Call–Fleming syndrome, primary thunderclap headache, migrainous vasospasm, benign angiopathy of the central nervous system, post-partum angiopathy and drug-induced arteritis) but was called reversible cerebral vasoconstriction syndrome by Leonard Calabrese in 2007 [2]. Both the vasoconstriction and headache result from innervation of cerebral blood vessels with sensory afferents from the trigeminal nerve (Va) and dorsal root of C2.

Epidemiology of RCVS

Reversible cerebral vasoconstriction syndrome peaks in the early 40s and is more common in women than in men. It has been reported in patients from 10 to 76 years of age. Incidence of RCVS has been estimated at 3 per million per year [3]. Recognised triggers include the post-partum state, vasoactive drugs, catecholamine-secreting tumours such as phaeochromocytoma, intravenous immunoglobulin and red cell blood transfusion [1]. The importance of the diagnosis is a distinction from primary angiitis of the central nervous system, which almost certainly has been misdiagnosed in previous cases of RCVS.

Clinical Features of RCVS

A clinical feature of RCVS is an acute onset followed by a self-limiting course in most, but not all, patients. The syndrome is a cause of recurrent thunderclap headache. Recurrent thunderclap headache with a moderate headache can persist. Straining (e.g. during defecation or coughing) is a well-recognised headache trigger. Transient focal deficits (often visual) occur in about 10% of patients. Seizures can also occur. Imaging can show convexity subarachnoid haemorrhage, intracerebral haemorrhage, cerebral infarction and reversible brain oedema or posterior reversible encephalopathy syndrome; the first two features were present in our patient.

In our patient, the right basal ganglia haemorrhage appeared during the course of the illness (as it was not present on the initial CT brain scan following hospital admission). This delayed vascular complication has been previously reported. Indeed, intracerebral haemorrhage, convexity subarachnoid haemorrhage, posterior reversible encephalopathy syndrome and infarction can evolve over a number of days. Haemorrhagic events can occur in over 40% of patients with RCVS. Calibre irregularities can affect anterior and posterior circulations. The arterial calibre changes can fluctuate and indirect methods may have only 70% sensitivity of catheter angiography. Maximal vasoconstriction of middle cerebral artery branches occurs 16 days after onset.

Diagnostic Criteria for RCVS

Proposed diagnostic criteria for RCVS [1] include acute and severe headache (often thunder-clap) with or without focal deficits or seizures. It is usually monophasic in that new symptoms do not develop more than one month after onset. Angiography demonstrates segmental vaso-constriction of cerebral arteries with no evidence of aneurysmal subarachnoid haemorrhage. Cerebrospinal fluid may be normal (as in our patient) or near normal (<15 white cells/μL, CSF protein of <1g/L). The criteria also stipulate complete or substantial normalisation of arterial vasoconstriction within 12 weeks of clinical onset [1].

An RCVS$_2$ (recurrent/carotid/vasoconstrictive/sex and subarachnoid haemorrhage) score has been devised and validated to discriminate RCVS from other large or medium-sized vessel intracranial arteriopathies. The scores range from –2 to +10 (see Table 12.1). A score of ≥ 5 had a specificity of 99% and a sensitivity of 90% for RCVS while an RCVS$_2$ score ≤ 2 had 100% specificity and 85% sensitivity for excluding RCVS. Our patient's score was 7. There are, however, inherent shortcomings of applying scoring systems to individual patients. As RCVS$_2$ scores of 3 or 4 are not very discriminatory, a clinical approach alone (such as recurrent thun-derclap headache in isolation or normal brain imaging with a recognised trigger – vasocon-strictive drug, post-partum or orgasm) are highly specific features of RCVS. In these settings, neurologists should consider RCVS and obtain vessel imaging.

Table 12.1 RCVS$_2$ score values and patient score

Criteria	Score value	Patient score
Recurrent or single thunderclap headache		
Present	5	5
Absent	0	
Intracranial carotid artery affected		
Affected	-2	
Not affected	0	0
Vasoconstrictive trigger		
Present	3	
Absent	0	0
Sex		
Female	1	1
Male	0	
Subarachnoid haemorrhage		
Present	1	1
Absent	0	
Total		**7**

Adapted from Rocha et al. [4] with permission from Wolters Kluwer.

Reversible cerebral vasoconstriction syndrome is almost certainly under-recognised in clinical practice. It is frequently associated with posterior reversible encephalopathy syndrome; 85% of patients with posterior reversible encephalopathy syndrome have multifocal vasoconstriction. Convexity sulcal subarachnoid haemorrhage has many causes; in the older patient, cerebral amyloid angiopathy can present with transient focal neurological deficits with sulcal haemorrhage and less prominent headache.

Management

Management of RCVS is not well standardised other than supportive care, partly because it has an excellent prognosis for the majority of patients and has a low incidence, which may be due to under-recognition of the condition. Reversible cerebral vasoconstriction syndrome has a spectrum of clinical severity. Severe vasospasm may prompt more aggressive treatment (e.g. verapamil). Future research will aim to identify which patients require timely and effective interventions.

References

1. Ducros A. Reversible cerebral vasoconstriction syndrome. *Lancet Neurol.* 2012;11(10):906–17.
2. Calabrese LH, Dodick DW, Schwedt TJ, Singhal AB. Narrative review: reversible cerebral vasoconstriction syndromes. *Ann Intern Med.* 2007;146(1):34–44.
3. Magid-Bernstein J, Omran SS, Parikh NS et al. RCVS: symptoms, incidence, and resource utilization in a population-based US cohort. *Neurology.* 2021;97:e248–53.
4. Rocha EA, Topcuoglu MA, Silva GS, Singhal AB. RCVS2 score and diagnostic approach for reversible cerebral vasoconstriction syndrome. *Neurology.* 2019;92(7):e639–47.

Learning Points

- Reversible cerebral vasoconstriction syndrome often presents with recurrent thunderclap headache, which may be the only symptom.
- Triggers for RCVS include the postpartum state, vasoactive or recreational drugs and catecholamine-secreting tumours.
- Complications of RCVS include subarachnoid bleeding, intracerebral haemorrhage, acute infarction and posterior reversible encephalopathy syndrome.
- Reversible cerebral vasoconstriction syndrome can appear radiologically similar to cerebral vasculitis but the clinical distinction is important to avoid unnecessary long-term immunosuppression.

Patient's Perspective

1. **What was the impact of the condition?**

   a. Physical (e.g. job, driving, practical support)
   Lack of energy, felt unfit as I could normally have walked three miles daily before my attack.

   b. Psychological (e.g. mood, future, emotional well-being)
   My mood was low and I had a short course of anti-depressants. I felt tearful at times. As I was also dealing with a bleed in the front of my brain, I can't be certain which caused the low mood.

   c. Social (e.g. meeting friends, home)
   Socially I was not confident for a few weeks, but that gradually improved.

2. **What could you not do because of the condition?**
   I felt at the time that it was not safe for me to drive my car. But with encouragement from my family, I overcame the fear of perhaps having another attack whilst on the road driving. I now drive with confidence.

3. **Was there any other change for you due to the condition?**
    Well, I suppose I live with the fear that a sudden cough or sneeze might trigger another attack. I am aware of the back of my head when straining for any reason.

4. **What is/was the most difficult aspect of the condition for you?**
    The most difficult aspect was the chronic pain in my head, which was hard to diagnose. Having a lumbar puncture was horrific. Again, the fear of it recurring is another difficult aspect.

5. **Was any aspect of the experience good or useful? What was that?**
    The only good aspect was getting a reason for the pain in my head after many tests for other possible causes.

6. **What do you hope for in the future for people with this condition?**
    I would hope that scans taken in hospital would be made available to a neurologist straight away so as an early diagnosis could be made, not as in my case much later.

History

While a passenger in a car, a 50-year-old woman experienced a sudden severe headache. The headache peaked instantaneously. She was very nauseated and started to shake. She did not lose consciousness. An ambulance was called and she was taken to a local hospital. Because of hospital bed scarcity and/or because she usually resided in another trust, arrangements were made to transfer her to her local hospital; no neuroimaging was performed at the first hospital.

Past medical history included urticaria, perianal abscess/fistula and renal stones. She was an ex-smoker of cigarettes. She drank less than 14 units of alcohol/week.

At her local hospital, a CT scan of brain was performed at 16:10 hrs on the following day (more than 25 hours after the headache onset). The CT brain scan was reported as normal. A lumbar puncture was performed on the next day, 50 hours after the onset of the headache. The cerebrospinal fluid (CSF) spectroscopy graph (Figure 13.1) showed an elevated net bilirubin absorbance (>0.007 absorbance unit or AU) consistent with subarachnoid haemorrhage [1].

While waiting for a CT angiogram and transfer to a regional neurosurgery centre, another thunderclap headache occurred six days after the first headache. Emergency transfer to the regional neurosurgery centre was arranged following a CT scan of the brain.

Examination

Initial neurological examination demonstrated mild neck stiffness. Pulse rate was 80 beats per minute and blood pressure was 124/74 mmHg. Visual acuity was 6/6 and funduscopy was normal.

Subsequent examination after the second thunderclap headache revealed a right third nerve palsy (pupil enlarged with eye deviated down and out). She also had concentration, processing and memory problems.

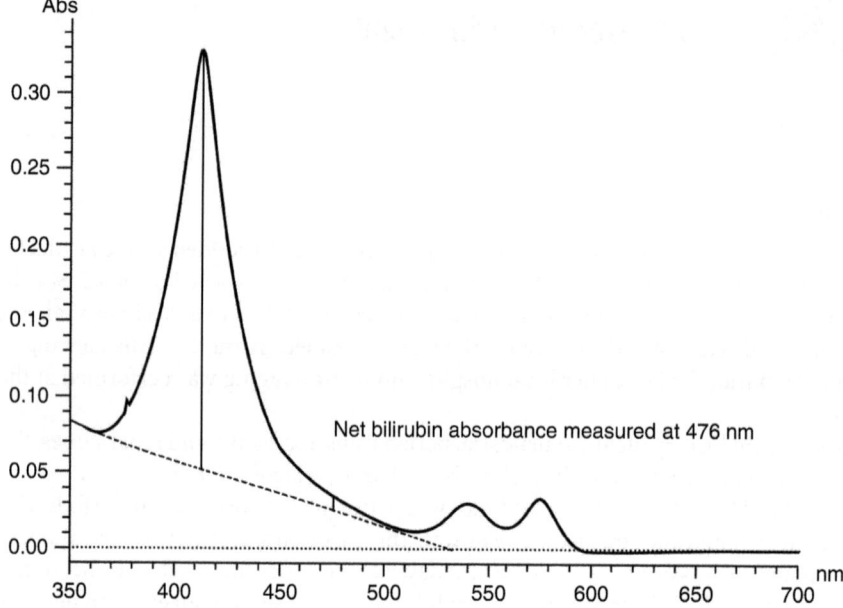

Figure 13.1 Cerebrospinal fluid spectroscopy showing dominant oxyhaemoglobin peak but also elevated net bilirubin absorbance at 476 nm.

Diagnosis: Aneurysmal Subarachnoid Haemorrhage

Investigations

After the second thunderclap headache and a clinical right third nerve palsy a CT scan of brain showed subarachnoid haemorrhage (SAH) in the suprasellar and interpeduncular cisterns with early hydrocephalus (Figure 13.2A).

A catheter angiogram was performed before and after coiling of a right posterior communicating artery aneurysm (Figures 13.2B and 13.2C).

Management

Coiling of the right posterior communicating artery aneurysm was successfully performed. Brain injury sequelae followed with headache, concentration and memory difficulties. She was referred to a community brain injury team.

Comment

Epidemiology and Management of Aneurysmal SAH

Aneurysmal SAH is not rare. About 1 in 50 (18 of 847 patients) patients presenting to a hospital emergency department with acute onset of headache have had an SAH. Aneurysmal SAH predominantly affects young people (peaking in the 40s and 50s), more often women than men (3:2 ratio) and has a very high mortality and disability burden. Perimesencephalic SAH makes up 5–10% of all SAHs, which is thought to arise from a venous bleed.

The global incidence of aneurysmal SAH has declined from 10.2 to 6.1 per 100,000 per year from 1980 to 2010, probably reflecting decreases in blood pressure and smoking prevalence [2]. Following publication of the International Subarachnoid Aneurysm trial (ISAT) [3], most patients with aneurysmal SAH are managed by interventional neuroradiologists who perform endovascular coiling of aneurysms.

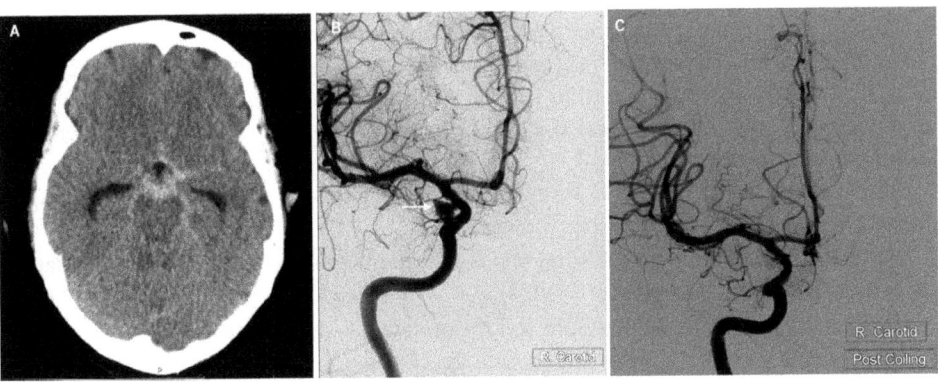

Figure 13.2 (A) A CT brain scan showing diffuse SAH and prominent temporal horns of the lateral ventricles suggestive of early hydrocephalus. (B) A catheter angiogram showing a 7 mm right posterior communicating artery aneurysm (arrow). (C) After coiling there is an occluded right posterior communicating artery aneurysm.

Diagnostic Delay in Aneurysmal SAH

Between 6 and 17% of all hospital inpatients experience an adverse event. Aneurysmal SAH remains a common cause of misdiagnosis. This condition requires interaction of multiple disciplines (acute physician/emergency doctors, radiologists, neurosurgeons and neurologists) and knowledge of limitations and interpretations of the relevant investigations.

The Ottawa subarachnoid rule helps guide clinicians on when a lumbar puncture is required. An online version is available that provides the risk of an underlying aneurysmal SAH from a combination of different clinical features (www.mdcalc.com/ottawa-subarachnoid-hemorrhage-sah-rule-headache-evaluation). Careful selection of patients for lumbar puncture is important to improve the positive predictive value of CSF spectroscopy. Using CSF spectroscopy without applying the Ottawa rule or even when a thunderclap headache has not occurred will decrease the positive predictive value of the test.

Why Not Just Proceed to Angiography in Patients Fulfilling Ottawa Criteria?

The prevalence of cerebral aneurysms is approximately 3.2%. Most of these cerebral aneurysms will not rupture (the <7mm anterior circulation aneurysm rupture rate is very low). Identifying all patients with small cerebral aneurysms may adversely affect their psychological well-being and prospects of life assurance.

Cerebrospinal fluid spectroscopy is used in the UK to identify aneurysmal SAH in patients who present with a thunderclap headache but have had a CT of the brain, which does not show any evidence of haemorrhage [1]. There is evidence that a minority of patients with aneurysmal SAH continue to be diagnosed using the combined clinical assessment, a negative CT brain scan and CSF spectroscopy performed at least 12 hours after and within two weeks of thunderclap headache onset. With emphasis on ruling out SAH, there is evidence that a CT brain scan using modern scanners will detect subarachnoid blood in all patients with aneurysmal SAH if performed within six hours of onset of a thunderclap headache.

Re-bleeding Risk

Neurosurgical literature has documented early or imminent risk of re-bleeding in patients with aneurysmal SAH. Even in modern-day neurosurgical centres, a 10% risk of in-hospital re-bleeding prior to aneurysm repair has been reported. The frequency of re-bleeding increases with the Hunt and Hess grade – a grade based on symptoms and signs, which predicts mortality. However, re-bleeding can occur in all grades of the Hunt and Hess scale: from grade 1 (asymptomatic, mild headache and slight nuchal rigidity) to grade 5 (coma and decerebrate posturing, moribund).

For a district general hospital, several opportunities exist to reduce delays in managing patients with thunderclap headache. These include:

1 Performing a CT brain scan as soon as possible after a patient with a new thunderclap headache arrives in hospital.
2 Performing urgent CT angiography if non-traumatic SAH is confirmed.
3 Appropriate use of CSF spectroscopy with the UK National External Quality Assessment Service (UKNEQAS) threshold for subarachnoid blood [1] 12 hours after headache onset to select patients for CT angiography.

4 Effective communication and teamwork in order to streamline the diagnostic pathway and achieve an early and accurate diagnosis.

5 Urgent transfer to a neurosurgical centre once a patient is diagnosed with aneurysmal SAH, as the risk of re-bleeding is imminent and can occur in 10% of patients.

References

1. Cruickshank A, Auld P, Beetham R et al. Revised national guidelines for analysis of cerebrospinal fluid for bilirubin in suspected subarachnoid haemorrhage. *Ann Clin Biochem.* 2008;45:238–44.

2. Etminan N, Chang HS, Hackenberg K et al. Worldwide incidence of aneurysmal subarachnoid hemorrhage according to region, time period, blood pressure, and smoking prevalence in the population: a systematic review and meta-analysis. *JAMA Neurol.* 2019;76(5):588–97.

3. Molyneux AJ, Kerr RSC, Yu L-M et al. International subarachnoid aneurysm trial (ISAT) of neurosurgical clipping versus endovascular coiling in 2143 patients with ruptured intracranial aneurysms: a randomised comparison of effects on survival, dependency, seizures, rebleeding, subgroups, and aneurysm occlusion. *Lancet.* 2005 Sep.;366(9488):809–17.

Learning Points

- Aneurysmal SAH is a medical emergency with a high morbidity and mortality.
- A patient with a thunderclap headache needs to be thoroughly and urgently evaluated and investigated to exclude an underlying aneurysmal SAH.
- Management of patients with thunderclap headache requires clinical suspicion and a multidisciplinary algorithm with local and regional multidisciplinary teamwork.
- Careful selection of patients with thunderclap headache for lumbar puncture increases the positive predictive value of CSF spectroscopy.

Patient's Perspective

1. **What was the impact of the condition on you?**

   a. Physical (e.g. job, driving, practical support)
   I am able to walk unaided but I need help crossing roads and stepping off pavements as I am now blind in one eye. My speech is affected; I have a stutter which gets worse when I am tired. I need help buttoning tops and trousers as my co-ordination is affected.

   b. Psychological (e.g. mood, future, emotional well-being)
   I have become a different person; my mood swings have increased. I am a lot more impatient and need people to stick to set plans or I become frustrated. Being unable to do everyday tasks alone has left me depressed, angry and also at times I felt it was my fault it happened.

   c. Social (e.g. meeting friends, home)
   I only go to social events if my husband and daughter are with me as I become very confused when people are talking in groups. I am unable to sit in company if people are behind me as it throws my co-ordination off.

2. **What can or could you not do because of the condition?**
   I am unable to take care of my grandchildren alone as I get tired a lot. I am forgetful and leave things on the cooker too long. I am unable to cross the road myself as I have to think about too many things all at once. I'm unable to pack a suitcase for holidays as I have to think ahead and plan, and I find this difficult.

3. **Was there any other change for you due to this condition?**
   Since my bleeds, my friends and family have said I am a lot more snappy and need things to go my way. When I get confused and upset, I would hit myself in the face, which upsets my family. Whatever my mind is thinking, my mouth now speaks it. I feel my brain takes time to catch up with my mouth.

4. **What is/was the most difficult aspect of the condition for you?**

   The changes to my personality and the fact I had to depend on other people for everyday tasks. I don't like the way I am happy one minute and can become upset the next. I wish I could be the independent person I was before and have the ability to care for my family the way I once did.

5. **Was any aspect of the experience good or useful? What was that?**

   It has shown me that life is for living. I have grown a very close bond with my daughter as she is the one that cares for me and tries her best to understand my condition.

6. **What do you hope for in the future for people with this condition?**

   That there is more aftercare outside of the hospital setting. That more people come to realise that it is a hidden injury. Also, for bleeds to be picked up faster from the onset, more people trained in recognising the condition so they know how to care and support people like myself.

Headache and Fever

History

A previously healthy 45-year-old woman was found by her family unresponsive and incontinent of urine. She had been talking with her family 10 hours earlier at 07:30. She had been headachy all day and had vomited. She was sleepy and went to bed. She had complained of lower back pain for the previous two days.

An ambulance was called. Her Glasgow Coma Scale was 11/15 – recorded as E4 (spontaneous eye opening), V1 (no verbal response) and M6 (obeyed commands). A capillary blood glucose was 12.2 mmol/L, temperature 40.0°C, respiratory rate 16 breaths per minute, pulse 87 beats per minute and blood pressure was 161/57 mmHg. Her oxygen saturation was 97%. She was agitated and seemed to have bitten her tongue.

Past medical history was unremarkable except for excision of a right axillary sebaceous cyst. She had no history of coeliac disease or diabetes mellitus. She had had no recent foreign travel and no history of a tick bite. She did not smoke cigarettes and drank two or three gins every three months. She had one brother and two sisters, who had no neurological illnesses.

Examination

In hospital, her Glasgow Coma Scale improved to 13 – E3 (eye opening to speech), V4 (confused verbal response) and M6 (obeyed commands). Her pupils were equal, of normal size and reactive to light. She had a regular breathing pattern. Full Outline of UnResponsiveness or FOUR score was E4 (eyelids open, tracking or blinking to command), M4 (thumbs up, fist or peace sign), B4 (pupil and corneal reflexes present) and R4 (not intubated and has regular breathing pattern) or 16/16. She was disorientated, photophobic and had neck stiffness. She had word-finding difficulties.

Investigations

Her haemoglobin was 141 g/L, white cell count 27.57×10^9/L (neutrophils 27.2) and platelets 227×10^9/L. Her CRP was 19.3 mg/L (and 114.4 mg/L two days later). Her glucose was 12.1 mmol/L and lactate 7.6 mmol/L. Electrolytes and liver function tests were normal. A pregnancy test was negative. HIV testing was negative. A COVID-19 PCR test was negative. A mid-stream specimen of urine was negative.

A CT of the brain and abdomen were reported as showing no abnormality.

A lumbar puncture was performed 24 hours after hospital admission; there was cloudy cerebrospinal fluid (CSF), 35 red cells/µL, 2,875 white cells/µL (90% polymorphs), CSF protein of 2.22 g/L and CSF glucose of 3.5 mmol/L with a serum glucose of 6.1 mmol/L.

Cerebrospinal fluid demonstrated PCR-positive *Streptococcus pneumoniae*. The *S. pneumoniae* cycle threshold was 31.88. A *Neisseria meningitidis* PCR was negative and *Haemophilus influenza* PCR was negative. Enterovirus, varicella zoster virus and herpes simplex virus 1 and 2 PCRs were all negative.

Subsequent blood culture grew Gram-positive cocci, *S. pneumoniae* serotype 10A sensitive to penicillin.

Diagnosis: Streptococcal Meningitis

Management

She received 14 days of intravenous ceftriaxone. Within a day of treatment, improvement began. However, six months later, she still had concentration difficulties. An audiogram was normal.

Comment

Diagnosis of Bacterial Meningitis

The classical features of meningitis – fever, headache, neck stiffness and altered mental status – were all present in this patient; not all such features may be present in patients with bacterial meningitis. The classic triad of fever, neck stiffness and altered consciousness may be present in less than 50% of patients with bacterial meningitis. Kernig's sign (pain in lower back and resistance to movement with passive extension of the knee on the flexed thigh in the recumbent patient) and Brudzinski's neck sign (passive flexion of the neck bringing the head onto the chest is accompanied by flexion of the legs) cannot be relied upon for the diagnosis. In strongly suspected bacterial meningitis, guidelines recommend antibiotic treatment in the community if there is likely to be more than a one-hour delay in reaching a hospital as there is evidence that early antibiotic treatment reduces mortality [1].

Once admitted to hospital, guideline recommendations for suspected bacterial meningitis are patient stabilisation (airway, breathing, circulation etc), consciousness assessment, blood cultures, lumbar puncture (if safe to perform) and antibiotic treatment within one hour of hospital arrival. Delay in lumbar puncture should not delay treatment despite the drop off in culture rate, particularly four hours after starting antibiotics.

When Is It Safe to Proceed to Lumbar Puncture without a Brain Scan?

A lumbar puncture in a patient with suspected bacterial meningitis can reveal inflammatory cells, identify the infecting pathogen and guide antimicrobial therapy. Although brain imaging in most patients with bacterial meningitis is normal, a CT scan of the brain can identify patients with mass effect who may be at risk of brain herniation. Brain imaging before lumbar puncture is recommended for patients with certain features – being 60 years or older, being immunocompromised, having a history of central nervous system disease and a history of seizure within a week of presentation (Table 14.1). Specific neurological features that prompt CT brain scanning prior to lumbar puncture include an abnormal level of consciousness, an inability to answer two consecutive questions correctly or to follow two consecutive commands, gaze palsy, abnormal visual fields, facial palsy, arm drift, leg drift and language disturbance. The language disturbance and presumed seizure in our patient indicated that a CT brain scan was required before lumbar puncture. Absence of all such clinical features predicts a normal scan with a high (97%) negative predictive value for an abnormality [2].

Epidemiology of Bacterial Meningitis

Bacterial meningitis is rare, with less than 10 laboratory-confirmed cases per year in most district general hospitals or 1 per 100,000 per year. Conjugate vaccines have reduced the incidence of the three major causes of bacterial meningitis (*S. pneumoniae*, *N. meningitidis* and *H. influenza*) [3]. Delays in diagnosis and treatment can be catastrophic. Pneumococcal

Table 14.1 Some contraindications to lumbar puncture in adults

Category	Clinical features
Neurological features suggesting raised intracranial pressure	Reduced or fluctuating level of consciousness (Glasgow coma scale less than 9 or a drop by 3 or more) Bradycardia or hypertension Focal neurological signs (as listed in the main text) Abnormal posture or posturing Unequal, dilated or poorly responsive pupils Papilloedema (permitted in idiopathic intracranial hypertension as no pressure gradient) Seizures
Systemic features	Shock, extensive purpura, respiratory insufficiency
Haematology issues	Abnormal coagulation results Platelet count $<100 \times 10^9$/L Receiving anticoagulant therapy Immunocompromised
Superficial infection or developmental abnormality at the lumbar puncture site	Myelomeningocele

meningitis mortality approaches 30% and increases with age. Pneumococcal meningitis is more common in the over 50s, may be due to a skull fracture/CSF leak, is often associated with an upper respiratory tract infection and, like both *N. meningitidis* and *H. influenza*, is more likely in asplenic or functionally asplenic individuals.

Recommended investigations by UK joint specialist societies include the following [1]:

1 Blood for culture, pneumococcal and meningococcal PCR, storage for serological testing, glucose, lactate, procalcitonin, full blood count, electrolytes, liver function tests and coagulation screen.

2 CSF opening pressure, CSF glucose with plasma glucose, CSF protein, lactate, microscopy, culture and sensitivities. CSF PCR for pneumococci and meningococci plus storage for later tests.

3 Posterior nasopharyngeal swab for meningococcal culture.

4 Any significant bacterial isolates should be sent to relevant national reference laboratory.

Treatment Algorithm of Streptococcal Meningitis

For Gram-positive diplococci (likely to be *S. pneumoniae*), 2 g ceftriaxone intravenously 12-hourly or 2 g cefotaxime intravenously six-hourly is recommended. In countries where penicillin resistance is common, vancomycin or rifampicin (in renal failure) are recommended. If *S. pneumoniae* is identified and is cephalosporin-sensitive, treatment can be stopped at 10 days if the patient has recovered. If not recovered, 14 days of treatment is recommended. For patients with penicillin- or cephalosporin-resistant pneumococcal meningitis, 14 days of treatment is required.

In suspected meningitis, 10 mg of dexamethasone intravenously six-hourly should be started on hospital admission either shortly before or at the same time as starting antibiotic therapy. Steroid therapy can decrease cytokine release. Although not all of the evidence is supportive, a Cochrane review concluded that corticosteroid treatment was associated with a small reduction in mortality for patients with pneumococcal meningitis. There was also a reduction in hearing loss and short-term neurological sequelae without an increase in harm. The British Infection Association recommends dexamethasone in patients with suspected bacterial meningitis before or up to 12 hours after starting antibiotics. If *S. pneumoniae* is identified, steroid treatment should continue for four days [1].

Intubation is recommended when the Glasgow coma scale is 12 or less. Sepsis treatment and intracranial pressure management may also be required. All patients with meningitis should have an HIV test. Regardless of aetiology, all cases of meningitis should be notified to the relevant public health authority. Close contacts of patients diagnosed with pneumococcal meningitis are not usually at increased risk of infection and do not require prophylaxis (unlike meningococcal infection for which ciprofloxacin or rifampicin are given to all close contacts).

Complications of Bacterial Meningitis

Complications of bacterial meningitis include hearing loss, hydrocephalus, seizures and a range of cerebrovascular complications. Co-existing septic shock is a predictor of poor outcome. Declining consciousness should prompt imaging to look for hydrocephalus, empyema, evolving abscess or infarction. Seizures and non-convulsive seizures need to be considered and treated. Pneumococcal meningitis in particular is associated with cerebrovascular complications – brain infarction in up to 30%. Cerebral venous sinus thrombosis and intracerebral haemorrhage may occur in up to 9% of patients [3]. Extensive delayed infarcts days to weeks after initial recovery is a rare complication (1.1% in the Netherlands in the years 2006–12) related to a hyper-inflammatory syndrome that can be particularly devastating. Adjunctive dexamethasone and elevated complement C5a were associated with delayed cerebral thrombosis. Case fatality rates for pneumococcal meningitis (10–37%) and listerial meningitis (up to 35%) are higher than other forms of bacterial meningitis.

Other neurological sequelae can include subtle cognitive deficits. Neuropsychological assessment and support are important. Fatigue, sleep disorders and emotional difficulties are frequent, occurring weeks to months after discharge.

Recurrence and Vaccination

The risk of a recurrent episode of pneumococcal meningitis is 5%. Risk factors for pneumococcal meningitis include a persistent CSF leak, immunodeficiency, asplenism or hyposplenism. In a quarter of patients with a recurrence, no risk factor has been identified. The European Society of Clinical Microbiology and Infectious Diseases (ESCMID) recommends that all patients with pneumococcal meningitis should be vaccinated with both pneumococcal polysaccharide vaccine (PPV) 23 and pneumococcal conjugate vaccine (PCV)13, although this has not been endorsed in all guidelines.

The 23-valent PPV is recommended for all adults 65 years and over. In younger age groups (2–64 years) at risk, the same 23-valent vaccine is recommended in patients with asplenia or splenic dysfunction, patients with chronic respiratory disease, chronic heart disease, chronic renal disease, chronic liver disease, diabetic patients, immunosuppressed patients, patients with a cochlear implant and in patients at risk of CSF leak.

Hypoglycorrhachia

Hypoglycorrhachia is low CSF glucose, usually defined as a CSF glucose of <2.2 mmol/L. It has been recognised since the 1930s. Under homeostatic conditions, the CSF/serum glucose ratio should be >0.6. It is not an unusual finding in bacterial, viral, fungal and tuberculous meningitis. Hypoglycorrhachia is also found in patients with stroke, malignancy, neurosarcoidosis, neurosyphilis and cerebral toxoplasmosis and glucose transporter 1 (GLUT 1) deficiency due to mutations in the *SCL2A1* gene. GLUT 1 protein is responsible for the transport of glucose from the blood into the brain. GLUT 1 deficiency causes epilepsy, microcephaly, developmental delay, paroxysmal choreathetosis with spasticity and paroxysmal exercise-induced dyskinesia.

Up to a quarter of patients with bacterial meningitis have hypoglycorrhachia. Patients with bacterial meningitis and hypoglycorrhachia are more likely to have been immunosuppressed, have a petechial rash, nausea or vomiting, nuchal rigidity, sinusitis or otitis media, an abnormal mental state and focal neurological deficits compared to patients with bacterial meningitis but without hypoglycorrhachia. Unsurprisingly, a finding of hypoglycorrhachia is also associated with a worse prognosis.

Inhibition of glucose entry into the subarachnoid spaces due to changes in the blood–brain barrier is one hypothesis for hypoglycorrhachia. Glucose is transported into the CSF via the choroid plexus as well as the ventricular and subarachnoid capillary system. Other hypotheses include increased glycolysis by leucocytes and increased rate of glucose transport across the arachnoid villi.

References

1. McGill F, Heyderman RS, Michael BD et al. The UK joint specialist societies guideline on the diagnosis and management of acute meningitis and meningococcal sepsis in immunocompetent adults. *J Infect*. 2016;72(4):405–38.

2. Hasbun R, Jekel J, Quagliarello V. Computed tomography of the Head before lumbar puncture in adults with suspected meningitis. *N Engl J Med*. 2001;345:1727–33.

3. van de Beek D, Brouwer MC, Koedel U, Wall EC. Community-acquired bacterial meningitis. *Lancet*. 2021;398(10306):1171–83.

Learning Points

- Clinical suspicion of bacterial meningitis is important even if all of the classical features of headache, fever, neck stiffness and altered consciousness are not present.
- Pneumococcal meningitis and listeria meningitis have a high mortality. Urgent assessment and empirical treatment of bacterial meningitis can be life-saving.
- CT brain scanning is indicated before lumbar puncture if there are risk factors or clinical signs that may indicate raised intracranial pressure.
- Bacterial meningitis is a notifiable disease.

Patient's Perspective

1. **What is the impact of the condition on you?**

   a. Physical (e.g. job, driving, practical support)
   For the first few months when I came home from hospital all I could do for myself was take a shower; my mother did everything else for me.

   b. Psychological (e.g. mood, future, emotional well-being)
   I was very anxious and worried that I may get sick again.

   c. Social (e.g. meeting friends, home)
   Being social drains me because when three or four people are talking, I lose a lot of the conversation. I can't hear or concentrate on some of the conversation.

2. **What can you not do because of the condition?**
I couldn't do anything physical because I was too tired and found it difficult to concentrate for long on anything.

3. **Has there been any other change for you due to this medical condition?**
My hearing has got bad.

4. **What is/was the most difficult aspect of the condition for you?**
The headaches for the first four months were daily and sometimes really bad. Now I only get about one headache a week. The tiredness is still bad. I don't have the energy to do much. Memory and concentration are still not good.

5. **Was any aspect of the experience good or useful? What was that?**
No.

6. **What do you hope for in the future for people with this condition?**
I hope that anyone who gets meningitis is treated as quickly as I was and recovers.

Brain Infection

History

A 42-year-old right-handed woman developed a persistent moderately severe headache, most severe behind her right eye. Within two days, she felt weak and nauseated. Bending over exacerbated her headache. She described a few involuntary shaking episodes, feeling very cold and sweating, suggestive of rigors. She also described an episode of contiguous spreading pins and needles down her left side.

Her GP arranged admission to hospital. Prior to a neurological assessment, she had been on trimethoprim 200 mg twice a day and had been given one dose of gentamicin 300 mg.

Examination

She was alert but pyrexial, 39°C. She had marked neck stiffness and limited straight leg raising bilaterally. Limb examination revealed no abnormality except for an extensor left plantar response.

Investigations

A CT brain scan was reported as normal. Blood investigations were unremarkable.

A lumbar puncture revealed an opening pressure of 14 cm of cerebrospinal fluid (CSF). The CSF had 22 white cells/μL (70% lymphocytes), no red cells/μL, protein of 0.20 g/L and glucose of 4.1 mmol/L. Serum glucose was 6.1 mmol/L.

An MRI scan of the brain showed signal change in the left temporal lobe with mass effect and to a lesser extent the right temporal lobe (Figure 15.1).

An EEG had a background of mixed activity of periodic lateralised epileptiform discharges of the right posterior regions spreading to both sides.

A diagnostic test was performed.

Cerebrospinal fluid yielded a positive PCR result for herpes simplex virus (HSV) type 1.

Management

She was treated on admission with intravenous aciclovir 10 mg/kg tid for two weeks. She received phenytoin but this was switched to valproate due to deranged liver function tests.

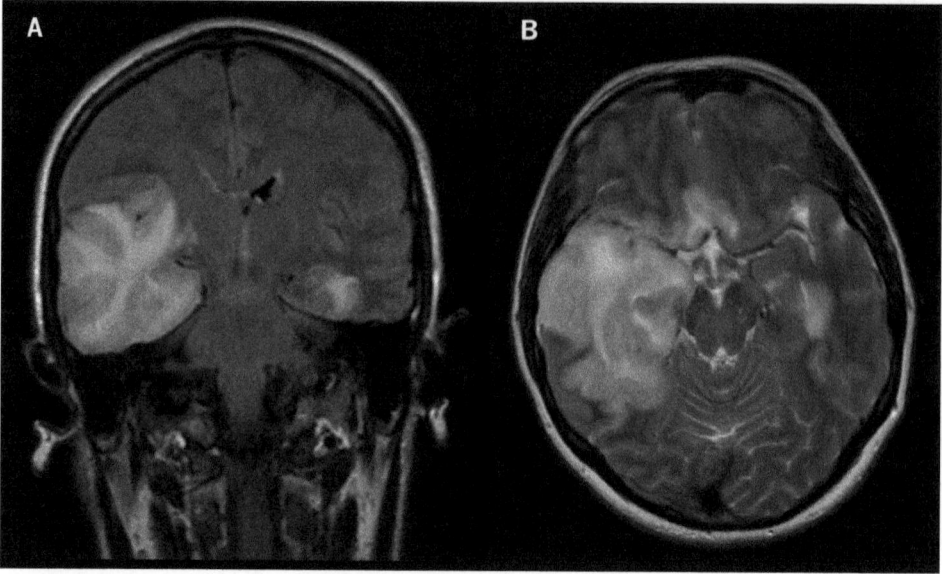

Figure 15.1 (A) Coronal FLAIR and (B) axial T2 MRI scan of the brain demonstrating high signal and mass effect predominantly in right temporal lobe and to a lesser extent cingulate gyrus and subcortical left temporal lobe.

Diagnosis: Herpes Simplex Meningoencephalitis

Management

At follow-up, she had difficulty recognising faces. She was referred to neuropsychology as fatigue, concentration and prosopagnosia were present. She was also referred to neuro-occupational therapy.

After four months, sodium valproate was withdrawn and at one year, she was able to drive. Thirteen months after her presentation, she was discharged from neurology follow-up.

Comment

Definitions

Encephalitis is inflammation of the brain. While this is strictly a pathological diagnosis, CSF pleocytosis and neuroimaging are used to make a clinical diagnosis.

Encephalopathy is an altered mental status and is a frequent presenting feature of encephalitis. However, our patient had little evidence of encephalopathy.

Meningoencephalitis, infection or inflammation of the meninges (headache, fever, neck stiffness) and brain (fever, focal seizures) was present in our patient.

Prosopagnosia is an inability to recognise previously known human faces and to learn to recognise new ones. Unilateral nondominant lesions in the fusiform gyrus have been associated with prosopagnosia.

Epidemiology of Encephalitis

Fever, focal neurological deficits and CSF lymphocytosis are inclusion criteria for all causes of encephalitis. With the identification of an increasing number of autoimmune encephalitides, the incidence of viral and autoimmune causes of encephalitis are similar. The incidence of acute encephalitis is 12.6 per 100,000 per year, with the highest incidence in children. Some causes of infective and autoimmune encephalitis are listed in Table 15.1. The other main differential diagnoses include septic encephalopathy, which can occur in 50–70% of septic patients and non-convulsive status epilepticus.

Herpes Simplex Encephalitis

Herpes simplex virus encephalitis is the most commonly diagnosed viral encephalitis in industrialised countries, with an estimated incidence of 2–4 per million per year. Most cases (90%) are due to HSV type 1. Herpes simplex virus type 2 is a more common cause of meningitis and neonatal meningoencephalitis than HSV type 1.

Fever and headache are the most common features of encephalitis and indeed any infection of the central nervous system. Altered behaviour or disorientation, personality change, focal (as in our patient) and generalised seizures, motor deficit and aphasia are presenting features that should prompt consideration of encephalitis. There are no pathognomonic symptoms or signs of herpes simplex encephalitis. However, some features may suggest an antibody-mediated encephalitis such as a subacute presentation over weeks or months, facio-brachial dystonic seizures poorly responsive to anti-epileptic medication, choreoathetosis and hyponatraemia.

Table 15.1 Some causes of infective and autoimmune encephalitis

Infective causes of encephalitis	Antibody identified in autoimmune causes of encephalitis
HSV 1 and 2	N-methyl D-aspartate receptor
Varicella zoster virus	Leucine-rich glioma inactivated 1
Enteroviruses	Gamma-aminobutyric acid-B receptor
Adenovirus	Contactin-associated protein 2
Parechovirus	Gamma-aminobutyric acid-A receptor
Measles virus	Myelin oligodendrocyte glycoprotein
HIV	Glycine receptor
Zika – Africa, India, South and Central America, Texas and Florida	α-amino-3-hydroxy-5-menthyl-4-isoxazolepropionic acid receptor
Chikungunya – Africa, South Asia, and Central and South America	Dipeptidyl-peptidase-like protein-6
Japanese encephalitis virus – Asia and northern Australia	IgLON5
Septic encephalopathy	No associated antibody

Investigations for Suspected Herpes Simplex Encephalitis

A definitive diagnosis of herpes simplex encephalitis requires an HSV-specific positive PCR test or viral antigen or nucleic acid detection from brain biopsy (now rarely performed) or autopsy.

Cerebrospinal fluid pleocytosis (10–1,000 cells/μL) is present in 95% of PCR-positive cases of herpes simplex encephalitis. Herpes simplex virus PCR testing has high sensitivity (98%) and specificity (94%) compared to biopsy in herpes simplex encephalitis. These test characteristics prompt the clinician to consider Bayesian decision analysis (useful tutorial at https://edhub.ama-assn.org/jn-learning/video-player/18117478). A negative test in the setting of a high pre-test likelihood of herpes simplex encephalitis does not exclude herpes simplex encephalitis. In this scenario, it is not advisable to stop aciclovir with a single negative PCR for herpes simplex.

Cerebrospinal protein is often moderately elevated and CSF glucose is usually normal. Investigative guidelines from the British Society of Infection recommend checking N-methyl D-aspartate receptor (NMDAR) antibody not only because NMDAR encephalitis can mimic herpes simplex encephalitis but also because NMDAR encephalitis can follow herpes simplex encephalitis. Increasingly, an infective panel is being requested accompanied by a panel for serum and CSF autoimmune antibodies.

An MRI of the brain is a more sensitive investigation for encephalitis than a CT of the brain. Temporal lobe abnormalities are suggestive of encephalitis. A stroke-like presentation can prompt CT brain imaging, which may be negative. It is important to consider herpes simplex encephalitis in the differential diagnosis, as further investigation (MRI and lumbar puncture) and aciclovir treatment should not be delayed. An EEG can add further support of temporal lobe dysfunction.

Aciclovir

Aciclovir is a guanosine nucleoside analog and is converted into its triphosphate form, which then competitively inhibits viral DNA polymerase. This terminates the growing viral DNA chain and inactivates the viral DNA polymerase. Aciclovir is a highly specific anti-herpes viral drug. A pivotal trial demonstrating the benefit of aciclovir was published in 1984 [1]. Aciclovir greatly improved six-month survival, 50% in the vidarabine group compared to 81% in the aciclovir group.

Even with aciclovir treatment, there is a 10–15% mortality rate among patients with herpes simplex encephalitis. Severe neurological and neuropsychiatric sequelae can occur in approximately 50% of patients.

Aciclovir nephrotoxicity (either crystal-induced nephropathy or rarely interstitial nephritis or direct tubular necrosis) mandates careful renal monitoring. Aciclovir neurotoxicity can manifest with a broad range of symptoms including disorientation, decreased level of consciousness, hallucinations, agitation, dysarthria, seizures, myoclonus and encephalopathy. Patients with end-stage renal failure are most at risk of aciclovir neurotoxicity, even with a renal dose of aciclovir. Measurement of serum 9-carboxymethoxymethylguanine (CMMG) and aciclovir (measured in Bristol, UK) can confirm aciclovir neurotoxicity.

Guidelines for Investigating Suspected Encephalitis

The Association of British Neurologists (ABN) and British Infection Association (BIA) guidelines for the investigation and management of patients with suspected encephalitis were published in 2012 [2]. The guidelines promote early recognition and treatment of encephalitis (including testing for autoimmune encephalitis) in order to reduce the devastating consequences of a delayed diagnosis. The ABN/BIA guidelines have an algorithm that outlines the clinical features of encephalitis, contraindications to lumbar puncture, starting aciclovir within six hours and appropriate neuroimaging. Immunosuppressed adults receive 21 days of aciclovir (10 mg/kg tid with renal adjusting if required). If not immunosuppressed, 14 days of aciclovir is required for patients with herpes simplex encephalitis. If a CSF PCR has confirmed herpes encephalitis (herpes simplex or varicella zoster), then a repeat lumbar puncture is advised after completing aciclovir. If CSF is still PCR positive, a further seven days of aciclovir is recommended.

Post Herpes Simplex NMDAR Encephalitis

N-methyl D-aspartate receptor encephalitis is an autoimmune encephalitis first recognised around 2007. Early prominent psychiatric or behavioural symptoms occur before speech dysfunction, seizures, movement disorder (dyskinesias, rigidity or abnormal posture) decreased level of consciousness and autonomic dysfunction or central hypoventilation may ensue. The median age of occurrence is 21 years and the female to male ratio is 4:1. Two recognised triggers of NMDAR encephalitis are tumours (mostly ovarian teratomas) and herpes simplex encephalitis [3]. In a Danish study, 9 out of 55 cases of NMDAR encephalitis developed after herpes simplex encephalitis. There is evidence that a relapsing clinical picture after herpes simplex encephalitis (types 1 and 2) may be due to NMDAR encephalitis developing 2–16 weeks after herpes simplex encephalitis [3]. In children four years and younger, choreoathetosis, decreased level of consciousness and frequent seizures or infantile spasms occurred, while older children and adults manifested mostly behavioural and psychiatric symptoms, sometimes accompanied by seizures.

References

1. Skoldenberg B, Forsgren M. Acyclovir versus vidarabine in herpes simplex encephalitis. *Lancet.* 1984;2(8405):707–11.

2. Solomon T, Michael BD, Smith PE et al. Management of suspected viral encephalitis in adults – Association of British Neurologists and British Infection Association national guidelines. *J Infect.* 2012;64(4):347–73.

3. Armangue T, Spatola M, Vlagea A et al. Frequency, syndromes, risk factors, and outcome of autoimmune encephalitis following herpes simplex encephalitis: a prospective observational study and a retrospective analysis of cases. *Lancet Neurol.* 2018;17(9):760–72.

Learning Points

- Herpes simplex virus type 1 is the most frequent cause of viral encephalitis in industrialised countries.

- Aciclovir has dramatically improved survival from herpes simplex encephalitis.

- National UK guidelines from the ABN and the BIA for suspected encephalitis aid early diagnosis and management.

- N-methyl D-aspartate receptor encephalitis can follow herpes simplex encephalitis.

Patient's Perspective

1. **What is/was the impact of the condition?**

   a. Physical (e.g. job, driving, practical support)

   Fatigue was a big issue initially and in order to get through the day I would take what I called resting periods to recharge. I would go off in a room to be on my own without any distraction for 10 to 15 minutes or however long it took until the fatigue passed.

   I could not be left alone as initially I was unable to look after myself. Physically I had to be retrained and monitored to do everyday tasks. At times I may have had the memory of what to do, but co-ordinating and doing the job at the same time was difficult. I may start a job but then get distracted and then forget to finish what I was doing.

   b. Psychological (e.g. mood, future, emotional well-being)

   Losing my independence did affect my own confidence as simple daily tasks often proved challenging and I was always looking for reassurance and checking if I was doing it right. I ended up doubting my ability a lot.

   Fatigue did have an impact on me psychologically. When feeling tired any job or even holding a conversation took a lot more effort. At times when everything became too much, I just ignored everyone and took a rest, but this did affect my mood and manners around people. Family tried to understand and work with me but because I looked ok and normal, visitors and friends did not see the issues.

   Coming to terms and coping with prosopagnosia/face blindness also had an impact on me emotionally as it turned my whole world upside down.

   c. Social (e.g. meeting friends, home)

   I only went out because I could not be left alone at home. When I did go out, I stayed away from people and any interaction. My memory for faces was exceptionally good before encephalitis, but not recognising even my own family members made it challenging. The fatigue also affected my manner around people.

2. **What could you not do because of the condition?**

   Look after myself, think for myself, remember conversations, remember faces, go out on my own as my sense of direction was affected and I would get lost very easily even in previously very familiar locations. I could not go to the shop on my own. I had an aversion to loud or repetitive noises. Background music in shops prevented me from even going in, following TV programmes or films. I could not drive.

3.   **Was there any other change for you due to your medical condition?**

The biggest change was the loss of facial memory. Initially I was also forgetful regarding conversations. I might ask a question and then a few minutes after having the conversation I might ask the same question again.

Remembering appointments and dates proved difficult.

4.   **What is/was the most difficult aspect of the condition for you?**

One of the hardest things to deal with is that when people meet me or see me out, I look normal as if nothing is wrong with me. If a conversation began sometimes, I got a bit of information that helped me connect to who they were. Often if I meet people and don't recognise them, I would ask "open" questions, nothing very specific. Over time I have got more open about my problem and now would just ask people I meet who they are and those that know me better now tell me their name when I meet them.

5.   **Was any aspect of the experience good or useful? What was that?**

Unable to work and having to take things a lot easier gave me a lot of time on my hands. I stayed with my children then seven and eight when they went to the swimming pool. At the time the club was looking for more support. Having time on my hands I volunteered my services. I completed a Level 1 – swim teacher course and started helping. I am still involved in the club and have completed Level 2 Swim Teacher and Level 1 Swim Coach.

I don't recognise the kids I teach but when they arrive, I make a note of their name and then beside their name put something they are wearing, pink spotty hat, green goggles, striped costume, which enables me to recognise them. All other coaches are aware of my problem and are supportive but not many of the kids I teach would know about it. I don't get involved in administration, as even connecting kids to parents would be impossible for me.

6.   **What do you hope for in the future for your condition?**

Although given the name of what I had in hospital and some explanation, I had very little understanding of the consequences, what to expect and how to deal with the changes. There was some follow-up after returning home but from my recollection and what my husband has said the nurse only seemed to check my medical condition making sure I was taking medication. No neurological support or follow-up was given to me, or advice to members of the family supporting me. Once I left hospital, we really felt we were left to fend for ourselves. It was hard enough coming to terms with the changes that we did not have the ability or time to see what other resources were available to us and very little was offered. A lot of the medical support we meet had very little understanding of what encephalitis was and the real consequences.

I have since had treatment for cancer and the level of support I received when receiving and after treatment was overwhelming in comparison to what I received after encephalitis. When I returned home after the encephalitis, I discovered the Encephalitis Society and it was this that really gave us a lot of support and helped us deal and cope with the consequences and changes from encephalitis. I know time has passed and I would like to hope that there would be a better understanding of encephalitis, its consequences and more resources made available for support and guidance for all affected.

16 Headache and Droopy Eye

History

A 51-year-old right-handed man developed new onset of pulsing right-sided headache. Three days later, his wife noticed that his right eyelid was drooped. He had attended a gym three days per week as usual where he often stretched his limbs and neck during his programme. His headache persisted and he thought his right face felt different from his left face.

Past medical history was unremarkable. He took no medication except paracetamol for the new onset headache.

Examination

He was alert, orientated and systemically well. His pulse rate was 66 beats per minute and his blood pressure was 145/94 mmHg. He had a right ptosis and miosis with an apparent enophthalmos (Figure 16.1). Visual acuity was 6/4 on the right and 6/5 on the left, both unaided. There was no other abnormality detected.

Investigations

An ophthalmologist applied 1% apraclonidine (an alpha-2 adrenergic receptor agonist with weak alpha-1 receptor agonist activity), which produced an upper lid retraction and a normal pupil size.

A chest X-ray was normal. Full blood count, CRP, electrolytes and liver function tests were all normal.

Neuroimaging

A CT of the brain performed at another hospital showed high signal in the wall of the right internal carotid artery (Figure 16.2A).

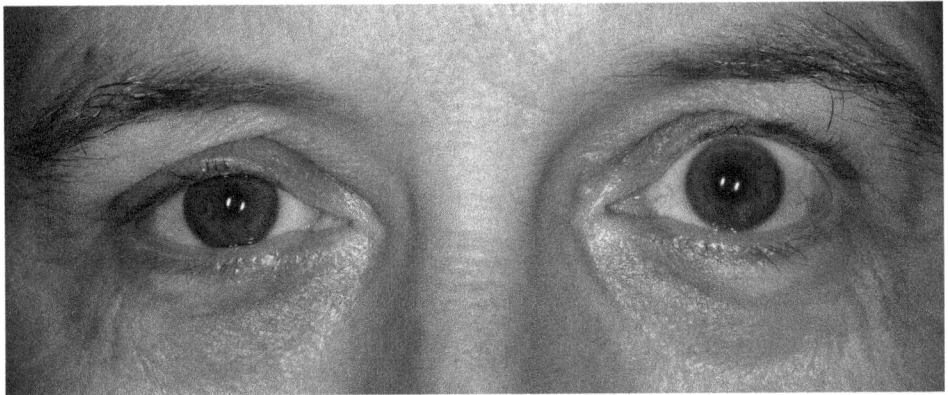

Figure 16.1 Right miosis and ptosis.

An MRI scan of the brain was performed. Fat-suppressed T1 axial images showed high signal consistent with a false lumen in the right internal carotid artery (Figure 16.2B). Sagittal T1 showed the same classical appearance of a right internal carotid artery dissection (Figure 16.2C).

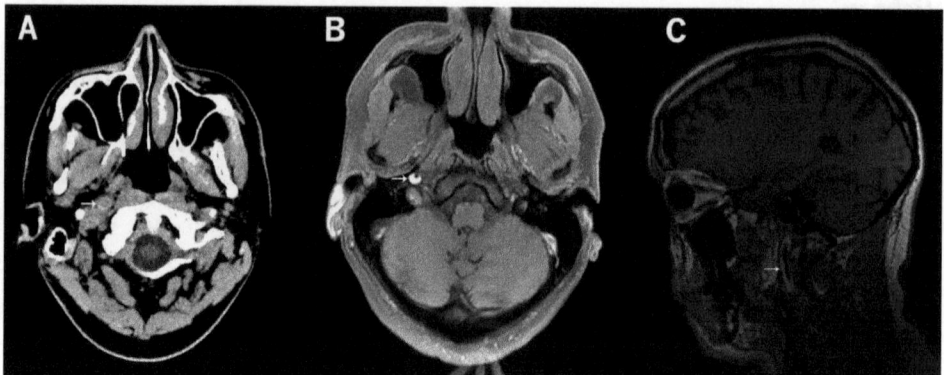

Figure 16.2 (A) A CT of the brain showing high signal in the wall of the right internal carotid artery (arrow). (B) A fat-suppressed T1 axial MRI of the brain showing high signal consistent with a false lumen in the right internal carotid artery (arrow). (C) A sagittal T1 MRI of the brain showing the same classical appearance of a right internal carotid artery dissection (arrow).

Diagnosis: Right Internal Carotid Artery Dissection

Management
He was treated with aspirin.

Follow-up MR angiography was performed to ensure that a pseudo-aneurysm had not developed. The lumen gradually returned to normal with no stenosis and no mural irregularity 18 months later.

No other neurological deficit developed.

Comment
Cervical Sympathetic Pathway
The cervical sympathetic pathway begins in the hypothalamus and is made up of three neurones. From the hypothalamus, the first neurone passes down through the brainstem to the lateral grey column of the cervicothoracic spinal cord to levels C8 to T2 and the ciliospinal centre of Budge. The second neurone joins the white rami of C8 and T1 nerve roots to synapse in the superior cervical ganglion. The third neurone leaves the superior cervical ganglion and enters the skull on the surface of the common and internal carotid artery via the carotid canal, which is located in the petrous portion of the temporal bone just superior to the jugular fossa.

Once in the cranial cavity, the third cervical sympathetic neurone innervates superior and inferior tarsus muscles of Müller (which assist in eye-opening) via the third cranial nerve, the blood vessels of the eye via vasomotor fibres in the nasociliary branch of the V cranial nerve and the ciliary ganglion, and the pupil via pupillodilator fibres on the nasociliary nerve passing around the eye as the long ciliary nerves. Damage to the oculosympathetic fibres along the internal carotid artery or removal of the superior cervical ganglion causes miosis (asymmetry of pupillary size or anisocoria that is more obvious within five seconds of darkness), ptosis, apparent enophthalmos or 'upside-down ptosis' due to lower lid elevation and abolition of sweating over one side of the face. The pattern of sweating loss may be useful in localising a lesion; central lesions usually impair sweating over the entire ipsilateral head, neck, arm and upper trunk. Lesions above the superior cervical ganglion may not cause anhydrosis at all because the sympathetic innervation of sweat glands and facial blood vessel is below the superior cervical ganglion.

Differential Diagnoses of Horner Syndrome
The anatomical pathway of the oculosympathetic chain renders it vulnerable to a long and diverse list of pathological processes (Table 16.1). There may be clinical clues to the aetiology and anatomical location of the Horner syndrome, which can be confirmed with pharmacological testing agents and strategic imaging.

Ipsilateral face, orbit or neck pain is a common presentation (in more than half of patients) with Horner syndrome due to internal carotid artery dissection. The classic Horner syndrome triad (miosis <2 mm, ptosis and anhydrosis) may not be present and the findings may be subtle. Old photographs for comparison may help confirm a clinical suspicion of Horner syndrome.

Table 16.1 Causes of Horner syndrome

Neuronal disorder	Location	Pathology	Associated clinical signs
First order (central)	Posterior hypothalamus	Pituitary tumour	
	Brainstem	Stroke – Wallenberg syndrome Demyelination	Vertigo Altered facial sensation Contralateral CN IV palsy Crossed motor/sensory signs Radicular signs
	Cervical cord intermediate grey substance C8 to T2	Arnold-chiari Cervical spondylosis Syringomyelia Neck trauma	
Second order (intermediate)	C8 to T2 ventral nerve roots	Cervical rib Brachial plexus injury	Neck/arm pain and weakness
	Apex of the lung	Tumours • Pancoast tumour • Mesothelioma	Signs of lung disease
	Mediastinum	Cardiothoracic surgery Aortic aneurysm or dissection	
	Cervical sympathetic chain	Subclavian artery aneurysm Thyroid tumour Posterior neck dissection	Vocal cord paralysis Anhydrosis of face and neck
Third order (post-ganglionic)	Superior cervical ganglion at C2 to C3	Jugular venous ectasia	
	Carotid artery	Carotid • dissection • aneurysm • arteritis	Facial pain Stroke Ocular ischaemia
	Cavernous sinus	Skull base tumour Inflammatory mass	Abducens palsy
	Orbit	Herpes zoster	

Adapted from Davagnanam et al. [1] with permission from Springer Nature.

Pharmacological Diagnosis of Horner Syndrome

Historically, topical cocaine was used to confirm the presence of Horner syndrome. Cocaine blocks the active re-uptake of noradrenaline by the sympathetic nerve endings, leading to dilatation of the normal pupil. In Horner syndrome, there is less noradrenaline and so the test is positive if cocaine increases the degree of resting anisocoria. There is failure of the ipsilateral pupil to dilate.

Topical hydroxyamphetamine, which releases noradrenaline, has been used to help localise a lesion in Horner syndrome. Should topical hydroxyamphetamine cause both pupils to dilate, then a first- (central) or second-order (pre-ganglionic) neurone lesion is confirmed.

Topical hydroxyamphetamine has no effect on a Horner pupil due to a third-order (post-ganglionic) neurone lesion.

The topical cocaine test has been superseded by the apraclonidine test. Apraclonidine, an alpha-2 adrenergic receptor agonist with weak alpha-1 receptor agonist activity causes dilatation of the Horner pupil due to denervation supersensitivity. A reversal of anisocoria is suggestive of Horner syndrome. There may be a mild pupillary constriction of the normal pupil due to down-regulation of noradrenaline release at the synaptic cleft. As the apraclonidine test relies on upregulation of alpha-1 adrenergic receptors on the dilator pupillae muscles, false negative results can occur within the first five to eight days. The apraclonidine test cannot localise the lesion.

Imaging in Horner Syndrome

In real-life practice, pharmacological tests are not as readily available as imaging [1]. Chest X-ray and carotid Doppler ultrasound lack sensitivity for detecting carotid artery dissection. As a first-order neurone, Horner syndrome is implicated with ataxic hemiparesis, an MRI scan of the brain is required. A first-order-neurone Horner syndrome without brain or brainstem signs also requires an MRI of the cervical and upper thoracic spine because of the course of the first-order neurone. A second- or third-order-neurone Horner syndrome requires a CT angiogram from the arch of the aorta (as low as T4 to T5) to the circle of Willis plus visualisation of the lung apices and orbits. Although longer to perform a fat-suppressed MRI scan and contrast-enhanced MR angiogram from the arch of the aorta to the circle of Willis may be used if iodinated contrast is contraindicated. Acute onset, pain and history of trauma or malignancy should prompt urgent imaging.

Cervical Artery Dissection

Cervical artery dissection is due to an intramural haematoma in the cervical portion of the internal carotid artery or vertebral artery. Dissection occurs because an endothelial breach allows blood into the inner intima where it tracks along the plane of the vessel wall (inner intima and outer fibrous adventitia separated by a muscular media layer). The haematoma may be predominantly subintimal or subadventitial (Figure 16.3); when subadventitial, it can cause a protrusion from the weakened vessel wall or pseudoaneurysm formation. Rupture of a pseudoaneurysm can cause subarachnoid haemorrhage if the dissection extends into intracranial vasculature. Dissection of the carotid and vertebral arteries accounts for 2–2.5% of all acute ischaemic strokes, but among young and middle-aged adults, cervical artery dissection can make up 25% of acute ischaemic strokes. The incidence of cervical artery dissection is 2.5–3.0 per 100,000 per year with dissection of the internal carotid artery occurring twice as frequently as vertebral artery dissection [2]. Acute ischaemic stroke is due to emboli arising from the endothelial flap or less frequently from the haemodynamic effect of vessel compromise/occlusion. Internal carotid artery dissection has been associated with a lower risk of ischaemic stroke in patients with Horner syndrome than in patients with internal carotid artery dissection but without Horner syndrome.

Complications of cervical artery dissection include formation of pseudoaneurysms, which can cause local mass effect on adjacent structures or promote distal thromboembolism. Depending on location, lower cranial nerve palsies may develop as in Collet–Sicard syndrome (unilateral palsy of cranial nerves IX, X, XI and XII) or Villaret syndrome (unilateral palsy of cranial nerves IX, X, XI and XII and Horner syndrome).

Subadventitial haematoma

Subintimal haematoma

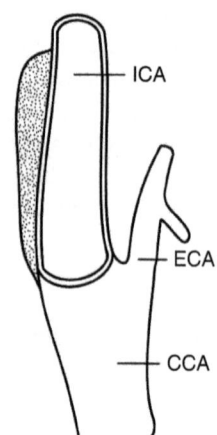

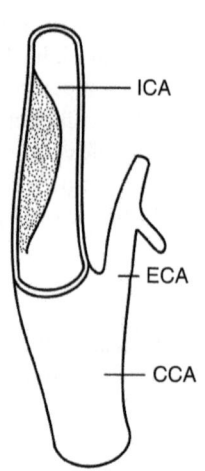

Figure 16.3 Schematic representation of internal carotid artery dissection with subintimal and subadventitial extension (CCA, common carotid artery; ECA, external carotid artery; ICA, internal carotid artery).

Radiological Diagnosis of Cervical Artery Dissection and Treatment

Prompt diagnosis and management of cervical artery dissection is important to minimise (further) stroke risk.

Digital subtraction angiography had been considered the gold standard for diagnosis but this investigation is invasive and only assesses the lumen without determining the arterial wall changes. A T1 fat-supressed MRI (as used in our patient) can demonstrate high-signal crescent-shaped mural haematoma and luminal narrowing (sensitivity reported at 95% and specificity 99%). The radiological differential diagnosis includes fibromuscular dysplasia, dysgenesis of the internal carotid artery, atherosclerosis, neck irradiation, Takayasu's arteritis, Behçet's disease and giant cell arteritis.

In the absence of any signal of harm, acute treatments for acute ischaemic stroke due to cervical artery dissection such as intravenous thrombolysis and endovascular revascularisation should be considered.

There is some evidence that antiplatelet therapy is protective against subsequent stroke (cervical artery dissection in stroke study or CADISS trial) as is vitamin K antagonist treatment (treatment in cervical artery dissection or TREAT-CAD trial). The studies had small numbers of clinical outcomes and, until better evidence becomes available, dual antiplatelet for 21 days is advocated for acute transient ischaemic attack and minor stroke with cervical artery dissection.

References

1. Davagnanam I, Fraser CL, Miszkiel K, Daniel CS, Plant GT. Adult Horner's syndrome: a combined clinical, pharmacological, and imaging algorithm. *Eye*. 2013;27(3):291–8.

2. Engelter ST, Lyrer P, Traenka C. Cervical and intracranial artery dissections. *Ther Adv Neurol Disord*. 2021;14:17562864211037238.

Learning Points

- The classical triad of internal carotid artery dissection includes Horner syndrome, facial/neck pain and ischaemic stroke.
- Patients with internal carotid artery dissection and Horner syndrome may have a lower risk of embolic stroke than patients with internal carotid artery dissection but without Horner syndrome.
- Patients with transient ischaemic attacks or acute ischaemic stroke due to internal carotid artery dissection can be treated with dual antiplatelet therapy, intravenous thrombolysis and mechanical thrombectomy.
- Complications of internal carotid artery dissection such as pseudo-aneurysm are not common.
- Internal carotid artery dissection can cause lower cranial nerve palsies such as Collet–Sicard syndrome (unilateral palsy of cranial nerves IX, X, XI and XII) or Villaret syndrome (unilateral palsy of cranial nerves IX, X, XI and XII and Horner syndrome).

Patient's Perspective

1. **What was the impact of the condition on you?**

   a. Physical (e.g. job, practical support, physical activity)
   Physically I managed everyday tasks but I limited myself due to uncertainty. My family offered practical support; however, I felt I could manage. Absent from work for a three-month period, returning on phased return. Difficult not being able to take part in physical activity in the same capacity as before.

   b. Psychological (e.g. mood, emotional well-being)
   Affected confidence initially. Feeling of vulnerability – worry, especially for family. Put life in perspective, but tried to remain upbeat, stay positive. Thankful for support of family and medical staff. Generally, fear of the unknown- what might have been. Lucky!

   c. Social (e.g. meeting friends, home)
   No real impact overall. Subtle changes to home life, restricting certain tasks. Mostly concern from family and friends.

2. **What could you not do because of the condition?**
   Physically I felt limited – no gym or training or swimming. Holiday planned so had to alter activities (adventure). Affected sleep patterns for a while. Worried about impact/posture on neck.

3. **Was there any other change for you due to your medical condition?**
   Physical appearance changed due to 'Horner's'. Impact of this. Could this be fixed? Would it remain? Long-term managing this aspect – confidence etc.

4. **What is/was the most difficult aspect of the condition for you?**
   Feeling limited. Vulnerable despite physically able to carry out everyday tasks. Waiting for diagnosis and potential impact of this.

5. **Was any aspect of the experience good or useful? What was that?**
   Perhaps a way of telling me to slow down. Less physical exertion (training).

6. **What do you hope for in the future for people with this condition?**
   Better awareness from medical profession and public. Early signs of detection. More education – impact psychologically of neurological conditions.

17 Facial Somatic Mosaicism

History

A 48-year-old right-handed man attended a neurology clinic. He had a long history of migraine with aura, hemiplegic migraine and glaucoma. He had always had poor vision from his left eye, which deteriorated further with a retinal detachment. When young, he had left buphthalmos (an enlarged eye – often a symptom of childhood glaucoma).

He once went for three years without a migraine. A typical migraine consisted of paraesthesia often starting over the right shoulder and moving down the right arm and right leg. Then he felt that he had loss of power in his right limbs with a facial hemisensory loss. His vision could be blurred and he would lose speech. The event usually lasted 30–45 minutes. A headache would then ensue and frequently persist into the next day.

He had had a left facial port-wine stain.

He had stopped drinking alcohol for over eight years. He did not smoke cigarettes.

An MRI scan of the brain was performed.

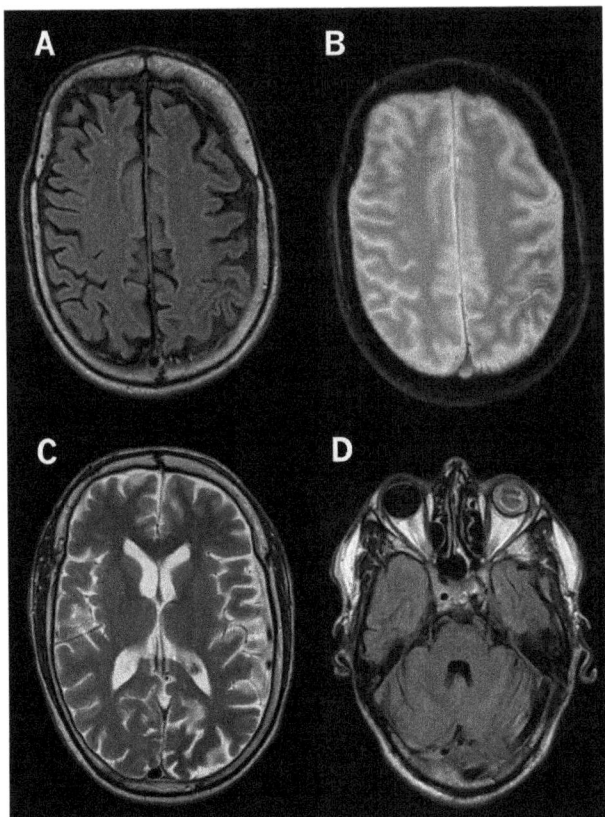

Figure 17.1 Axial MRI brain imaging of a patient with Sturge–Weber syndrome. FLAIR imaging shows (A) left hemiatrophy and left parietal cerebrospinal fluid high signal due to angiomatous lesion while (B) gradient echo imaging shows the overlying haemosiderin in left parietal region. (C) Enlarged left choroid plexus and (D) left eye changes.

Diagnosis: Sturge–Weber Syndrome

A diagnosis of Sturge–Weber syndrome was made when he was three months old. In later years, hemiplegic migraine and other migraine auras proved medically refractory. Migraine auras also affected his left arm but much less frequently.

Examination

He had widespread but mild facial capillary angiomatous lesions, more marked on the left than the right. The lesion involving the left V1 and V2 dermatomes consistent with a port-wine stain was more prominent. The left eye had no perception of light. Whitish Salzmann's nodular degeneration was present on the surface of the left eye. The remainder of the examination was normal.

Investigations

An MRI scan of the brain showed left hemiatrophy (Figure 17.1A), left parietal haemosiderin (gradient echo) consistent with prominence of vessels (Figure 17.1B), left hypertrophy of the trigonal choroid plexus (Figure 17.1C) and an abnormal left orbit (Figure 17.1D), all consistent with Sturge–Weber syndrome. There was no change over nine years.

Management

At the age of 26–7 years he had photoderm treatment for the capillary angiomatous lesions. A left cosmetic contact lens was fitted.

He tried a number of migraine prophylaxis agents including nortriptyline, propranolol and riboflavin, with variable effects.

Diagnosis: Sturge–Weber Syndrome Type 1

Comment

Migraine with and without Aura

Migraine, a leading cause of disability worldwide and often a chronic and lifelong disease, affects over 1 billion people. The one-year prevalence is 15%. Migraine affects women more than men (3:1 ratio) and peak prevalence occurs in the 30–50-year age groups. A new diagnosis of migraine after the age of 50 years should prompt consideration of a secondary headache cause.

Diagnostic Criteria

The third edition of the International Classification of Headache Disorders (ICHD-3) defines three main categories of migraine: migraine without aura, migraine with aura and chronic migraine (Table 17.1).

Table 17.1 ICHD-3 diagnostic criteria for migraine

Migraine without aura	Migraine with aura	Chronic migraine	Probable migraine
Criterion A			
At least five attacks fulfilling criteria B–D	At least two attacks fulfilling criteria B and C	Headache (migraine or tension type) on ≥15 days/month for >3 months, and fulfilling criteria B and C	Attacks fulfilling all but one of criteria A–D for migraine without aura, or all but one of criteria A–C for migraine with aura
Criterion B			
Headache attacks lasting 4–72 hours (when untreated or unsuccessfully treated)	One or more of the following fully reversible aura symptoms • visual • sensory • speech or language • motor • brainstem • retinal	Occurring in a patient who has had at least five attacks fulfilling criteria B–D for migraine without aura, or criteria B and C for migraine with aura	Not fulfilling ICHD-3 criteria for any other headache disorder
Criterion C			
The headache has at least two of the following four characteristics • unilateral location • pulsating quality • moderate or severe pain intensity • aggravation by or causing avoidance of routine physical activity (e.g. walking or climbing stairs)	At least three of the following six characteristics • at least one aura symptom spreads gradually over ≥5 minutes • two or more aura symptoms occur in succession • each individual aura symptom lasts 5–60 minutes • at least one aura symptom is unilateral	Any of the following are fulfilled on ≥8 days/month for >3 months • criteria C and D for migraine without aura • criteria B and C for migraine with aura • believed by the patient to be migraine at onset and relieved by a triptan or ergot derivative	Not better accounted for by another ICHD-3 diagnosis

Table 17.1 (cont.)

Migraine without aura	Migraine with aura	Chronic migraine	Probable migraine
	• at least one aura symptom is positive • the aura is accompanied, or followed within 60 minutes, by headache		
	Criterion D		
At least one of the following during a headache • nausea, vomiting or both • photophobia and phonophobia	Not better accounted for by another ICHD-3 diagnosis	Not better accounted for by another ICHD-3 diagnosis	
	Criterion E		
Not better accounted for by another ICHD-3 diagnosis			

Reprinted from Ashina et al. [1] with permission from Elsevier.

Hemiplegic migraine is defined as criteria similar to migraine with aura but with an aura that involves a fully reversible motor weakness and fully reversible visual, sensory and/or speech/language symptoms. The ICHD-3 criteria acknowledge that it can be difficult to distinguish weakness from sensory loss.

Treatments of Migraine

Early or acute treatments of migraine include non-steroidal anti-inflammatory drugs, triptans or a combination of both. Newer drugs include calcitonin-gene-related peptide receptor antagonists (gepants) and 5-hydroxytryptamine type 1F receptor agonists (ditans). Preventive treatments aim to reduce the frequency, duration and severity of migraine attacks. Migraine preventive drugs include beta-blockers (propranolol), anti-depressants (amitriptyline), calcium channel blockers (flunarizine in the USA) and anti-convulsants (topiramate and valproate), although teratogenicity should be borne in mind in prescribing for women of child-bearing age. Monoclonal antibodies to calcitonin gene-related peptide or its receptor (eptinezumab, erenumab, fremanezumab and galcanezumab) have shown efficacy in randomised controlled trials. Lifestyle interventions have been much less researched but have a growing body of evidence of efficacy with low risk of harm.

For the neurologist, consideration of migraine co-morbidities is important. There is a strong association of migraine with both depression and anxiety disorders. Depression can increase the risk of transformation to chronic migraine. Migraine is associated with chronic pain disorders (e.g. back pain), epilepsy and obesity.

History, Definition and Epidemiology of Sturge–Weber Syndrome

Sturge–Weber syndrome, also known as encephalofacial or encephalotrigeminal angiomatosis is a rare sporadic congenital vascular disorder in which there may be cutaneous capillary malformation in the trigeminal nerve distribution (port-wine stain) and/or abnormal capillary venous vessels in the choroid (vascular layer between the retina and the sclera) and

Table 17.2 Roach classification of Sturge–Weber syndrome

Type	Facial angioma	Leptomeningeal angioma	Glaucoma
1 (classical)	Present	Present	Can occur
2	Present	Absent	Can occur
3	Absent	Present	Usually not present

leptomeninges. Port-wine stains typically involve the ophthalmic (V1) and maxillary (V2) branches, or even all three trigeminal branches. A port-wine stain in the V1 territory confers a 15–20% risk of Sturge–Weber syndrome and a risk of ipsilateral glaucoma of 50%. Abnormal capillary venous vessels in the leptomeninges of the brain, ocular abnormalities including glaucoma (all present in this patient) and choroidal venous malformations can all occur in Sturge–Weber syndrome. The syndrome occurs in 1 in 20,000–50,000, affecting males and females equally. Up to a quarter of children born with a port-wine stain develop the other features of Sturge–Weber syndrome.

William Allen Sturge in 1879 and Parkes Weber in 1922 both described two cases of encephalofacial angiomatosis, or what has been subsequently termed the Sturge–Weber syndrome by Hilding Bergstrand in 1935 [2]. The Roach classification categorises Sturge–Weber syndrome based on the presence of facial angioma, leptomeningeal angioma and glaucoma (Table 17.2).

Clinical Features of Sturge–Weber Syndrome

Clinical manifestations of Sturge–Weber syndrome vary but include seizures, hemiparesis, headache, stroke-like episodes, behavioural problems, cognitive disability and visual field defects. Epilepsy (which can manifest with various types of seizures) occurs in 70% of patients with unilateral leptomeningeal capillary malformation and 90% of patients with bilateral disease. Myoclonic-astatic epilepsy may be exacerbated by carbamazepine. Sturge–Weber syndrome type 3 (leptomeningeal angioma without facial port-wine stain) is rare [3].

Imaging

Tram-line or tram-track calcifications on skull X-rays, atrophy and gyral calcification on CT brain scans are recognised features of Sturge–Weber syndrome. Appearances on MRI of the brain include hemiatrophy, leptomeningeal changes and enlarged ipsilateral choroid plexus, which are all features of encephaloangiomatosis (Figure 17.1).

Genetics: Somatic Mutation of *GNAQ*

Somatic mutations in signalling proteins involved in vascular development have been suspected in causing Sturge–Weber syndrome. In 2013, whole-genome sequencing of DNA in affected and unaffected tissue identified a somatic mutation in the *GNAQ* gene (RI83Q) on chromosome 9q21 as the cause of Sturge–Weber syndrome [4]. The average mutation frequency of *GNAQ* (R183Q) in Sturge–Weber syndrome brain endothelial cells is 18–27% compared to port-wine stain skin blood vessels of 7–8%. *GNAQ* encodes guanine nucleotide-binding protein subunit alpha (Gαq) that mediates signalling from G-protein-coupled receptors to downstream proteins. The RI83Q mutation impairs autohydrolysis of activated Gαq. The timing of the mutation during foetal development determines the extent of the involvement. More limited involvement follows later somatic mutation, which may result in isolated non-syndromic port-wine stain or isolated brain involvement without skin manifestation.

Another molecular development has been the recognition of somatic mutation in the PI3 K pathway in port-wine stains. Recognition of the dysregulation of the vascular signalling pathways of MAPK and PI3 K may herald future treatment potential.

Treatment of Port-Wine Stain

Port-wine stains are often treated with pulse dye laser providing selective photothermolysis. Pulse dye laser at 595 nm is preferentially absorbed by blood vessels less than 300 microns beneath the skin surface. Dynamic skin cooling minimises complications and adjacent tissue damage.

There have been some advances in our knowledge of the molecular contributors to Sturge–Weber syndrome and port-wine stains, but there are still gaps. In addition to molecular and animal models, standardised longitudinal studies and clinical trials are required to further improve our understanding of and outcomes from Sturge–Weber syndrome.

References

1. Ashina M, Terwindt GM, Al-Mahdi Al-Karagholi M et al. Migraine: disease characterisation, biomarkers, and precision medicine. *Lancet*. 2021;397:1496–504.

2. Sudarsanam A, Ardern-Holmes SL. Sturge–Weber syndrome: from the past to the present. *Eur J Paediatr Neurol*. 2014;18(3):257–66.

3. Siri L, Giordano L, Accorsi P et al. Clinical features of Sturge–Weber syndrome without facial nevus: five novel cases. *Eur J Paediatr Neurol*. 2013;17(1):91–6.

4. Shirley MD, Tang H, Gallione CJ et al. Sturge–Weber syndrome and port-wine stains caused by somatic mutation in *GNAQ*. *N Engl J Med*. 2013;368(21):1971–9.

Learning Points

- Migraine is a leading cause of neurological disability.
- Sturge–Weber syndrome is a neurocutaneous syndrome, with vascular malformations occurring on the face, choroid and leptomeninges.
- Clinical manifestations of Sturge–Weber syndrome include epilepsy, stroke-like episodes, migraine, glaucoma and developmental delay.
- Somatic mutations of *GNAQ* in Sturge–Weber syndrome and *PI3 K* in port-wine stain at low frequency implicate signalling proteins in the pathogenesis.

Patient's Perspective

1. **What was the impact of the condition?**
   a. **Physical (e.g. job, driving, practical support)**
   I have a residual weakness in my right arm, which improves with time.
   b. **Psychological (e.g. mood, future, emotional well-being)**
   Depressed – low mood at times. If invited out, I have to think whether this is safe for me, to know if I have someone there who knows my situation.
   c. **Social (e.g. meeting friends, home)**
   I am comfortable with friends and family.

2. **What could you not do because of the condition?**
   It only mattered if I was with strangers. I need to keep in my own environment to feel safe.

3. **Was there any other change for you due to your medical condition?**
    I have had to accept my limitations. Due to my circumstances, it was arranged that I am able to work closer to home.

4. **What is/was the most difficult aspect of the condition for you?**
    My appearance – blockages of my skin circulation.
    Secondly, not knowing when I will have a further attack, the unpredictability!

5. **Was any aspect of the experience good or useful? What was that?**
    I feel it has made me a stronger character and more accepting of problems as they arise.

6. **What do you hope for in the future for your condition?**
    I hope more is discovered about these conditions and that better treatment is available.

An Alarm Clock Headache

History

An 81-year-old left-handed man who still drove a car was referred to a neurology clinic because he had an eighteen-month history of nocturnal headaches. He explained that he was wakened most nights around 4 am with a global headache reaching 8 out of 10 in severity. He usually took 1 g of paracetamol and the pain eased over 30 minutes.

When he was in his 30s, he had migraines but this new headache was different. He was a non-smoker and occasionally drank half a pint of beer. There was no history of hypertension, diabetes mellitus, stroke or heart disease.

Past medical history included depression, pleural plaques, restrictive lung disease and gastro-oesophageal reflux. He had been exposed to asbestos when previously working in a power station.

Medication included inhalers (salbutamol and beclometasone/formoterol/glycopyrronium bromide), finasteride 5 mg/per day, omeprazole 20 mg/per day, fluoxetine 40 mg/per day, paracetamol as required and cetirizine 10 mg/per day.

Examination

He was alert and orientated with no cognitive deficit. His neck had a good range of pain-free movements. His blood pressure was 150/78 mmHg. Visual acuity was 6/9 on the right and 6/6 on the left with glasses. Apart from a slight decrease in hearing, he had no neurological deficit.

Investigations

His GP had already checked his thyroid status and had organised a CT scan of the brain (both normal). ESR and CRP were normal.

Diagnosis: Hypnic Headache

Management
A cup of coffee with caffeine was recommended before going to bed. This was associated with headache-free sleeping.

Comment

History of Hypnic Headache
First described in six patients by Neil Raskin in 1988, hypnic headache is a rare and benign sleep-related or 'alarm clock' primary headache disorder [1]. The lack of daytime attacks helps distinguish hypnic headache from many other causes of headache. A 30-year review of published cases highlighted an average of 7.6 years from headache onset to diagnosis [2]. In headache centres, hypnic headache accounts for only 0.1% of all headache patients. Accurate diagnosis can, however, be reassuring for the patient because of the benign nature of the headache and improving outcome with appropriate treatment with caffeine. Accurate diagnosis may also decrease health care costs.

Diagnostic Criteria of Hypnic Headache
The third edition of the International Classification of Headache Disorders (or ICHD-3) describes hypnic headache as frequently occurring headache attacks developing only during sleep, causing wakening and lasting up to four hours, without characteristic associated symptoms and not attributed to other pathology. Hypnic headache usually begins after the age of 50 years but can occur in younger people. It is more common in women.

Pain is bilateral in two-thirds of patients, often mild to moderate but severe in 20%. The onset of hypnic headache does not appear to be related to sleep stage. Neuroimaging volume reduction in hypothalamic grey matter has been reported in patients with hypnic headache.

In published cases, the only symptom reported was headache in 60% of patients. Nausea or vomiting (over 20%), photophobia and/or phonophobia (15%) and autonomic features (8%) including bilateral lacrimation or rhinorrhoea may also occur in patients with hypnic headache.

Differential diagnosis includes primary and secondary headaches. The clinical features can help distinguish such headaches (Table 18.1). Cluster headache, which is thought to be one of the most painful human experiences, can waken patients at night and last up to 180 minutes. The restlessness and ipsilateral autonomic features (facial parasympathetic activation) may distinguish cluster headache from hypnic headache. The other four trigeminal autonomic cephalalgias are rarer than cluster headache and also have diagnostically helpful autonomic features (conjunctival injection, lacrimation, nasal congestion, rhinorrhoea, eyelid oedema, forehead and facial sweating, miosis and/or ptosis). Hemicrania continua, which is more common in females with a mean age of 30 years, can last from hours to days, may cause restlessness or be aggravated by movement, and responds to indomethacin treatment.

Paroxysmal hemicrania has a duration of 2–30 minutes.

The shorter-lasting trigeminal autonomic cephalalgias – short-lasting unilateral neuralgiform headache attacks with conjunctival injection and tearing (SUNCT) and short-lasting

Table 18.1 Differential diagnosis of hypnic headache

Headache	Clinical features or associations
Primary	
Migraine	Recurrent headache disorder, attacks lasting 4–72 hours, unilateral, pulsating, moderate to severe, aggravated by physical activity and associated with nausea and/or photophobia and phonophobia
Cluster headache	Severe attacks, strictly unilateral temporal or (supra)orbital pain lasting 15–180 minutes occurring from once every other day to eight per day, often at night between 2 and 3 am, with ipsilateral autonomic features (ipsilateral conjunctival injection, lacrimation, nasal congestion, rhinorrhoea, forehead/facial sweating, miosis, ptosis and/or eyelid oedema) and/or restlessness/agitation
Paroxysmal hemicrania	Severe, strictly unilateral attacks of orbital, supraorbital or temporal pain lasting 2–30 minutes occurring several or many times per day and associated with autonomic features (ipsilateral conjunctival injection, lacrimation, nasal congestion, rhinorrhoea, forehead/facial sweating, miosis, ptosis and/or eyelid oedema). Absolute response to indomethacin
Hemicrania continua	Can last hours to days
Secondary	
Obstructive sleep apnoea	Morning headache usually bilateral lasting <4 hours and often associated with dry or sore throat. Resolves with successful sleep apnoea treatment
Medication over-use	Headache on 15 or more days per month with a pre-existing headache disorder and over-using regular analgesia for three months or more
Nocturnal seizures	Headache can be sole manifestation
Giant cell arteritis	Various headache features. Usually, continuous unilateral temporal headache
Nocturnal hypertension	Can mimic hypnic headache
Secondary cluster headache	Pituitary adenoma, meningioma and arteriovenous malformation
Phaeochromocytoma	Rapid onset, sometimes peaking within minutes or one minute (thunderclap) and usually lasting less than 15 minutes. May be associated with diaphoresis and palpitations

unilateral neuralgiform headache attacks (SUNA) – are less likely to be confused with hypnic headache as they both only last seconds to minutes and cause many more attacks per day.

Treatment of Hypnic Headache

Case series and case reports support the use of caffeine (tablet or drink) at bedtime, which proved effective in our patient.

Indomethacin 50 mg tid and melatonin have also been used with good results. Finally, lithium is a second-line agent. All of these agents have been reported in more than 20 patients and have had a 50% or more response rate. The same drugs may have some prophylactic role.

The pathophysiology of hypnic headache is not known. A chronobiological disorder, hypothalamic dysfunction or serotonin and melatonin dysregulation have been proposed. Although the condition can last for years in almost half of all patients, a similar proportion seem to have remission without recurrence [3]. However, the natural history of hypnic headache requires further study.

References

1. Raskin NH. The hypnic headache syndrome. *Headache J Head Face Pain*. 1988;28(8):534–6.
2. Silva-Néto RP, Santos PEMS, Peres MFP. Hypnic headache: a review of 348 cases published from 1988 to 2018. *J Neurol Sci*. 2019;401:103–9.
3. Liang JF, Wang SJ. Hypnic headache: a review of clinical features, therapeutic options and outcomes. *Cephalalgia*. 2014;34(10):795–805.

Learning Points

- Hypnic headache is a rare and benign sleep-related or 'alarm clock' primary headache disorder occurring mostly in patients over 50 years of age.
- Differential diagnosis of hypnic headache includes migraine and trigeminal autonomic cephalalgias, particularly cluster headache, which can occur nocturnally.
- Caffeine has proven effective treatment for hypnic headache and is the first-line treatment.
- Indomethacin, melatonin and lithium have some case series and case report evidence for efficacy in acute and preventive treatment of hypnic headache.

Patient's Perspective

1   **What was the impact of the condition on you?**

   a. Physical (e.g. sleep, activities of daily living)
   I was wakened out of sleep with a bad headache on my forehead, roughly around 4 am, which resulted in me being tired, fatigued all day as I could not get back to sleep.

   b. Psychological (e.g. mood, emotional well-being)
   It left me feeling emotional, brought me to tears, brought me into low mood. I didn't feel like going out during the day, left me uninterested in stuff.

   c. Social (e.g. meeting friends, home)
   I didn't feel like doing anything as I was so tired through the day. It left me in bad mood.

2.   **Did the headaches stop you from doing anything?**
   Yes, they stopped me from going about my daily duties.

3.   **Has there been any other change for you due to the condition?**
   My condition went on for 18 months before I got diagnosed. I thought I had a brain tumour, the pain was that bad.

4.   **What is/was the most difficult aspect of the condition for you?**
   Not being able to get a full night's sleep, left me tired and sleeping during the day.

5.   **Was any aspect of the experience good or useful? What was that?**
   Once I got diagnosed, they advised me to take a coffee late at night before bed and it is working. I am delighted.

6.   **What do you hope for in the future for your condition?**
   I hope people can get diagnosed earlier. I feel doctors didn't take me seriously, maybe because of COVID-19 I was delayed getting diagnosed.

CASE 19   Bleeding Brain

History

A 42-year-old man complained of a weak right leg of several months' duration. He had a history of deafness for more than five years and wore bilateral hearing aids.

In the past, he had misused drugs, including intravenous drugs from which he developed hepatitis C. He had been treated with pegylated interferon and ribavirin for one year; he was PCR-negative on follow-up. He had a history of hypertension, anxiety and depression.

He smoked cigarettes and drank excessive amounts of beer in a binge-like manner.

Examination

He was alert and orientated. Abnormalities in the neurological examination included deafness, increased tone in his legs, hip flexion weakness and brisk lower limb reflexes accompanied by a right extensor plantar response. Otherwise he had normal power but could not heel-toe walk.

Investigations

An MRI of the brain showed non-specific white matter changes, a left lacunar cystic infarct and a low signal rim in the cerebellum and brainstem consistent with haemosiderin (Figures 19.1A–19.D). An MRI scan of the spine showed that the spinal cord was coated in low signal. There was also an extradural cyst in the dorsal thoracic canal (Figure 19.1E).

A CT myelogram revealed an ovoid filling defect within the posterior spinal canal between T5 and T7 vertebrae. The cyst filled on the more delayed images, abutting the anterior margin of the cord and causing mild cord displacement. No evidence of block was identified.

Audiometry demonstrated bilateral deafness worse on the left (Figure 19.2).

HIV antibody screening, hepatitis B surface antigen and syphilis immunoassay were negative.

Cerebrospinal fluid (CSF) examined at the time of the myelogram was negative for oxyhaemoglobin and bilirubin (spectrophotometry). There were no white cells identified. Cerebrospinal fluid protein was elevated at 0.72 g/L and CSF glucose was 3.6 mmol/L (plasma glucose was 4.7 mmol/L).

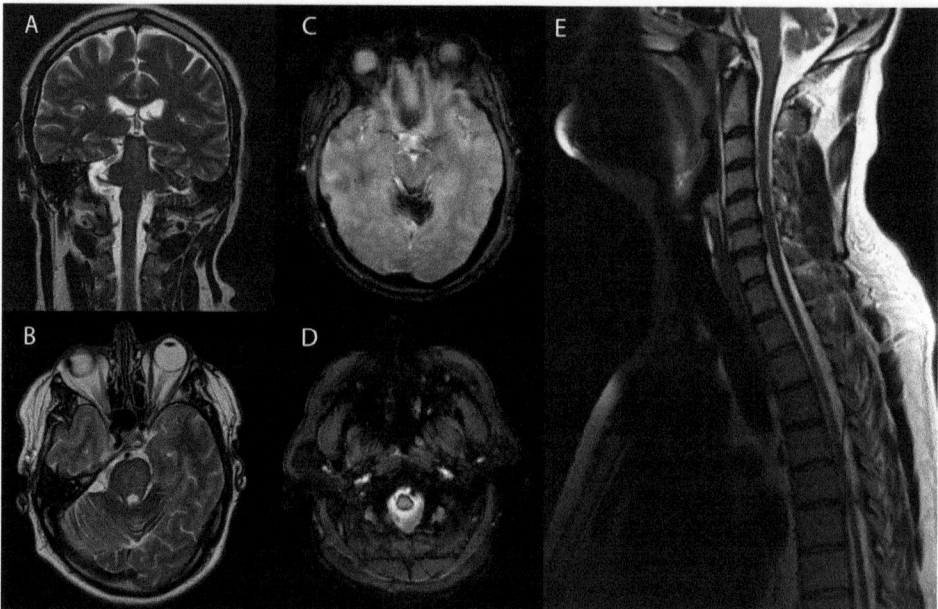

Figure 19.1 (A) A coronal T2 MRI scan of the brain showing low signal of haemosiderin coating the brainstem and upper cervical spine. (B) An axial T2 of the brain showing low signal in brainstem and cerebellar folia. (C and D) Axial T2* gradient echo scans of the brain confirming haemosiderin in the brainstem and cerebellum. (E) A sagittal T2 scan of the spine showing coating of haemosiderin and extradural dorsal thoracic spinal cyst at T6.

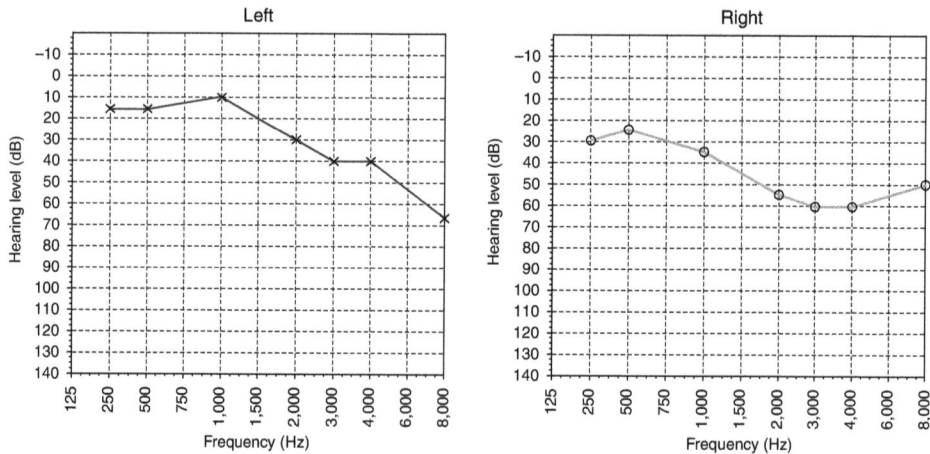

Figure 19.2 Audiometry showing bilateral deafness (i.e. hearing threshold beyond 25 dB). Hearing loss is worse on the right where it spans all hearing frequencies.

Diagnosis: Superficial Siderosis of the Central Nervous System

Management

He was advised about risks of alcohol consumption and prescribed baclofen for the leg spasticity. He attended for physiotherapy for a crutch and a push ortho ankle brace aequi (restricted ankle movement but allowing flexion). The role and evidence for deferiprone therapy were explained; he declined treatment.

Comment

Chronic low-grade bleeding into the subarachnoid space causes subpial accumulation of haemosiderin and superficial siderosis of the central nervous system [1]. The preferential involvement of the posterior fossa may be due to accelerated ferritin synthesis by cerebellar Bergmann glia and/or early irrigation or contact with haemorrhagic CSF. Superficial siderosis of the central nervous system may present with a classical triad of pyramidal signs, cerebellar ataxia and deafness (all present in this patient).

Multiple causes have been identified including trauma, arteriovenous malformation and posterior fossa tumours. Increasingly, intradural, extramedullary spinal cysts have been associated with superficial siderosis of the central nervous system (Table 19.1).

Classification and Investigation

Infratentorial superficial siderosis (iSS) is rare and occurs much less frequently than superficial siderosis due to cerebral amyloid angiopathy. Clinical presentations of classical iSS of the central nervous system fall into two groups: type 1 without any potential causal radiologically confirmed single spontaneous or traumatic intracranial haemorrhage (as in this case); and type 2 with a potentially causal radiologically confirmed spontaneous or traumatic intracranial haemorrhage [2]. The latter patients usually do not have hearing loss, myelopathy or ataxia. Intra-arterial digital subtraction angiography does not usually identify causal lesions for type 1 iSS. Rational investigation (including spinal MRI) frequently identifies the cause, including the more recently recognised intraspinal cysts.

Table 19.1 Recognised causes of superficial siderosis of the central nervous system

Aetiology of superficial siderosis	Comment
Spinal dural abnormality	Dural tear implicated in 18 of 30 patients from the Mayo Clinic, Rochester, MN and 40 of 65 patients from Queen Square, London Trauma Dural ectasia in Marfan syndrome, neurofibromatosis and ankylosing spondylitis
Tumours	Prior surgery or irradiation
Vascular malformation	Often incidental
Radiotherapy	Telangiectasia and cavernous angiomas may develop and cause chronic subarachnoid haemorrhage

Pathogenesis

Haemosiderin macrophages and iron-positive foamy structures have been observed in the neuropil of affected patients at post-mortem, particularly in the VIII cranial nerves and spinal cord. Heme oxygenase-1 immunoreactivity in macrophages exists in cerebellar folia. Iron and holoferritin concentrations are elevated. Bergmann glia of the cerebellum, which serve as a heme transporter, may explain cerebellar susceptibility. In addition, microglia are susceptible to injury. Bergmann glia and microglia are stimulated to synthesise heme oxygenase-1 and ferritin in the presence of heme. The plentiful exposure of the VIII cranial nerve (myelin and axons) to the subarachnoid space seems to render this cranial nerve susceptible to injury from free heme or its conversion to haemodiserin.

Duropathy

An emerging theme in superficial siderosis of the central nervous system has been the recognition that a duropathy is a cause of persistent subarachnoid bleeding. Intraspinal fluid-filled collections (often ventrally located – compared to our patient's dorsal cyst – and longitudinally extensive) may communicate with the subarachnoid space through a dural defect. Case series have suggested that this duropathy may play an aetiological role in the development of many cases of superficial siderosis of the central nervous system. The dura is most closely opposed to the dorsal surface of the vertebral bodies and intervertebral discs from C5 to T7, the location where high flow CSF leaks are most commonly seen. This may explain the association between intracranial hypotension and superficial siderosis of the central nervous system.

Therapeutic Management

Iron chelation has been advocated but many iron chelators do not cross the blood–brain barrier. However, deferiprone, a drug used to treat iron overload in thalassaemia has shown some preliminary evidence of benefit. An open label study found that a measurable reduction in MRI haemosiderin was achieved in 8 of 16 patients at a dose of 30 mg per kg per day for two years [3]. Two patients showed clinical improvement, ten stayed clinically stable and four worsened. However, neuronal injury in superficial siderosis of the central nervous system is due to unbound iron when the ferritin and haemosiderin biosynthesis capacity of microglia is overwhelmed. Clearance of protective haemosiderin may not be a biomarker of improved outcome. More data are required for effective intervention before routinely recommending the use of deferiprone in patients with superficial siderosis of the central nervous system [1].

References

1. Kumar N. Superficial siderosis: a clinical review. *Ann Neurol.* 2021;89(6):1068–79.
2. Wilson D, Chatterjee F, Farmer SF et al. Infratentorial superficial siderosis: classification, diagnostic criteria, and rational investigation pathway. *Ann Neurol.* 2017;81(3):333–43.
3. Kessler RA, Li X, Schwartz K et al. Two-year observational study of deferiprone in superficial siderosis. *CNS Neurosci Ther.* 2018;24(3):187–92.

Learning Points

- Superficial siderosis of the central nervous system has a classical triad of signs – myelopathy, ataxia and deafness.
- MRI scanning with blood-sensitive sequences has increased recognition of superficial siderosis of the central nervous system.

- Intraspinal cysts have been implicated in the aetiology of superficial siderosis of the central nervous system via a duropathy, which is thought to lead to episodic or chronic bleeding.
- Deferiprone, an iron chelator, which crosses the blood–brain barrier, has shown some preliminary imaging benefit for some patients.

Patient's Perspective

1. **What was the impact of the condition on you?**

   a. Physical (e.g. practical support)
   Everything. Difficulty walking because of balance. I can fall even when walking with my friend. It is very embarrassing as people think I am drunk.

   b. Psychological (e.g. mood, emotional well-being)
   I can spend all day in bed. No point in getting up to do anything because I am all over the place. Walking is not great.

   c. Social (e.g. meeting friends, home)
   I am more isolated. I cannot go and see them again because other people think I am drunk.

2. **What can you not do because of the condition?**
   I last worked in 2002. I cannot work. I used to do more at a gym. Now I just do weights.

3. **Was there any other change for you due to your medical condition?**
   Much reduced social life.
   I smoke more.

4. **What is/was the most difficult aspect of the condition for you?**
   The most difficult aspect is walking. I now get pain in my right hip and in my back.

5. **Was any aspect of the experience of the condition good or useful? What was that?**
   Nothing.

6. **What do you hope for in the future for people with this condition?**
   I hope they get a cure.

20 A Battery Issue

History

A 29-year-old woman was told by her optician that she had droopy eyelids. She had difficulty looking in both horizontal and vertical planes, but she had not been fully aware of the difficulty. There was also a history of longstanding constipation with her bowels opening once every two or three days. She had early satiety, poor appetite and marked fatigue. The optician had noted ptosis and ophthalmoplegia from at least the age of 18 years. At primary school she was a poor runner but could cycle.

She had no history of stroke, diabetes mellitus or deafness.

She smoked cigarettes and drank six or seven alcoholic drinks at the weekend. She had a six-year-old son. She had a family history of neurological illness; 5 of her 12 siblings had ptosis, progressive external ophthalmoplegia and proximal weakness (Figure 20.1). Memorial pictures of her parents showed no parental ptosis.

Examination

She weighed 53 kg, was 1.51 m tall, and had a BMI of 23.1 kg/m². Her pulse was 72 bpm and her blood pressure was 122/82 mmHg. She had marked bilateral ptosis, worse on the right than the left. Her pupils were equal and reactive to light. Visual acuity was 6/9 bilaterally. Her optic discs were normal and there was no evidence of a retinopathy. Her eye movement range was markedly restricted both horizontally and vertically (<30° downgaze). There was neck, truncal and proximal limb weakness (grade 4 power at shoulder abduction and hip flexion).

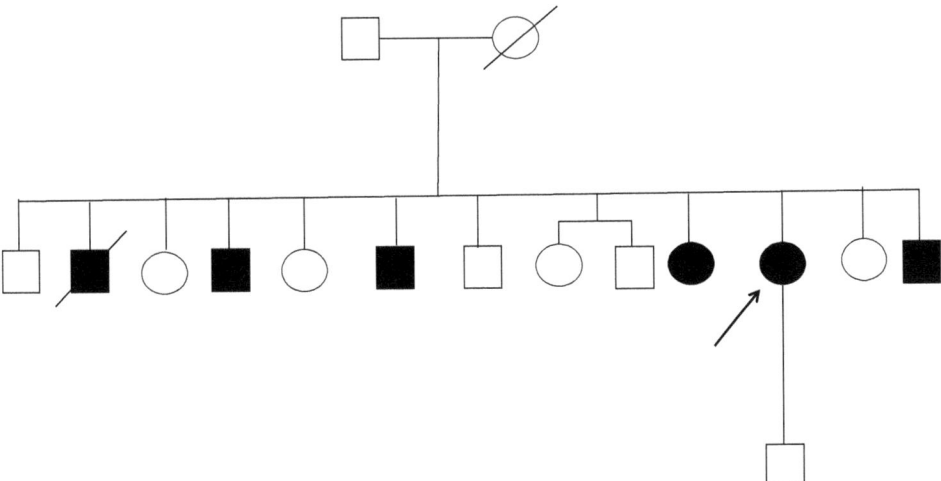

Figure 20.1 Family pedigree demonstrating individuals with ptosis, ophthalmoplegia and proximal weakness.

She had an adapted Gower's sign, hesitant tandem gait, normal reflees and sensation. She had a delayed swallow and tucked her chin in when sipping water.

Investigations

An ECG had shown normal sinus rhythm, QTc 416 ms. Creatine kinase was 73 U/L (normal range 25–200 U/L) and lactate was 2.6 mmol/L (normal range 0.5–2.2 mmol/L). She declined an EMG and muscle biopsy.

Gene mutation requests were sent for: *RRM2B, POLG, POLG2, SLC25A4* and *PEO 1* (now known as *C10ORF2*) in order to investigate progressive external ophthalmoplegia phenotype [1].

The Mitochondrial Unit in Newcastle, UK subsequently identified heterozygous mutations in *RRM2B* c.122G>A, p.(Arg41Gln) (seen in autosomal dominant disease) and c.817G>A, p.(Gly273Ser) (seen in autosomal recessive disease).

Diagnosis: Ribonucleotide Reductase M2B (*RRM2B*) Mitochondrial Disease

Management

She had subsequent ptosis correction with a brow suspension. Coenzyme Q10 was prescribed. Multidisciplinary management included dietetics, speech and language therapy and annual neurology follow-up. Five years later, her weight had fallen to 37.6 kg, with a BMI of 16.4 kg/m².

She declined assistance with enteral nutrition. She developed pneumonia and required admission to ICU for intubation and ventilation. She was treated with antibiotics and early parenteral nutrition. She improved. She accepted the need for enteral nutrition via a radiologically inserted gastrostomy. She was successfully treated and discharged just as the COVID-19 pandemic commenced.

Comment

Chronic Progressive External Ophthalmoplegia

Chronic, progressive, bilateral, typically symmetrical and external (sparing the pupil) ophthalmoplegia is usually a hereditary myopathy of the extraocular muscles and is often accompanied by progressive bilateral ptosis.

Sixty per cent of cases of mitochondrial chronic progressive external ophthalmoplegia (CPEO) are due to mitochondrial deletions. Nuclear DNA-related defects of mitochondrial DNA maintenance make up the remainder of cases.

Genetic Testing in Progressive External Ophthalmoplegia

Nuclear genes associated with progressive external ophthalmoplegia include *POLG*, *RRM2B*, *TWNK*, *SLC25A4*, *POLG2*, *TK2* and *RNASEH1*. Diagnosis can still be difficult as somatic mosaicism (a single variant occurring in two or more populations of soma cells in one individual) may occur, necessitating targeted next-generation sequencing with a high depth of coverage.

Our patient and her family were diagnosed genetically based on their phenotype. There was no requirement for muscle biopsy or EMG once a genetic diagnosis had been achieved. Advances in high-throughput genetic sequencing technologies have promoted genetics to an earlier level in diagnostic algorithms, reducing the need for other tests.

Causes of CPEO (defined as ophthalmopareis and ptosis) are outlined in Table 20.1

Mitochondrial Disorders

In 1988, the first pathogenic mutations of mitochondrial DNA were identified. Novel nuclear gene defects were subsequently found to cause mitochondrial disorders, known to make up over 20% of mitochondrial disorders, which together have a prevalence of 1 in 4,300 [3].

Biology of *RRM2B*

Ribonucleotide reductase *M2B* or *RRM2B* is a nuclear encoded maintenance gene for mitochondria, which encodes the p53-inducible small subunit (p53R2) of ribonucleotide

Table 20.1 Some causes of CPEO

Cause	Additional features
CPEO syndromes	Nuclear genes include *POLG, RRM2B, TWNK, SLC25A4, POLG2, TK2* and *RNASEH1*
Kearns–Sayre syndrome	Onset before 20 years of age, pigmentary retinopathy, cardiac conduction defect and cerebellar ataxia
Oculopharyngeal musculodystrophy	Autosomal dominant due to guanine-cytosine-guanine repeat expansion in polyalanine-binding protein-1 (PABP-1). Dysphagia, ptosis and proximal weakness
Myotonic dystrophy	Other ocular issues include lid lag, slow saccades and cataracts. Distal motor weakness, hand, face and tongue myotonia (delayed relaxation of contracted muscles)
Congenital fibrosis of extraocular muscles, Duane retraction syndrome and Mobius syndrome	Congenital cranial dysinnervation syndromes. Non-progressive
Ocular or generalised myasthenia gravis	Variable ptosis, impaired extraocular motility and diurnal variation
Sagging eye syndrome	Age-related acquired strabismus. Laxity of superior rectus-lateral rectus band, causing the lateral rectus to both abduct and depress the globe
Thyroid-associated ophthalmopathy	Eyelid retraction, conjunctival swelling and redness, and proptosis are distinguishing features
Ocular myositis	In addition to motility issue, there are orbital inflammatory signs, pain and acute onset
Progressive supranuclear palsy (PSP)	Vertical eye movement impairment (downwards more than upwards) prior to loss of horizontal eye movements. Oculocephalic reflex manoeuvres retained in PSP, which also has Parkinsonian features
Chronic nucleoside reverse transcriptase inhibitor	Used in HIV
Statin drugs	Possible cause of ophthalmoparesis

Reprinted by permission from Springer Nature Customer Service Centre GmbH: Springer. Copyright 2016 [2].

reductase [4]. This enzyme, a heterotetrameric structure, catalyses de novo synthesis of deoxynucleotide triphosphates by direct reduction of ribonucleoside diphosphates.

$$\text{Ribonucleoside diphosphates} \longrightarrow \text{Deoxyribonucleoside diphosphate}$$

The so-called mitochondrial depletion syndromes develop because *RRM2B* disease affects mitochondrial DNA synthesis. Human disease from *RRM2B* was first reported by Alice Bourdon et al. in 2007, manifesting as a multisystem disease with early infant mortality. Adult disease was subsequently recognised. *RRM2B* has emerged as the third most common multiple mitochondrial deletion syndrome in adults after *POLG* and *PEO1* (now called *C10ORF2*). Deafness, gastrointestinal symptoms and bulbar weakness (dysarthria, dysphagia, dysphonia, neck and facial weakness) are more common in *RRM2B* disease and suggest that *RRM2B* disease is more likely than *POLG* or *C10ORF2* disease in patients with a progressive external ophthalmoplegia phenotype.

The transcription of *RRM2B* is tightly regulated to the p53 tumour suppressor gene. However, it is not known if the *RRM2B* mutations are oncogenic. Our patient and her affected sister both subsequently developed breast carcinoma and two cancers were reported in a review of 31 patients with *RRM2B* disease [4].

RRM2B Mutations

RRM2B disease manifests as both autosomal recessive and autosomal dominant disease. This family had a compound heterozygous pattern from a dominant mutation – c.122G>A, p.(Arg41Gln) – and a known recessive mutation – c.817G>A, p.(Gly273Ser). Recessively inherited compound heterozygotes result in earlier age of onset and more severe and more multisystem disease than single heterozygous mutations [4]. The compound heterozygous mutations exist in *trans*.

Four phenotypes of the *RRM2B* mitochondrial DNA maintenance defects (MDMDs) have been described. *RRM2B* mutations are leading causes of paediatric and adult-onset mitochondrial disease due to disruption of mitochondrial maintenance.

1 *RRM2B* encephalomyopathic MDMD manifests as hypotonia, poor feeding requiring hospitalisation. This is the most severe phenotype, which often presents shortly after birth and also often involves other systems including sensorineural hearing loss, renal tubulopathy and respiratory failure.

2 *RRM2B* autosomal dominant progressive external ophthalmoplegia usually has an adult onset and includes ptosis, bulbar dysfunction, fatigue and muscle weakness.

3 *RRM2B* autosomal recessive progressive external ophthalmoplegia often has a childhood onset of myopathic progressive external ophthalmoplegia with ptosis, proximal muscle weakness and bulbar dysfunction.

4 *RRM2B* mitochondrial neurogastrointestinal encephalopathy-like phenotype with progressive ptosis, ophthalmoplegia, gastrointestinal dysmotility, cachexia and peripheral neuropathy.

Management

Management involves surveillance for multisystem involvement and supportive measures particularly nutrition.

A lipid-soluble antioxidant and electron carrier in the mitochondrial respiratory chain coenzyme Q10 is often recommended in mitochondrial disorders. While coenzyme Q10 is thought to be beneficial in mitochondrial disorders, there is currently no randomised clinical trial evidence.

The Mitochondrial Unit in Newcastle, UK is a specialist mitochondrial disease centre with experience of the diverse phenotype from adult *RRM2B* disease. Enteral nutrition is important in the long-term management of *RRM2B* disease, particularly because of the vulnerability to aspiration pneumonia in the presence of bulbar dysfunction and weight loss as occurred in our patient.

References

1. Fratter C, Raman P, Alston CL et al. *RRM2B* mutations are frequent in familial PEO with multiple mtDNA deletions. *Neurology*. 2011;76(23):2032–4.

2. McClelland C, Manousakis G, Lee MS. Progressive external ophthalmoplegia. *Curr Neurol Neurosci Rep*. 2016;16:53.

3. Gorman GS, Schaefer AM, Ng Y et al. Prevalence of nuclear and mitochondrial DNA mutations related to adult mitochondrial disease. *Ann Neurol*. 2015;77(5):753–9.

4. Pitceathly RDS, Smith C, Fratter C et al. Adults with *RRM2B*-related mitochondrial disease have distinct clinical and molecular characteristics. *Brain*. 2012;135(11):3392–403.

Learning Points

- Progressive external ophthalmoplegia – usually defined as a progressive and diffuse reduction in ocular motility accompanied by progressive bilateral ptosis – is a common finding in mitochondrial myopathy.

- Nuclear encoded mitochondrial disorders may have autosomal recessive and dominant inheritance in contrast to mitochondrial DNA disorders, which usually have maternal transmission pedigrees.

- Mitochondrial DNA depletion syndrome is usually a severe disorder of infancy or childhood due to a lack of mitochondrial DNA.

- In patients with a progressive external ophthalmoplegia phenotype, ptosis and proximal myopathy, deafness, gastrointestinal symptoms and bulbar weakness (dysarthria, dysphagia, dysphonia, neck and facial weakness) are more common in *RRM2B* disease than *POLG* or *C10ORF2* disease.

- *RRM2B* disease compound heterozygotes result in earlier age of onset, more severe and more multisystem disease than single heterozygous mutations.

Patient's Perspective

1. **What is/was the impact of the condition?**
    a. Physical (e.g. job, driving, practical support)
    I am always tired. My legs feel weak. I lose my appetite. I have poor balance.
    b. Psychological (e.g. mood, future, emotional well-being)
    I am always worried that I will fall. I am annoyed that I can't eat solid food.
    c. Social (e.g. meeting friends, home)
    I never socialise now. I used to go to pubs and shopping with my sister, but I cannot do those activities now.

2. **What can you no longer do?**
    I can't eat big meals, go out by myself or visit family.

3. **What is/was the change for your family/partner?**
    I lost weight. I have poor vision and poor balance. My arms and legs have become weaker. I have become more prone to chest infections.

4. **What was/is the most difficult aspect of the condition?**
    When I fell, I was embarrassed because it happened in public. I can't do anything without feeling tired and having to rest.

5. **Was any aspect of the experience good or useful? What was that?**
    No, I wish I did not have this condition.

6. **What do you hope for in the future for your condition?**
    I hope there is a cure found for this condition one day so all the people with this condition can live normal lives.

Symptoms Took Years to Develop

History

A 56-year-old man presented with a gradual onset of swallowing difficulty. He described swallow fatigue. In addition to the need for extra care when swallowing, dental visits had become an anxious experience for him.

Past medical history included high-frequency hearing loss on the right for at least 10 years. He had a history of right vocal cord palsy for 20 years. In 1988, almost 30 years before his neurological assessment, he underwent a right superficial parotidectomy for a pleomorphic adenoma. He was treated with localised radiotherapy. Five years, later a right neck neurofibroma was removed.

He had a history of depression and hypertension.

Examination

He was alert, orientated and had normal blood pressure. He was dysarthric with evidence of right hypoglossal nerve palsy (i.e wasting and fasciculating right tongue which deviated to the right on protrusion). Despite right sternocleidomastoid atrophy, he had intact head rotation power. Right-sided deafness was confirmed. He had no other neurological deficit.

Investigations

Acetylcholine receptor and MUSK antibodies were negative. An MRI of the brain showed tongue atrophy. An MRI of the brain with contrast showed no perineural infiltration. EMG demonstrated repetitive discharges in the right sternocleidomastoid muscle. There were neurogenic changes in the right side of the tongue but no spontaneous activity. EMG revealed no neurogenic changes in the arms and legs.

Diagnosis: Late-Radiation-Associated Dysphagia with Lower Cranial Neuropathy

Management
He was provided with supportive management and an explanation of late-radiation-associated dysphagia with lower cranial neuropathy after localised radiotherapy.

Comment
Late dysphagia after radiotherapy treatment has been recognised in long-term survivors of head and neck cancer [1]. This late effect can progress and is commonly associated with lower cranial nerve palsies (IX, X and XII). Late-radiation-associated dysphagia is uncommon with modern treatment of head and neck cancer. There is evidence that the mean radiation dose to the superior pharyngeal constrictor may predict late-radiation-associated dysphagia [2].

Causes of Hypoglossal Nerve Palsy
Although hypoglossal nerve palsy is rare, there are many causes that can be considered via a segmental approach to the entire course of the nerve [3]. Stroke and demyelination may compromise the medullary aspect of the XII cranial nerve, while vascular causes such as vertebrobasilar ectasia or aneurysm have been implicated in cisternal XII cranial nerve palsy. Examination of the skull base is important for tumour (particularly metastasis) and synovial cysts. Carotid dissection may result in XII cranial nerve palsy (e.g. Collet–Sicard syndrome or ipsilateral IX, X, XI and XII cranial nerve palsies). A sublingual segment XII cranial nerve palsy may be due to carcinoma (Figure 21.1). The differential diagnosis underscores the

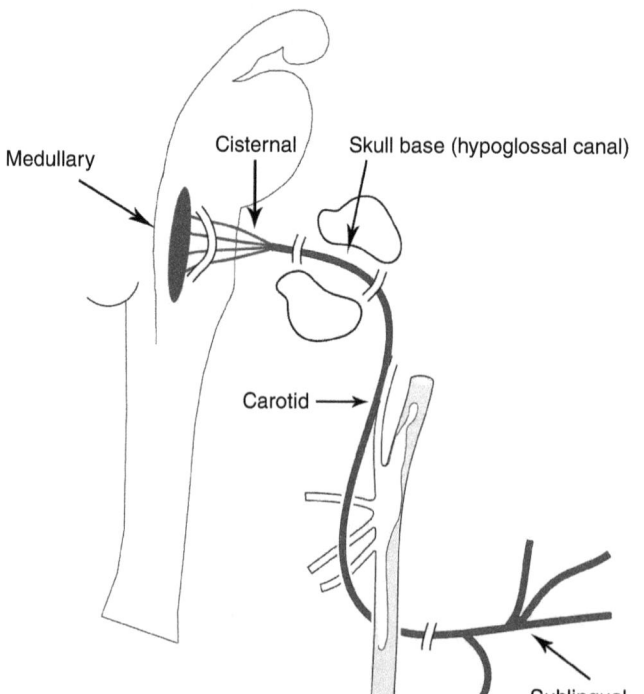

Figure 21.1 Schematic view of anatomical segments of the hypoglossal nerve.

Medullary

Cisternal

Skull base (hypoglossal canal)

Carotid →

Sublingual

importance of adequate imaging in identifying a structural cause of XII cranial nerve palsy. Idiopathic hypoglossal cranial nerve palsy is also recognised.

Delayed Effects of Neck Radiation

Baroreflex failure, carotid stenosis/occlusion and cranial nerve palsies are all recognised delayed complications of neck radiotherapy. While baroreceptor failure can occur after carotid surgery (carotid endarterectomy, carotid stenting and carotid body excision), it is thought that baroreceptor failure may be underdiagnosed in patients with head and neck surgery and/or radiation. The combination of baroreceptor failure and bulbar palsy has been recognised in the same patient.

Dysphagia, xerostomia and neck fibrosis are frequently present at long-term follow-up of patients who have had radiotherapy for head and neck cancer. It is important to note that swallowing questionnaires or patients' dysphagia perspectives are only weakly correlated with swallowing impairment and aspiration. Intensity-modulated radiation therapy reduces xerostomia and can improve quality of life compared to conventional radiotherapy.

Radiotherapy of the head and neck is associated with more than 50% carotid stenosis at 12 months in 4% of patients, at 24 months in 12% and at 36 months in 21% of patients. Carotid stenting has been performed for radiation-induced stenosis.

References

1. Hutcheson KA, Lewin JS, Barringer DA et al. Late dysphagia after radiotherapy-based treatment of head and neck cancer. *Cancer.* 2012;118(23):5793–9.

2. Awan MJ, Mohamed ASR, Lewin JS et al. Late radiation-associated dysphagia (late-RAD) with lower cranial neuropathy after oropharyngeal radiotherapy: a preliminary dosimetric comparison. *Oral Oncol.* 2014;50(8):746–52.

3. Thompson EO, Smoker WR. Hypoglossal nerve palsy: a segmental approach. *Radiographics.* 1994;14(5):939–58.

Learning Points

- Although a rare presentation, hypoglossal nerve palsy has many possible causes.
- Tumour is the most frequent cause of hypoglossal nerve palsy.
- Dysphagia and lower cranial neuropathies can be a late complication of radiotherapy for head and neck cancer.
- Baroreceptor failure and carotid stenosis/occlusion are recognised complications of head and neck radiotherapy.

Patient's Perspective

1. **What was the impact of the condition?**

    a. Physical (e.g. job, driving, practical support)
    Due to the difficulty in swallowing my sleep was stressful; the feeling of not being able to breathe led to very disrupted sleep.

    b. Psychological (mood, future, emotional well-being)
    This has had a major impact. I suffered from a lack of confidence from not being able to form my words clearly. This has led to regular spells of deep depression.

    c. Social (e.g. meeting friends, home)
    I stopped 99% of any social meetings outside my family. I closed my business, stopped attending church, funerals, weddings, birthday parties etc. I was ashamed of my voice.

2. **What can or could you not do because of the condition?**
    It is not possible to eat many foods because of choking. When my voice was so broken, my wife had to make phonecalls for me, all very embarrassing.

3. **Was there any other change for you due to your medical condition?**
    I feared the quiet of bedtime sleep due to the restriction I feel in my throat.

4. **What is/was the most difficult aspect of the condition for you?**
    Swallowing difficulty and the distortion of my tongue means that my words are not formed properly. I have a constant feeling of phlegm in the back of my throat due to a lack of mobility of my muscles in that area.

5. **Was any aspect of the experience good or useful? What was that?**
    It has made me more reflective as I speak as little as possible. I am much more aware of others with issues (medical conditions) that do not present themselves in any outwardly visible way.

6. **What do you hope for in the future for people with this condition?**
    A quicker diagnosis may to drill down to what the problem really is. I am thankful to neurologists.

High-Frequency Improvement

History

A 49-year-old male non-smoker was referred to neurology with fatigue. He recounted a sudden onset of pain followed by weakness while lying on a sofa. He described an 'electrocution in slow motion' feeling. He was subsequently exhausted after even mild exercise, noticing fatigue mostly in his thighs. He had intermittent visual difficulty with focusing, knee buckling (with a fall on one occasion), a feeling of unsteadiness, difficulty gripping when trying to open screwtops and erectile dysfunction. On one occasion, a droopy eyelid may have been witnessed. Previously, he had been very fit, competing at a very high level of kickboxing. He had a dry mouth but no associated weight loss.

He had coeliac disease and kept to a gluten-free diet.

There was a family history of autoimmune disorders, with rheumatoid arthritis in his mother and polymyalgia rheumatica in his father. A rheumatologist had declined assessment, attributing his symptoms to chronic fatigue.

Examination

He was alert and orientated. Cranial nerves were normal with no evidence of ptosis. His eye movements were normal. Limb examination was normal except for mild proximal leg weakness with slight difficulty rising from a squatting position. Examination later in the afternoon demonstrated more weakness (shoulder abduction grade 4/5, hip flexion grade 4/5). Reflexes were diminished but present and plantar responses were flexor. Sensation was intact.

A diagnostic test was performed.

Investigations

Thyroid profile (TSH 1.16 mU/L, freeT4 18.0 pmol/L) and creatine kinase (193 U/L) were normal.

Myasthenia gravis antibodies (acetylcholine receptor and muscle tyrosine kinase) were negative. Voltage-gated calcium channel (VGCC) antibodies were positive on three occasions (667 pmol/L, 539 pmol/L and 448 pmol/L).

Nerve conduction studies demonstrated small compound motor action potentials in ulnar and motor nerves with normal motor conduction. Repetitive nerve stimulation at 3 Hz produced 30% reduction in motor amplitude. Repetitive nerve stimulation at 20 Hz for 50 stimulations demonstrated facilitation of approximately 250%, a feature of Lambert–Eaton myasthenic syndrome (LEMS), demonstrated in Figure 22.1.

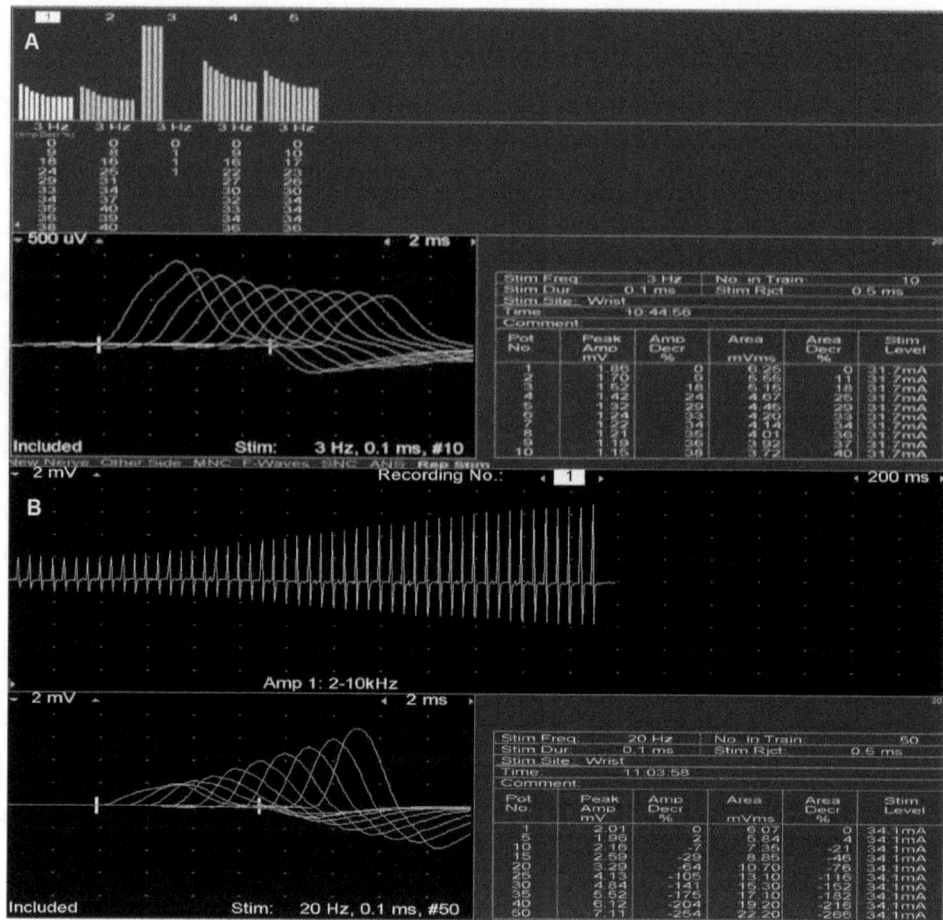

Figure 22.1 Repetitive nerve stimulation in a patient with Lambert–Eaton myasthenia gravis. (A) A low-frequency stimulation at 3 Hz produced a 30% reduction in motor amplitude. (B) A high-frequency stimulation at 20 Hz for 50 stimulations demonstrated facilitation with the amplitude of the motor response.

Diagnosis: Lambert–Eaton Myasthenic Syndrome

Further investigations included a CT of the chest abdomen and pelvis, and a PET scan on three occasions, all reported as showing no evidence of malignancy.

Risk stratification revealed a Dutch–English LEMS Tumour Association Prediction (DELTA-P) score [1] of 1 (Table 22.1).

Management
Pyridostigmine had mild benefit for the fatigue. Attempts to secure funding for 3,4-diaminopyridine were unsuccessful despite evidence of efficacy and guidelines recommending its use [2].

Comment
History and Clinical Features of LEMS
This type of myasthenic syndrome was first described by Edward Lambert, Lee Eaton and Edward Rooke in 1956 [3]. Unlike the more common form of myasthenia syndromes (often acetylcholine receptor antibody mediated), LEMS usually affects the trunk, shoulder, pelvic girdle and legs, which become weak and fatigable. Ptosis, diplopia, dysarthria and dysphagia are unusual in LEMS. Tendon reflexes are often diminished. Autonomic features such as dry mouth, constipation and erectile dysfunction are frequent accompaniments to problems with walking or rising from a chair. The response to cholinesterase inhibitors is poor. The neurological examination tends to under-estimate the weakness of LEMS as the post-tetanic potentiation can deliver good power, but this does not reflect ongoing power capacity. Most reports suggest an insidious onset of weakness in LEMS, but our patient was alerted to the problem with sudden weakness from rest.

Lambert–Eaton myasthenic syndrome is a rare neuromuscular disorder, more than 40 times less prevalent than myasthenia gravis. Prevalence of LEMS has been estimated to be 2.8–3.8 per million. Sixty per cent of patients have small-cell lung carcinoma. However, this proportion may decline as smoking prevalence is decreasing (45% of adults smoked in the 1950s but less than 20% in the 2020s). Other associated cancers include breast, prostate, stomach, rectum and lymphoma.

Table 22.1 DELTA-P score in Lambert–Eaton myasthenia gravis syndrome

Category	Outcome
D – Dysarthria, dysphagia, chewing, neck weakness, bulbar weakness	Absent (0) or present (1)
E – Erectile dysfunction	Male – Absent (0) or present (1)
L – Loss of weight	Absent <5% (0) or ≥5% (1)
T – Tobacco use at onset	Absent (0) or present (1)
A – Age at onset	Age ≥ 50 years (1) or age < 50 years (0)
P – Karnofsky performance score	70–100 (0) or 0–60 (1)
DELTA-P score	**0–6 Patient score = 1**

Patient's scores underlined

Adapted from Titulaer et al. [1] with permission from Wolters Kluwer.

Pathophysiology

In LEMS, antibodies (P/Q-type VGCC antibodies) impair the presynaptic release of acetylcholine. About 85% of patients with LEMS have antibodies against the P/Q-type VGCC. Rarely, antibodies against the N-type VGCC have been found in patients with malignancy-associated LEMS. In the first report, Lambert, Eaton and Rooke noted an association of LEMS with lung cancer. The expression of antigens on the tumour induces the autoantibody production, which then cross-reacts with the presynaptic VGCC. There is evidence that small-cell lung cancer-associated LEMS confers a survival advantage over small-cell lung cancer patients without LEMS even if they have VGCC antibodies; the presence of P/Q-type VGCC antibodies does not always associate with LEMS.

Non-tumour LEMS is associated with HLA-B8 (class I) and HLA-DR3 and -DQ2 (class II). These same HLA genotype associations are found with other autoimmune disorders, including myasthenia gravis but not in LEMS associated with small-cell lung carcinoma.

The VGCC is a large transmembrane protein, which mediates the influx of calcium into the nerve terminal to release stored vesicles of acetylcholine. The released acetylcholine binds to postsynaptic acetylcholine receptors (the target of antibody in most cases of seropositive myasthenia gravis). Rapid entry of cations depolarises the endplate region of the muscle fibre to generate an action potential and muscle contraction. The acetylcholine in the synaptic cleft is rapidly degraded by acetylcholinesterase.

Eaton and Lambert reported low compound muscle action potential (CMAP) amplitude at rest, a decremental response at low-frequency repetitive nerve stimulation (e.g. 3 Hz), and an incremental response at high-frequency stimulation (e.g. 20 Hz) over 200% or more. Repetitive muscle contractions and high-frequency repetitive nerve stimulation cause increased flux of calcium in the presynaptic membrane. The build-up of calcium enables release of acetylcholine by binding to multiple vesicles. Lambert's sign is an increasingly powerful grip on repeated evaluation of strength. The post-exercise or high-frequency facilitation is a temporary phenomenon as mitochondria clear the excess calcium. Current recommended standard electrodiagnostic testing requires 10 seconds of exercise or high-frequency repetitive nerve stimulation to elicit an incremental response of 60% in the CMAP [2].

Single-fibre EMG shows increased jitter (as also occurs in myasthenia gravis) and transmission blocking that is often improved at increased firing rates. Single-fibre EMG is more sensitive than repetitive nerve stimulation but repetitive nerve stimulation is more widely available and is better at distinguishing LEMS from myasthenia gravis.

Screening for Malignancy

A diagnosis of LEMS prompts an urgent search for underlying malignancy. CT chest and PET scanning are undertaken every six months for up to two years. The DELTA-P score (Table 22.1) is used to risk stratify the association with small-cell lung carcinoma in LEMS patients and guide the screening for underlying malignancy [1]. Scores of 0–1 have been associated with <2% risk of small-cell lung carcinoma; a score of 2 had a 30% risk of small-cell lung carcinoma; and DELTA-P scores 3–6 were associated with 90% risk of harbouring small-cell lung carcinoma [1]. Our patient's low DELTA-P score of 1 suggested a non-tumour LEMS diagnosis.

Differential Diagnosis

Myasthenia gravis, myopathies and polyneuropathy must all be considered in the differential diagnosis of LEMS. However, LEMS can usually be distinguished by the presence of areflexia, autonomic dysfunction and post-exercise facilitation.

Treatment

3,4-diaminopyridine has been used to treat LEMS since 1983. Evidence for the efficacy of 3,4-diaminopyridine in LEMS comes from published trials in which the base formulation was used.

Pricing of orphan drugs emerged as an issue for the 3,4-diaminopyridine phosphate salt. In the UK and USA, a legal attempt to enhance development of drugs for rare conditions severely limited availability of 3,4-diaminopyridine. An exclusivity licence for the much more expensive phosphate salt of 3,4-diaminopyridine restricted patient access to treatment.

References

1.   Titulaer MJ, Maddison P, Sont JK et al. Clinical Dutch–English Lambert–Eaton Myasthenic Syndrome (LEMS) Tumor Association Prediction score accurately predicts small-cell lung cancer in the LEMS. *J Clin Oncol.* 2011;29(7):902–8.

2.   Oh SJ. Neuromuscular junction disorders beyond myasthenia gravis. *Curr Opin Neurol.* 2021;34(5):648–57.

3.   Titulaer MJ, Lang B, Verschuuren JJGM. Lambert–Eaton myasthenic syndrome: from clinical characteristics to therapeutic strategies. *Lancet Neurol.* 2011;10(12):1098–107.

Learning Points

- Lambert–Eaton myasthenic syndrome may present with proximal weakness, fatigue, impotence and dry mouth.
- Lambert–Eaton myasthenic syndrome may be a paraneoplastic condition or an autoimmune (non-tumoural) neuromuscular disorder.
- Repetitive nerve stimulation findings are more specific for LEMS than the presence of the P/Q-type VGCC antibody.
- The DELTA-P score can risk stratify a cancer search with PET imaging and CT scanning, looking particularly for small-cell lung carcinoma.

Patient's Perspective

1.   **What was the impact of the condition on you?**

   a. Physical (e.g. practical support, ability to work)
   Ability to work has been severely curtailed and some elements I've had to stop completely.

   b. Psychological (e.g. mood, emotional well-being)
   Over time I've noticed that my psychological well-being has deteriorated. Restrictions on my ability to do any exercise has had a detrimental effect.

   c. Social (e.g. meeting friends, interacting with others)
   Previously I didn't have to consider any possibilities arising out of social events, but now I either have to cancel meeting people or friends or abstain from certain activities.

2.   **What can or could you not do because of the condition?**
   I can do the basics of managed and controlled movements but only at a very low level of exertion. I can no longer do any exercise or sports. I was a competitive kickboxer, I also played squash and went skiing.

3.   **Was there any other change for you due to your medical condition?**
   I am constantly having to explain my condition to friends and strangers! Dealing with sceptics, social isolation, forward planning, learning medical terminology.

4.   **What is/was the most difficult aspect of the condition for you?**
   Frustration at being denied known treatments, navigating the health care system. I've gone from never really being in the health care system to never being out of it! Having to accept a completely different lifestyle. Apprehension about my future.

5. **Was any aspect of the experience of the condition good or useful? What was that?**
    For me, I haven't seen any positives, apart from opening my eyes to the limitations of the system and the frustrations of those affected and those trying to help them.

6. **What do you hope for in the future for people with this condition?**
    I hope that people can get the diagnosis quicker and receive the treatment that they may need. It would also be nice if research into all autoimmune conditions was carried out by individuals or institutions who are not involved with the pharmaceutical industry.

Singling Out Dermatomes

History

A 75-year-old woman developed a vesicular rash on her left neck, pinna and face. She had left neck pain in the week preceding the rash. Left facial weakness ensued (Figures 23.1A–2.31C). There was no alteration of her taste or hearing.

Past medical history included obesity, diabetes mellitus and obstructive sleep apnoea. She had anxiety and was not keen on accessing medical help because of this.

Examination

There was a left lower motor neurone facial weakness with an unfurrowed forehead on the left, widened left palpebral fissure and drooping of the left mouth due to weakness of orbicularis oris (Figure 23.1A). The lower eyelid was sagged. On attempted closure of both eyes there was incomplete closure of the left eye (Figure 23.1B). visible rolling up of the left globe. There was a rash involving the left C2 dermatome (neck and pinna) as well as the left Vc dermatome (Figure 23.1C). Hearing, tested using the finger rub test, was intact.

Investigations

No investigations were performed.

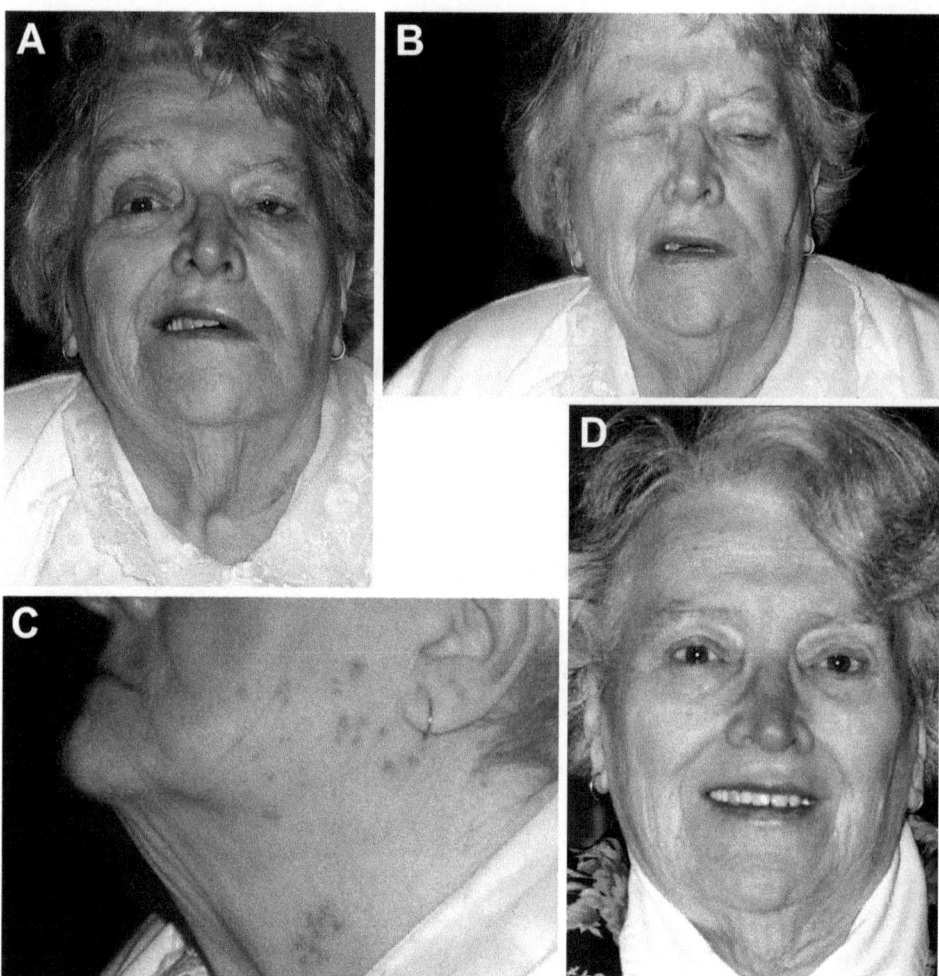

Figure 23.1 Features of Ramsay Hunt syndrome type 2. (A) An unfurrowed left forehead, widened left palpebral fissure due to sagging of left lower eyelid and drooping of the left mouth due to weakness of orbicularis oris. (B) Incomplete closure of the left eye. (C) Vesicular rash involving the left C2 dermatome (neck and pinna) as well as the left Vc dermatome. (D) Full recovery of facial nerve function after two months

Diagnosis: Ramsay Hunt Syndrome Type 2 (i.e. Herpes Zoster of the Left Geniculate Ganglion)

Management

Artificial tears and advice to tape the eye shut at night were provided to protect the cornea. Famciclovir 750 mg bd and prednisolone 40 mg per day were prescribed for 10 days.

Two months later, full recovery (Figure 23.1D) had occurred with no suggestion of post-herpetic neuralgia.

Comment

Nomenclature

James Ramsay Hunt (1872–1937) was an American neurologist, who graduated from the University of Pennsylvania School of Medicine in 1893. He described three syndromes, the best-known being Ramsay Hunt syndrome type 2.

Ramsay Hunt syndrome type 1 is a cerebellar syndrome involving myoclonic epilepsy, progressive ataxia, tremor and dementia. Ramsay Hunt syndrome type 3 is an occupationally induced neuropathy of the deep palmar branch of the ulnar nerve.

Ramsay Hunt syndrome type 2 is the reactivation of herpes or varicella zoster in the geniculate ganglion, as described for this patient. Typically, ipsilateral ear pain is followed by facial paralysis and vesicles within two to three days. Ramsay Hunt syndrome type 2 also frequently causes tinnitus, hearing loss, nausea, vomiting, vertigo and nystagmus, indicating involvement of the VIII cranial nerve in the bony facial canal [1]. Multiple cranial neuropathies may occur (cranial nerves IX, X, XI and XII). In up to 28% of presentations, neither pain nor rash are present.

Epidemiology of Herpes Zoster and Bell's Palsy

The incidence of herpes zoster is 3.2–4.2 per 1,000 per year. Lifetime incidence of zoster is about 30% and it is most frequent after 50 years of age. Women are affected more than men. Facial nerve involvement occurs in 1% of cases.

The incidence of Bell's palsy increases with age, with an overall incidence of 15–30 per 100,000 per year, accounting for 60–75% of all cases of unilateral facial weakness.

Modified House–Brackmann Grading of Facial Weakness

Facial weakness severity can be clinically assessed with a number of grading systems. The original House–Brackmann grading system reported in 1985 ranges from grade 1 (normal function) to grade VI (no movement at all). The House–Brackmann grading scale or its modification with regional assessment and secondary movements or synkinesis (facial nerve grading scale 2.0) is used to measure the extent of facial weakness. Grade IV and higher grades are associated with incomplete eye closure.

Neurological Manifestations of Varicella Zoster Virus

Varicella zoster virus has a number of neurological manifestations (Table 23.1), which increase in frequency with age.

Table 23.1 Clinical manifestations of varicella zoster virus infection reactivation

Clinical manifestation
Zoster sine herpete (radicular pain or facial palsy without rash)
Postherpetic neuralgia
Meningitis/meningoencephalitis
Ramsay Hunt syndrome type 2
Polyneuritis cranialis
Cerebellitis
Vasculopathy
Myelopathy
Ocular disorders (such as acute retinal necrosis or progressive outer retinal necrosis)

Adapted with permission from Springer Nature Customer Service Centre GmbH: Springer. Gilden et al. [1]. Copyright 2013.

The failure to close the eye on the paretic side elicits Bell's phenomenon (visible rolling up of the eye globe). In herpes zoster ophthalmicus, involvement of the nasociliary nerve can be predicted from vesicles on the tip of the nose (alae nasae) due to involvement of the anterior ethmoidal nerve, which is a terminal branch of the nasociliary nerve. This sign, known as Hutchinson's sign, can predict ocular involvement as the nasociliary nerve also innervates the ciliary body, iris, cornea and conjunctiva. Importantly, although much less frequent, an absent Hutchinson's sign does not exclude eye involvement.

Eye protection is crucial in both Bell's palsy and Ramsay Hunt syndrome type 2. Even if the eye is not infected, the cornea is not protected; failure to close the eye risks corneal scarring. The eye should be taped closed at night. During the day, regular washing of the eye with artificial tears is recommended.

Anatomy of the VII Cranial Nerve

Facial nerve clinical-anatomical correlation suggests that the facial nerve in our patient was injured in the stylomastoid foramen (Figure 23.2). A lesion more proximal than the stylomastoid foramen above the junction with the chorda tympani but below the geniculate ganglion causes ipsilateral loss of taste over the anterior two-thirds of the tongue (not present in our patient). Similarly, the nerve to the stapedius muscle was spared. Nervus intermedius, a sensory and parasympathetic division of the facial nerve, can cause a neuralgia (stabbing pain in the lower jaw) as a complication of Ramsay Hunt syndrome type 2.

When multiple cranial nerves are involved in Ramsay Hunt syndrome type 2, this has been termed Ramsay Hunt plus syndrome. Motor paresis in zoster is also seen in other areas as myotome weakness.

In Ramsay Hunt syndrome type 2 and Bell's palsy adjacent dermatomes are frequently involved (as present in our patient). Many patients have additional features (Table 23.1). Ramsay Hunt syndrome type 2 has a worse prognosis then Bell's palsy. Zoster in a skin graft is particularly dangerous as there is a risk of losing the graft.

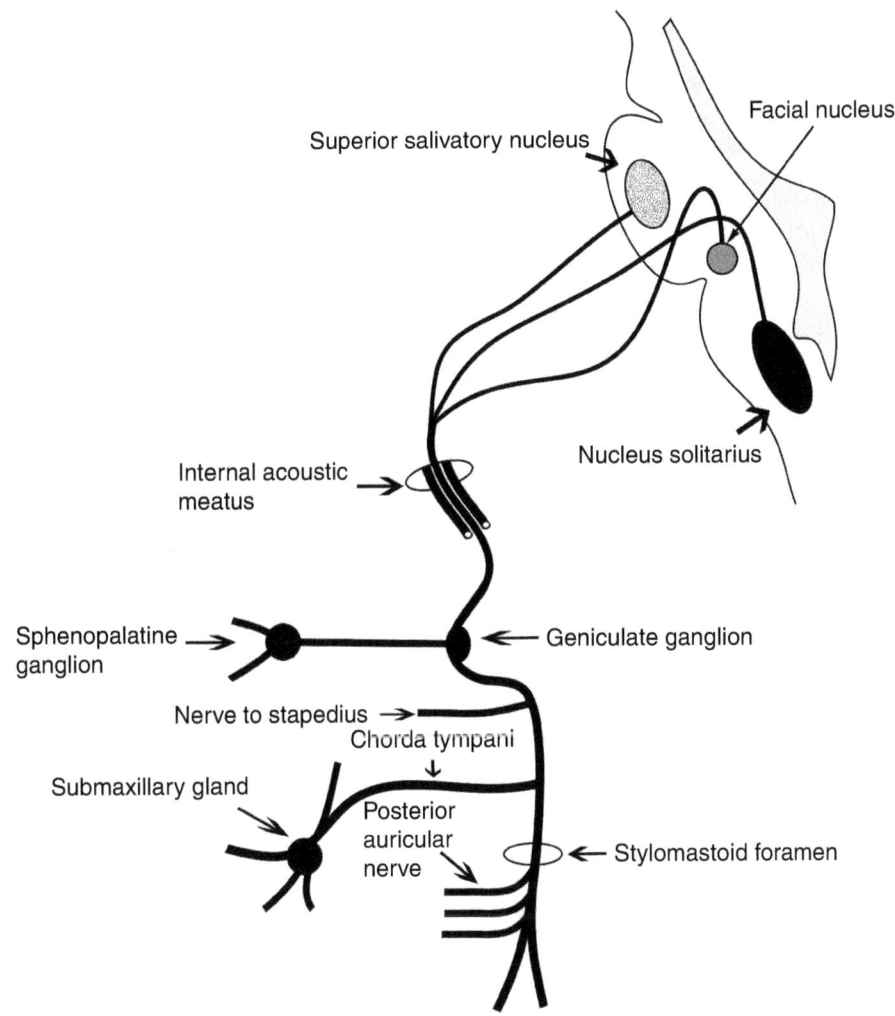

Figure 23.2 Schematic drawing of facial nerve anatomy

Pathogenesis of Ramsay Hunt Syndrome Type 2

Bell's palsy may be caused by reactivation of latent herpes viruses (herpes simplex and herpes zoster). Herpes simplex-1 DNA has been isolated from endoneurium of the facial nerve during the acute phase of Bell's palsy.

Varicella zoster virus, a double-stranded DNA virus, is transmitted by direct contact or inhalation of aerosols. Varicella zoster travels retrogradely along sensory neurone fibres to spinal dorsal root ganglia, autonomic and cranial ganglia and remains dormant until specific immunity wanes with age, cellular immunodeficiency, genetic susceptibility, systemic disease such as diabetes mellitus (as in our patient), stress, or trauma and fatigue. Zoster represents reactivation of the chickenpox virus from the geniculate ganglion. This then spreads via neurotropism to innervated targeted tissues such as skin, cornea and laryngeal mucosa. The rash eruption of shingles makes the clinical diagnosis of Ramsay Hunt type 2. Zoster sine herpete is difficult to diagnose in that no vesicular lesions accompany the facial nerve palsy due to zoster virus.

Zoster also has an arterial tropism, which may play a role in triggering giant cell arteritis and zoster vasculopathy.

Investigation for Varicella Zoster

A clinical diagnosis of Ramsay Hunt syndrome type 2 may not require investigation. An MRI scan in both Bell's palsy and Ramsay Hunt syndrome type 2 may show increased enhancement of the facial nerve. However, it is important to know that facial nerve enhancement is not an unusual finding in the absence of facial weakness (i.e. can be a normal finding).

Swabs, saliva, cerebrospinal fluid (CSF) and blood can all be tested for varicella zoster DNA via PCR. In patients with zoster sine herpete, rising anti-varicella zoster virus antibody titres in the serum or CSF can confirm active viral infection. Reduced ratios of serum/CSF varicella zoster virus immunoglobulin G (IgG) can reflect intrathecal synthesis of anti-varicella zoster virus IgG.

Management

Current management of Bell's palsy is the same as that for Ramsay Hunt syndrome type 2 (corticosteroids and antiviral medication) as Bell's palsy may result from Ramsay Hunt syndrome sine herpete. If treatment with corticosteroids and an antiviral drug (aciclovir, valaciclovir or famciclovir) is started within three days, four to seven days or eight days and later for Ramsay Hunt syndrome type 2, paresis resolves in 75%, 48% and 30% of patients, respectively. A literature review has shown similar benefit from steroid use combined with antiviral treatment [2]. As already stated, the importance of protecting the cornea is crucial to avoid corneal scarring.

Vaccination

Acute complications of zoster are recognised in immunocompetent individuals, including zoster dissemination, hospitalisation and death. The risk increases further in adults over 50 years of age. Since 2008, a single live attenuated herpes zoster vaccine (Zostavax) has been advised for immunocompetent people over 60 years of age as a means of reducing herpes zoster and post-herpetic neuralgia. However, vaccine efficacy may decrease with time from vaccination. A subsequent development (to enhance CD4 T cell immune response) with two doses of HZ/su improved efficacy and duration of effect. Vaccination in the UK has been rolling out for patients over 70 years of age since 2013 [3] as incidence of shingles increases with age. In the 70–9 year-old age group, the incidence of shingles is 790–880 cases per 100,000 per year. In addition, post-herpetic neuralgia increases with age (9% of the 60–4-year-old age group and 52% in individuals over 85 years) [3]. In England, the vaccine prevented an estimated 40,500 GP consultations and 1,840 hospitalisations in the first five years of the vaccination programme.

A second vaccine, Shringix, is a recombinant vaccine, which contains varicella zoster virus glycoprotein E antigen and is given as a two-dose schedule. Since 2021, Shringix is offered to individuals who are not eligible for the live vaccine (Zostavax).

References

1. Gilden D. The variegate neurological manifestations of varicella zoster virus infection. *Curr Neurol Neurosci Reports.* 2013;13(9):374.

2. Da Costa Monsanto R, Bittencourt AG, Bobato Neto NJ et al. Treatment and prognosis of facial palsy on Ramsay Hunt syndrome: results based on a review of the literature. *Int Arch Otorhinolaryngol.* 2016;20(4):394–400.

3. Public Health England. Shingles (Herpes Zoster): The Green Book. chapter 28a. 2021. 1–15 p. Available from: https://assets.publishing.service.gov.uk/government/uploads/system/uploads/attachment_data/file/1012943/Green_book_of_immunisation_28a_Shingles.pdf.

Learning Points

- Ramsay Hunt syndrome type 2 causes ipsilateral facial paralysis, otalgia and vesicles near the ear and auditory canal due to the reactivation of varicella zoster virus in the geniculate ganglion.

- Facial weakness in Ramsay Hunt syndrome type 2 is less likely to recover than a Bell's palsy facial weakness.

- If facial weakness prevents the eye from closing (House–Brackmann grade IV severity and above), the eye should be taped closed at night and treated regularly with artificial tears to prevent corneal scarring.

- Famciclovir, aciclovir or valaciclovir and prednisolone are recommended for Ramsay Hunt syndrome type 2 and Bell's palsy.

- Varicella zoster virus vaccination can reduce herpes zoster and post-herpetic neuralgia.

Patient's Perspective from Nephew

1. **What was the impact of the condition?**
   Apart from the transient facial asymmetry and anxiety concerning possible hospital admission for treatment, my aunt really had no other issues. She was very anxious about hospitals. She was reassured by the good prognosis, suffered no pain and was content that she did not have to go to hospital.

2. **What was the most difficult aspect of the condition?**
   She found it difficult to apply the eye patch correctly and needed help to do this.

3. **Was any aspect of the experience good or useful? What was that?**
   She was so grateful to avoid an admission to hospital. She had been assessed at home and her GP quickly started treatment. She had no sequelae such as corneal scarring or post-herpetic neuralgia. She lived for a further 10 years with full recovery in her facial movements.

4. **What would your aunt hope for in the future for this condition?**
   More opportunities for local care at home, which can be achieved with a high level of satisfaction for patient and doctor.

CASE 24 Asthmatic Neurology

History

A 54-year-old man developed tingling in his right toe and the dorsum of his right foot. A few days later, he had a numb sensation in his left calf. He then noticed pain from his left thigh to left ankle without back pain. Two days later, his right leg was similarly affected. After another two days, he was aware of numbness in his right index finger and right thumb. Within minutes, his right hand and forearm were weak; he was unable to reach for a cup of coffee. He was admitted to a stroke ward in his local hospital. That evening, his right arm and hand improved but he was aware of numbness in the dorsum of his left hand.

Daily neurological developments occurred in hospital. Numbness spread over the right foot. The left leg numbness receded to the calf and foot. On the day of his neurological assessment, he had left hand numbness and weak left wrist extension. By now he had difficulty dressing and described his walking as 'clunky'.

He had no headache and no bladder or bowel sphincter disturbance. He had no swallowing or visual difficulties.

Past medical history included asthma and nasal polyps.

Medication included montelukast, budesonide inhaler and mometasone furoate nasal spray.

Examination

Higher mental function was normal. He had no rash. He was cardiovascularly stable. Cranial nerves were normal with visual acuity 6/9 bilaterally unaided. Optic discs were normal. Tone was normal in all limbs. Left wrist extension was weak (grade 3/5). There was also weakness at right hip flexion (grade 4/5), right knee flexion (grade 4/5) and bilateral ankle dorsiflexion (grade 4/5). Ankle jerks were absent. There was decreased pinprick sensation in the dorsum of the left hand (the anatomical snuffbox area), consistent with left radial nerve palsy. There was decreased pinprick sensation in the right lower leg and lateral right foot.

Clinical Impression

Mononeuritis multiplex (including left radial nerve palsy) with confluent peripheral neuropathy.

Investigations

Full blood count revealed an eosinophilia peaking at 13.8×10^9/L (Figure 24.1). C-antineutrophil cytoplasmic antibody (ANCA) titre was 20. Myeloperoxidase (MPO) or perinuclear ANCA 80. Creatine kinase was 644 U/L (normal range 22–198 U/L).

Chest X-ray was normal. High-resolution CT of the chest revealed no interstitial disease and no significant mediastinal or hilar lymphadenopathy. Echocardiography was normal.

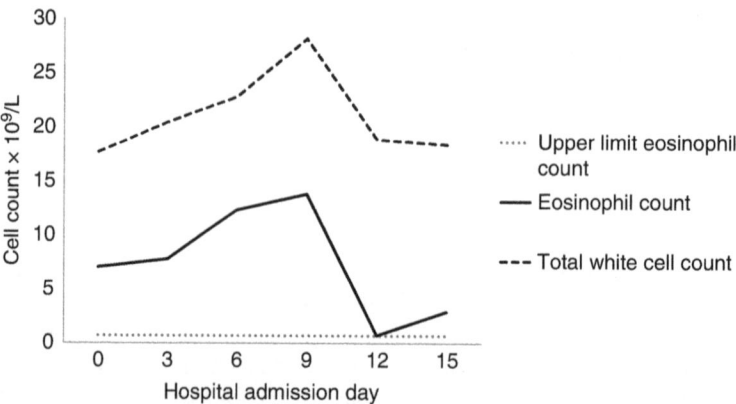

Figure 24.1 Eosinophil and total white cell counts during hospital admission.

A CT scan of the sinuses showed sinusitis and marked thickening of the nasal mucosa, with polypoidal soft tissue projecting into the nasal cavity (Figure 24.2).

A lumbar puncture demonstrated normal cerebrospinal fluid (CSF) cell count, protein and glucose. Nerve conduction studies (Tables 24.1 and 24.2) demonstrated a patchy, length-dependent, probably axonal loss or mixed peripheral neuropathy involving the motor and sensory fibres. The right peroneal F wave was unrecordable and the left peroneal F wave was prolonged at 54.4 ms.

Nasal polypectomy was performed after starting treatment. Polyp histology showed oedematous subepithelial connective tissue with lymphoplasmacytic inflammatory infiltrate containing eosinophils.

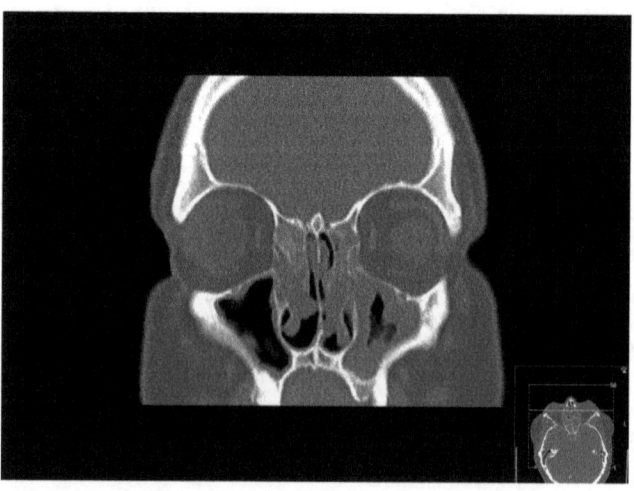

Figure 24.2 A coronal non-contrast CT scan of the sinuses showing extensive nasal polyps and sinusitis.

Table 24.1 Sensory nerve conduction study

Nerve and site	Peak latency (ms)	Amplitude (µV)	Normal amplitude (µV)
Peroneal right Ankle	NR	NR	
Sural right Lower leg	3	**3.5**	≥4
Median right Palm	1.8	42	≥10
Ulnar right Palm	1.8	21	≥10
Radial right Anatomical snuffbox	1.6	37	≥18
Peroneal left Ankle	2.5	6	
Sural left Lower leg	3.5	**2**	≥4
Median left Palm	1.8	55	≥10
Ulnar left Palm	1.7	31	≥10
Radial left Anatomical snuffbox	1.7	28	≥18

NR: not recordable
Abnormal results in bold

Table 24.2 Motor nerve conduction study

Nerve and site	Latency (ms)	Amplitude (µV)	Segment	Conduction velocity (m/s)
Peroneal right				
Ankle	3.8	**0.0**	Ankle-fibula (head)	39
Fibula (head)	11.8	**0.0**	Fibula (head)-popliteal fossa	33
Popliteal fossa	14.5	**0.1**		
Tibial right				
Ankle	3.7	3.8	Ankle-popliteal fossa	45
Popliteal fossa	13.3	**2.3**		
Median right				
Wrist	3.4	7.5	Wrist-elbow	52
Elbow	8.2	7.3	Elbow-axilla	63
Axilla	10.3	7.1		

Table 24.3. (cont.)

Ulnar right				
Wrist	2.9	7.6	Wrist-below elbow	59
Below elbow	6.3	7.3	Below elbow-above elbow	59
Above elbow	8.4	7.0	Above elbow-axilla	63
Axilla	10.5	6.8		
Peroneal left				
Ankle	4.8	**0.6**	Ankle-fibula head	42
Fibula (head)	12.0	**0.4**	Fibula (head)-popliteal fossa	40
Popliteal fossa	14.3	**0.4**		
Tibial left				
Ankle	4.0	**2.8**	Ankle-popliteal fossa	41
Popliteal fossa	14.8	**2.3**		
Median left				
Wrist	3.2	6.1	Wrist-elbow	57
Elbow	7.7	6.1	Elbow-axilla	61
Axilla	9.9	6.7		
Ulnar left				
Wrist	2.7	7.1	Wrist-below elbow	66
Below elbow	5.6	6.6	Below elbow-above elbow	59
Above elbow	7.7	6.7	Above elbow-axilla	60
Axilla	9.5	6.3		

Abnormal results in bold

Initial Diagnosis: Eosinophilic Granulomatosis with Polyangiitis (MPO-ANCA-Associated Vasculitis)

Management

Steroid treatment was started with intravenous methylprednisolone 500 mg/day for five days and then prednisolone 50 mg per day. His eosinophil count dropped (Figure 24.1). Prednisolone was then tapered with the introduction of azathioprine. However, azathioprine had to be stopped due to deranged liver function tests. Mycophenolate was then used. He developed diabetes mellitus on steroid therapy.

The neuropathy had almost fully resolved, but ongoing asthma issues prompted boosts of steroid therapy. In 2020, nearly nine years after his neurological presentation, benralizumab, a monoclonal antibody to interleukin 5 (which depletes eosinophil counts) was introduced to decrease his steroid requirement. After one year of benralizumab treatment and with an almost unrecordable peripheral blood eosinophil count (Figure 24.3), he was weaned off prednisolone. Four months later and three days after a third COVID-19 vaccine, he developed new numbness and pain in his left thigh. Two weeks later, he had pins and needles in the right leg with numbness in his ring and little fingers bilaterally. Over a 10-day period, he noticed numbness in his upper legs, dorsum of his right hand, numb feet, a 'fuzzy feeling' in his legs and left ankle weakness and 'floppy feet'.

Examination demonstrated a distal asymmetrical motor weakness, pinprick sensory loss in his left median nerve territory and decreased pinprick sensation in lower legs and feet. Initially, ankle jerks were present before becoming absent.

Further Investigations

Full blood count was normal except eosinophil count was 0.00×10^9/L (Figure 24.3). CRP was 16 mg/L. HbA1c, B12, folate, liver function tests, thyroid profile were normal. Plasma protein electrophoresis revealed a faint paraprotein band in the gamma region. Kappa (37) and lambda (36) light chains were mildly elevated with a normal ratio. Tests for HIV, treponema

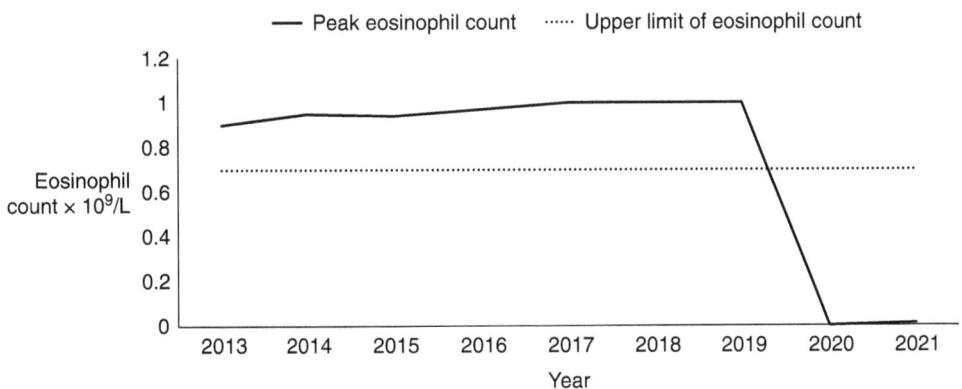

Figure 24.3 Annual peak eosinophil counts before and with benralizumab treatment (from 2020 onwards).

pallidum, and hepatitis B and C were negative. MPO-ANCA, which had been negative on three occasions over the preceding nine years, became positive at 107.6 IU/mL (normal range 0–5.9 IU/mL) with p-ANCA 320. Immunoglobulin E (IgE) (42kU/L, normal range 0–81 kU/L) and immunoglobulin G4 (IgG4) (9.39 g/L, normal range <1.3 g/L) were elevated. Complement C3 and C4 were normal. Rheumatoid factor was positive (19). A 24-hour urinary protein collection was 0.55 g/L (normal range 0–0.1 g/L).

A CT of the chest, abdomen and pelvis and a PET scan revealed no evidence of malignancy. Echocardiogram was again normal. Repeat CSF was normal (0 white cells/μL, 9 red cells/μL, CSF protein of 0.3 9g/L, CSF glucose of 4.2 mmol/L and serum glucose of 5.7 mmol/L). No malignant cells were seen.

Nerve conduction studies were repeated six weeks after the recurrence of neurological symptoms. The sensory responses were absent in the peroneal and sural nerves on both sides. Median, ulnar and radial responses were small. Motor nerve conduction showed that the response was absent in the right peroneal nerve and extremely small in the left peroneal nerve. Tibial responses were also very small, especially on the left. The right median response was attenuated and the left median response was absent. Ulnar motor responses were borderline in amplitude. There was no conduction block. F waves were unrecordable at right and left peroneal nerves, left tibial and left median nerves. At EMG, tibialis anterior and vastus lateralis were silent at rest on both sides. Occasional unsustained positive waves were noted in the right tibialis anterior. Some prolonged polyphasic motor units were activated with slightly reduced interference patterns in all except right tibialis anterior, which had no motor unit activity. The findings were consistent with a severe, length-dependent probably axonal peripheral neuropathy, acknowledging that a mononeuritis multiplex may have become confluent.

Nerve biopsy confirmed axonal neuropathy with secondary demyelination (Figure 24.4). No eosinophils and no IgG4 cells were seen. Electron microscopy showed loss of myelinated axons and secondary axonal proliferation. No plasma cell infiltrate was identified.

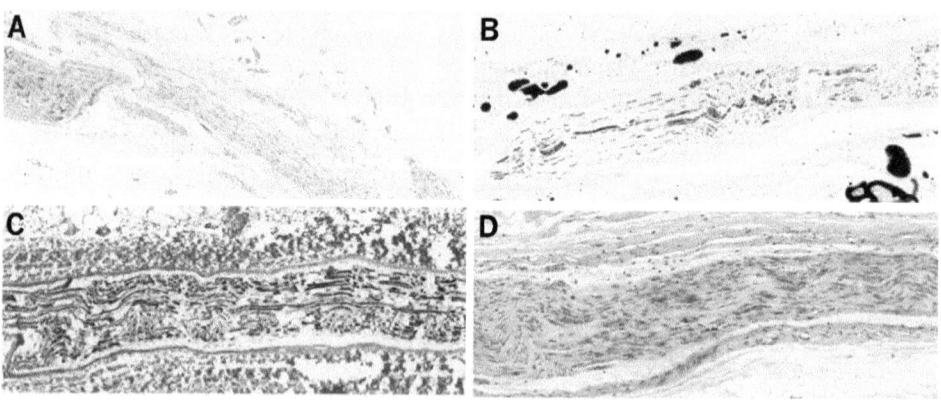

Figure 24.4 Sural nerve biopsy. (A) A longitudinal section of the sural nerve showing axonal loss. (B) Myelin stain shows secondary myelin loss. (C) Immunohistochemistry for neurofilament protein shows axonal loss and fragmentation. (D) A histochemical stain, luxol fast blue, confirms little residual myelin.

Subsequent Diagnosis: Neurologically Restricted MPO-ANCA Vasculitic Neuropathy

Comment

ANCA-Associated Vasculitis

ANCA-associated vasculitis has a prevalence of 200–400 per million. There is granulomatous and neutrophilic tissue inflammation with antibodies (leukocyte proteinase 3 or PR3 and myeloperoxidase or MPO), which target neutrophil antigens. Necrotising inflammation and fibrinoid necrosis in the walls of small to medium-sized blood vessels are the hallmarks of ANCA-associated vasculitis. There are three categories of ANCA-associated vasculitis: 1. granulomatosis with polyangiitis; 2. microscopic polyangiitis; and 3. eosinophilic granulomatosis with polyangiitis (EGPA) [1].

ANCA-associated vasculitides affect many organ systems including lung, kidney, skin and the nervous system. Improving knowledge of pathogenesis (genetics, environment, innate and adaptive immune systems) and targeted treatment has improved outcomes.

Mononeuritis Multiplex Differential Diagnosis

Mononeuritis multiplex is a distinctive clinical presentation of progressive motor and sensory deficits in the distribution of specific peripheral nerves. Pain is frequent and may be neuropathic or in the affected sensory loss area. Causes of mononeuritis multiplex include diabetes mellitus, rheumatoid arthritis, systemic lupus erythematosus, HIV, Lyme disease, leprosy and amyloidosis. Our patient gave a history very suggestive of a rapidly evolving mononeuritis multiplex. Causes of vasculitic mononeuritis multiplex are shown in Table 24.3.

Radial Nerve Palsy (and Posterior Interosseus Nerve Palsy)

Clinically, a left radial nerve palsy was identified in our patient. Arising from the posterior cord of the brachial plexus, the radial nerve has fibres from C5, C6, C7, C8 and T1 roots. It winds around the proximal part of the humerus on its medial side to innervate the triceps muscle. It lies on the spiral groove of the humeral shaft to enter the anterior compartment between brachialis and brachioradialis. Distally, it passes anterior to the lateral humeral condyle. At the elbow, the radial nerve supplies branches to brachioradialis, extensor carpi radialis longus and anconeus. Depending on anatomical variation, the extensor carpi radialis brevis is innervated by the radial nerve or its deep branch, the posterior interosseus nerve.

Proximal to the elbow, the radial nerve divides into the superficial (purely sensory) and deep branch – the posterior interosseus nerve. The posterior interosseus nerve innervates the supinator muscle and most of the forearm and hand extensors – extensor carpi ulnaris, extensor digitorum communis, extensor digiti minimi, extensor indicis propius, extensor pollicis longus, abductor pollicis longus and extensor pollicis brevis.

With triceps weakness, an upper lesion of the radial nerve may be implicated. Radial nerve injury only affects extension in the metacarpophalangeal joints, as interphalangeal extension is performed by the interossei and lumbrical muscles innervated by the ulnar nerve.

Radial nerve injuries can occur from humeral fractures, elbow dislocations and fractures, tight casts and from causes of mononeuritis multiplex.

Table 24.3 Some vasculitic causes of mononeuritis multiplex

Disease
Primary systemic vasculitis
Predominantly small vessel
EGPA
Granulomatosis with polyangiitis (formerly known as Wegener's granulomatosis)
Microscopic polyarteritis
Predominantly medium vessel
Polyarteritis nodosa
Predominantly large vessel vasculitis
Giant cell arteritis
Secondary systemic vasculitis
Connective tissue diseases (rheumatoid arthritis, systemic lupus erythemosus, Sjögren syndrome)
Infections (hepatitis B, hepatitis C-induced cryoglobulinaemia, HIV, Lyme disease, human T-lymphotropic virus 1)
Neurosarcoidosis
Behcet's disease
Drugs
Malignancy
Inflammatory bowel disease
Non-systemic vasculitic neuropathy
Diabetic and non-diabetic radiculoplexus neuropathy
Wartenberg's migrant sensory neuritis

Adapted from Collins et al. [2] with permission from Wiley, Copyright 2010.

Eosinophilic Granulomatosis with Polyangiitis

Eosinophilic granulomatosis with polyangiitis, formerly known as Churg Strauss syndrome (when Jacob Strauss and Lotte Strauss identified the condition in 1951), most commonly presents with asthma, nasal and sinus symptoms and a peripheral neuropathy. It is a rare chronic inflammatory systemic disease occurring in patients with bronchial asthma and is associated with blood and tissue eosinophilia. Other manifestations may include weight loss, fever, myalgia, arthralgia, skin involvement (tender subcutaneous nodules on extensor surfaces), pulmonary opacities, cardiomyopathy, kidney disease (progressive renal insufficiency, proteinuria or microscopic haematuria) and gastrointestinal involvement (eosinophilic gastroenteritis).

Diagnostic Criteria of EGPA

Diagnostic criteria for EGPA were updated in 2022 by the American College of Rheumatology and the European Alliance of Associations for Rheumatology. The criteria use a scoring system for clinical and laboratory features (Table 24.4); a score of six or more has a sensitivity of 85% and specificity of 99%.

Table 24.4 2022 American College of Rheumatology/European Alliance of Associations for Rheumatology Classification criteria for EGPA

Clinical criteria	Score	Patient score
Obstructive airway disease	+3	+3
Nasal polyps	+3	+3
Mononeuritis multiplex	+1	+1
Laboratory and biopsy criteria		
Blood eosinophil count ≥1 × 10⁹/L	+5	+5
Endovascular eosinophilic predominant inflammation on biopsy	+2	
Positive test for cytoplasmic antineutrophil cytoplasmic antibodies (cANCA) or anti-PRS antibodies	-3	-3
Haematuira	-1	
Total		9

A diagnosis of small- or medium-vessel vasculitis could be classified as having EGPA if the cumulative score was ≥6 points

Adapted from Grayson et al. [3] with permission from John Wiley and Sons. Copyright 2022.

Stratification of Patients with EGPA

Measuring the Five Factor Score can predict survival [4]. In this risk stratification, each feature is awarded a point. The features include age over 65 years, cardiac insufficiency, renal insufficiency (stabilised peak creatinine of 150 μmol/L), gastrointestinal involvement and absence of ear, nose and throat manifestations. A Five Factor Score of 0 has none of the factors present, a Five Factor Score of 1 has just one factor present, and a Five Factor Score of 2 has two or more factors present; higher scores are associated with decreased survival.

Management of EGPA

All patients with EGPA usually receive systemic glucocorticoid therapy. Patients with a Five Factor Score of 2 often also receive cyclophosphamide. Rituximab has induced and sustained remission in EGPA. Maintenance immunosuppressant with many other agents is not unusual. Benralizumab has shown efficacy in eosinophilic asthma, is well tolerated and facilitates oral corticosteroid reduction [5]. Our patient had a Five Factor Score of 0 and had done well before he developed neurologically restricted MPO-ANCA vasculitic neuropathy.

Restricted Forms of EGPA

Interleukin 5 inhibition with drugs such as mepolizumab and benralizumab have shown benefit in EGPA patients particularly, like our patient, for asthma. However, the breakthrough in neurological disease with upstream activation of lymphocytes (IgE, IgG4, ANCA-MPO inflammatory biomarkers) demonstrates that eosinophils are not necessary for some forms of EGPA. Indeed, other forms of EGPA (arthralgia and rash) may also manifest in patients taking benralizumab for eosinophilic asthma. With increasing use of interleukin 5 blockade neurologists may see more such patients.

References

1. Almaani S, Fussner LA, Brodsky S, Meara AS, Jayne D. ANCA-associated vasculitis: an update. *J Clin Med.* 2021;10(7):1446.

2. Collins M, Dyck P, Gronseth G et al. Peripheral nerve society guideline on the classification, diagnosis, investigation, and immunosuppressive therapy of non- systemic vasculitic neuropathy: executive summary. *J Peripher Nerv Syst.* 2010;15:176–84.

3. Grayson PC, Ponte C, Suppiah R et al. 2022 American College of Rheumatology/European Alliance of Associations for Rheumatology Classification criteria for eosinophilic granulomatosis with polyangiitis. *Arthrit. & Rheumatol.* 2022;74(3):386–92.

4. Guillevin L, Pagnoux C, Seror R et al. The five-factor score revisited: assessment of prognoses of systemic necrotizing vasculitides based on the french vasculitis study group (FVSG) cohort. *Medicine (Balt).* 2011;90(1):19–27.

5. Guntur VP, Manka LA, Denson JL et al. Benralizumab as a steroid-sparing treatment option in eosinophilic granulomatosis with polyangiitis. *J Allergy Clin Immunol.* 2021;9(3):1186–93.

Learning Points

- Eosinophilic granulomatosis with polyangiitis is a multisystem disorder due to a small-to-medium sized vasculitis.

- Eosinophilic granulomatosis with polyangiitis can affect any organ system. The most common presenting features are asthma, nasal and sinus symptoms and peripheral neuropathy.

- Eosinophilic granulomatosis with polyangiitis is the least common of ANCA-associated vasculitides, although MPO-ANCA may only be positive in 40–60% of patients.

- Neurological manifestations of EGPA include mononeuritis multiplex and polyneuropathy.

- Interleukin 5 inhibition depletes eosinophils but may not prevent restricted forms of eosinophilic granulomatosis.

Patient's Perspective (on Initial Presentation)

1. **What was the impact of the condition on you?**

   a. **Physical (e.g. practical support)**

   I first noticed symptoms, of what I later found out to be Churg Strauss syndrome, in December 2011. I became aware of a small patch of skin on the top of my foot which had 'pins and needles'. I thought no more about it but soon after I started to get severe pain through the centre of both my legs. My GP diagnosed a form of sciatica and prescribed pain relief meds. These had no effect whatsoever on my pain which was constant throughout the day and night.

   On Monday 6th February 2012, whilst at my desk at work, I lost the power in my right arm and was admitted to hospital with a suspected stroke or TIA. All the normal tests for these conditions performed on admission were negative.

   My condition was getting worse literally by the hour. I experienced a whole range of nerve sensations including pain, numbness and extreme sensitivity of the skin. These sensations started in my feet and spread progressively up through my legs towards my waist whilst at the same time starting in my fingers and spread up through my arms. The sensations of pain, numbness, cold and extreme sensitivity seemed to be on a continuous cycle and they changed from one to the next every 20 seconds or so.

   I still had the severe pain through the core of the bones in my legs. I likened it at the time to someone putting a hot poker through the very centre of the bones in my legs. This persisted both day and night. The extremely sensitive skin meant that I couldn't even have a sheet over me whilst in bed as the touch of it on my skin was literally unbearable. I had now lost the power not only in my right arm but also in my left leg and both feet as well as my sense of balance. My condition continued to deteriorate as the week progressed and I was getting increasingly worried as the medical team in the stroke ward were unable to provide a diagnosis.

I was eventually referred to the hospital Neurology department on Friday 10th February and it was only when I spoke with the consultant neurologist, that I was at last able to get an accurate diagnosis of my condition. He very quickly diagnosed Churg Strauss syndrome and my treatment was started within the hour. The diagnosis was both very worrying, as it was obviously a very serious and rare condition, but it was also a great relief to finally have an understanding of what was wrong with, me and a plan to deal with it.

I spent a number of weeks in hospital and slowly began to recover some power in my limbs. I struggled to rebuild the muscle strength and the balance was even slower to return. My fine motor skills were severely impaired and I found great difficulty using my fingers to lift things.

When I was discharged from hospital, I had severe pain in my feet and legs. I had suffered a lot of muscle wastage and could not climb stairs. It took a lot of effort to get myself washed and dressed each day. My recovery was tough at first and I struggled with simple daily tasks. Everything took me longer to do than before. I was very lucky to have a loving wife and family who helped me so much at that difficult time. I could not have gotten through it without their tremendous support.

b. Psychological (e.g. mood, emotional well-being)
I went through a range of emotions on my journey with Churg Strauss. Obviously at first the uncertainty of what was wrong with me caused huge turmoil. I had not considered that I would have such a rare condition such that medical teams would have difficulty diagnosing it. The longer the uncertainty of not knowing what was wrong the more my mood became down.

When I was eventually diagnosed, I felt very worried because of the serious nature of the condition but I also felt a sense of relief at finally knowing. The medical team now inspired confidence and this undoubtedly rubbed off on me as my mood lifted and I found a sense of positivity. I decided at this time that the only way to deal with this was to meet it head on and I set about my long road to recovery. I sourced as much reference material as I could, in order to better understand how to start to rebuild my life. I kept pushing myself to do more, to walk further in the hope that I would improve my physical strength and my gross and fine motor skills.

c. Social (e.g. meeting friends, home)
I have to say that my condition was a complete unknown to me and everyone of my family and friends. It felt strange and somewhat awkward being ill. I would perhaps even go so far as to say I was embarrassed. I had lots of love and support from everyone and this undoubtedly helped me to remain positive. My physical weakness made it challenging to do many things such as going out with friends and I consciously avoided social meetings at the beginning. When I began to feel more confident again then I started to become more outgoing again.

2. **What can or could you not do because of the condition?**
There were lots of things that I could not do immediately after contracting Churg Strauss. I took ages to do the most simple of things. There were many physical daily tasks that were very difficult at first and these were a source of frustration on more than one occasion. I lost my sense of balance overnight. Putting my trousers on whilst standing up without falling over was impossible. Slipping my feet into my slippers was impossible at first because I had no feeling in the bottom of my feet. When out walking to build muscle strength in my legs I found it impossible to walk across a slope in the footpath without falling over. I still struggle with buttons when using my right hand even today. I was unable to drive for many months because I could not feel the pedals in the car and found the clutch difficult to judge. When I did start to drive again, I hated traffic queues because of the constant stopping and starting and using the clutch. One of the biggest problems with my condition was my total inability to concentrate on anything for more than a few minutes at a time. This was very frustrating and made for some very long days and sleepless nights.

3. **Was there any other change for you due to your medical condition?**
Because of my medication I had a huge appetite and my lack of any formal sleep pattern together with poor concentration meant that many long nights were spent going on a continuous cycle between living room tv and kitchen fridge. This led to a lot of weight gain which I hated.

4. **What is/was the most difficult aspect of the condition for you?**
My inability to do lots of things I had taken for granted previously was difficult everyday but my sense of the uncertain future course of the condition was perhaps the most difficult aspect of my condition.

5.   **Was any aspect of the experience good or useful? What was that?**

A renewed appreciation for the simple things in life, which we all so easily take for-granted. During my Churg Strauss journey I came into contact with many brilliant members of the health service and I really came to appreciate their care and concern for my well-being. I will be forever grateful for their help and support throughout my illness.

On a lighter note, my condition meant I could no longer play golf and so I took up a new hobby, photography. I have found this to be both enjoyable and very rewarding and a great activity for maintaining physical and mental well-being.

6.   **What do you hope for the future for people with this condition?**

Early diagnosis and belief that with a positive attitude they can make significant improvements in their quality of life. Possibly access for patients to or information about others who have experienced similar conditions and how their recovery journey unfolded. That all disciplines within hospitals keep an open mind when trying to diagnose patients with rare and unusual presentations.

Neurological Consequences of Infection

History

One night, a 22-year-old left-handed electrician and driver had consumed excess alcohol. He started to vomit on the next day but had no diarrhoea. He had no flu-like symptoms. Four days later he noticed numbness in his hands and feet. His symptoms progressed over the next few days. He had seen his GP and then an out-of-hours GP service. By day 9, he struggled to lift his arms and by day 13, he had difficulty climbing stairs. He was then admitted to hospital.

He had an unremarkable past medical history. He had been taking no medication. He had no known drug allergies. He did not smoke cigarettes. He denied any illicit drug abuse. He drank alcohol in a binge-like manner, ten pints of beer twice a month.

Examination

He was alert and orientated. Heart rate was 78 bpm, blood pressure was 118/72 mmHg and respiratory rate was 14 breaths per minute. He had a right lower motor neurone facial weakness. Pupils were equal and reactive to light. Visual acuity was 6/6 bilaterally and eye movements were normal. Neck flexion was grade 4/5. He had proximal arm weakness (shoulder abduction grade 2/5, right elbow flexion grade 4/5, left elbow flexion weaker but also grade 4/5, elbow extension grade 3/5 bilaterally, wrist extension grade 3/5 bilaterally, right finger abduction grade 3/5 and left finger abduction grade 4/5). His legs were weak (right hip flexion grade 4/5, left hip flexion grade 4/5, knee flexion grade 4/5 bilaterally, right ankle dorsiflexion grade 4/5, left ankle dorsiflexion was stronger but also grade 4/5). He was areflexic. He had decreased pinprick sensation only on the soles of his feet. Proprioception and vibration were normal.

A number of investigations were performed.

Investigations

An MRI of the spine was reported as normal. A neuropathy screen (HbA1c, thyroid profile, B12, folate, plasma protein electrophoresis and immunoglobulins) was normal. Creatine kinase was normal.

Lumbar puncture was performed. Cerebrospinal fluid (CSF) had no white cells/μL and 415 red cells/μL. CSF protein was 0.86 g/L (normal range <0.45 g/L), CSF glucose was 3.5 mmol/L and serum glucose was 6.7 mmol/L.

The nerve conduction studies (Tables 25.1 and 25.2) showed that right radial, median and ulnar sensory nerve action potentials were reduced with preserved conduction velocities. There were prolonged distal motor latencies from right median nerve stimulation to abductor pollicis brevis and right ulnar nerve stimulation to abductor digit minimi. There was slowing of the right ulnar motor nerve conduction velocity across the elbow. There was a prolonged distal motor latency of right peroneal nerve stimulation to extensor digitorum brevis. The right peroneal motor nerve conduction velocities were within acceptable limits. The right tibial

Table 25.1 Sensory nerve conduction study

Sensory	Latency (ms)	Amplitude (µV)	Segment	Velocity (m/s)
Median right		Normal >10		
Thumb	2.1	**3**	Thumb-wrist	51
Middle	3.7	**9.2**	Middle-wrist	38
Ulnar right		Normal >10		
Little	2.5	**3**	Little-wrist	47
Radial right		Normal >18		
Forearm	2.0	**4**		**43**
Sural right		Normal >4		
Calf	2.2	17	Lateral malleolus-calf	51
Superficial peroneal right				
Midcalf	2.9	9	Ankle-mid calf	**34**

Abnormal results in bold

Table 25.2 Motor nerve conduction study

Motor nerve and site	Latency (ms)	Amplitude (µV)	Segment	Velocity (m/s)
Median right	Normal<4.2	Normal>3.5		Normal>48
Wrist	**5.9**	9.5		
Elbow	**10.6**	9.2	Wrist-elbow	53
Ulnar right	Normal<3.4	Normal>2.8		Normal>50
Wrist	**5.0**	8.2		
Below elbow	**8.5**	7.6	Wrist-below elbow	66
Above elbow	**12.4**	5.1	Below elbow-above elbow	**29**
Peroneal right	Normal<5.5	Normal>2.5		Normal>40
Ankle	**10.8**	4.4		
Fibula (head)	**19.7**	2.7	Ankle-fibula (head)	**37**
Popliteal fossa	**22.1**	2.1	Fibula (head)-popliteal fossa	**38**
Tibial right	Normal<5	Normal>2.6		
Ankle	**5.1**	6.3	Dispersed waveform	

Abnormal results in bold

motor nerve response from abductor hallucis was dispersed. Right median F wave (35.8 ms) and right ulnar F wave (39.5 ms) had normal latencies.

In summary, there was demyelinating (prolonged distal motor latencies) and axonal loss features (reduced action potentials), more prominent in the upper limbs than the lower limbs (similar to the clinical picture).

Viral screen was reported as showing cytomegalovirus immunoglobulin M reactive/positive (34.61 units). HIV and hepatitis B and C tests were negative.

Diagnosis: Guillain–Barré Syndrome

Management
The following management plan was implemented prior to nerve conduction studies.
1 Forced vital capacity monitoring
2 Intravenous immunoglobulin therapy started at 0.4 g/kg/day for five days.
3 ICU/critical care team and anaesthetic staff were informed of the patient.

A remarkable recovery ensued with return to work within six weeks.

Comment
Georges Guillain, Jean Alexandre Barré and André Strohl wrote their seminal paper in 1916. They reported two soldiers who had weakness with absent tendon reflexes and increased CSF protein concentration with a normal cell count. The condition is now frequently referred to as Guillain–Barré syndrome, an inflammatory disease of the peripheral nervous system.

Epidemiology
Guillain–Barré syndrome is the most common cause of acute flaccid paralysis. The crude incidence of Guillain–Barré syndrome varies from 0.8 to 1.9 per 100,000 per year. Unlike autoimmune conditions, Guillain–Barré syndrome occurs more frequently in men than women. The recurrence rate of Guillain–Barré syndrome is low but recurrence can occur. Human leukocyte antigen associations may indicate an increased susceptibility.

Diagnosis of Guillain–Barré Syndrome
Diagnostic features of Guillain–Barré syndrome include progressive limb weakness and areflexia [1]. The progressive phase of weakness lasts at most four weeks (usually two weeks) and the weakness is usually symmetrical. Bilateral facial weakness, autonomic disturbance and pain are other clinical features [1]. Elevated CSF protein in the absence of a pleocytosis is a common and diagnostically helpful finding. Nerve conduction studies, although not required to diagnose Guillain–Barré syndrome, add further support to the diagnosis. Typical findings include a sensorimotor polyradiculoneuropathy or polyneuropathy with reduced conduction velocities, reduced sensory and motor evoked amplitudes, abnormal temporal dispersion and/or partial motor conduction blocks.

The Brighton collaboration devised criteria for Guillain–Barré syndrome. The highest level of diagnostic certainty is level 1 and includes:

> bilateral and flaccid weakness of the limbs and decreased or absent deep tendon reflexes in weak limbs and monophasic illness pattern and interval between onset and nadir of weakness between 12 hours and 28 days and subsequent clinical plateau and cytoalbuminologic dissociation (i.e. elevation of CSF protein level above laboratory normal value and CSF total white cell count <50 cells/μL) and electrophysiologic findings consistent with Guillain–Barré syndrome and absence of an identified alternative diagnosis for weakness.

Differential Diagnosis of Guillain–Barré Syndrome
There is a wide differential diagnosis for weakness, some of which are listed here.
1 chronic (progressing >8 weeks) and sub-acute (four- to eight-week progression) inflammatory demyelinating polyradiculoneuropathy (CIDP)

2 nodo-paranodopathies

3 critical illness myopathy – motor syndrome post-steroids and neuromuscular blocking agent (+ neuropathy). Septic encephalopathy can cause critical illness myopathy.

4 nutritional – B1 deficiency causing Wernicke encephalopathy and B12 deficiency causing sub-acute combined degeneration of the spinal cord

5 vasculitic neuropathy – polyarteritis nodosa, eosinophilic granulomatosis with polyangiitis

6 transverse myelitis (as in neuromyelitis optics spectrum disorder or anti-myelin oligodendrocyte glycoprotein-associated disease)

7 epidural abscess or haematoma (spinal cord compression)

8 acute flaccid myelitis (polio, West Nile virus or enterovirus)

9 infection – tuberculosis, HIV myelopathy and Lyme disease

10 spinal stroke

11 spinal contusion

12 functional weakness.

Patients with nodo-paranodopathies present with a rapidly progressive neuropathy and these conditions are particularly important to consider in the differential diagnosis of Guillain–Barré syndrome as their treatment requires early escalation. Because such patients can meet diagnostic criteria for Guillain–Barré syndrome (nadir within four weeks) or previous criteria for CIDP (nadir within eight weeks), serological testing for paranodal/nodal antibodies (immunoglobulin G4 to nodal neurofascin 186 or paranodal neurofascin 155, contactin-1 and contactin-associated protein-1) is recommended ideally before treatment. Nodo-paranodopathies occur most frequently in adult men in their sixth decade with a severe and symmetrical motor-predominant and distal-predominant polyneuropathy.

A clinically progressive and relapsing-remitting course of nodo-paranodopathy can fulfil 2010 European Federation of Neurological Societies/Peripheral Nerve Society criteria for 'definite CIDP'. However, different pathology and treatments mean that these are now excluded from the CIDP definition in the 2021 European Academy of Neurology/Peripheral Nerve Society guideline on diagnosis and treatment of CIDP.

Nephrotic syndrome has been recognised in patients with contactin-1 antibodies. Patients with pan-neurofascin antibodies (cross-react with both neurofascin 155 and neurofascin 186) may have an underlying haematological disorder including Hodgkin's lymphoma, chronic lymphocytic leukaemia and myeloma. Patients with nodo-paranodopathies are less responsive to the usual treatments for inflammatory neuropathies – intravenous immunoglobulins and plasma exchange. While there may be a transient response to intravenous immunoglobulins (possibly due to an effect on complement-fixing immunoglobulin G1–G3 only), escalation to rituximab may be required.

For other differential diagnoses, it is important to be aware that spinal shock can initially cause depressed reflexes, and so an MRI scan of the spine in patients with weakness may be considered. A patient with cauda equina syndrome (urinary retention, saddle anaesthesia, back and/or leg pain and weakness) may have flexor plantar responses and absent ankle jerks. Guillain–Barré syndrome can present with early back pain. A conus lesion may cause brisk ankle jerks and extensor plantar responses.

Neurologists frequently look at scans and seek input from a neuroradiologist as the consequences from spinal cord disease can be devastating. MRI is not part of the diagnostic routine workup in Guillain–Barré syndrome but may be important to exclude structural differential diagnoses.

Electrophysiological Sub-types and Clinical Variants of Guillain–Barré Syndrome

Electrophysiological testing can distinguish sub-types of Guillain–Barré syndrome as acute inflammatory demyelinating polyradiculoneuropathy (AIDP), acute motor axonal neuropathy (AMAN) and acute motor sensory axonal neuropathy (AMSAN). In addition, clinically there are regional variants of Guillain–Barré syndrome (paraparetic, pharyngeal-cervical-brachial, bilateral facial palsy with paraesthesias, Miller Fisher syndrome and Bickerstaff brainstem encephalitis), which also probably reflect variations in the underlying pathology (Table 25.3). The best-known clinical variant is the Miller Fisher syndrome (ophthalmoplegia, ataxia and areflexia). About 90% of patients with the Miller Fisher syndrome have antibodies to a particular ganglioside, GQ1b. Oculomotor nerves are enriched with GQ1b. Such patients may become weak, resulting in a Miller Fisher – Guillain–Barré overlap syndrome. It is, however, well known that overlapping features are a frequent finding among patients with Guillain–Barré syndrome. Pure sensory or ataxic phenotypes do not strictly fulfil criteria for Guillain–Barré syndrome because of the lack of weakness.

Pathology

Molecular mimicry has been implicated from a preceding bacterial or viral infection although the pathogenesis is not fully understood. The dichotomy of Guillain–Barré syndrome into AIDP and AMAN suggests immune-mediated injury occurs at the myelin sheath

Table 25.3 Variants of Guillain–Barré syndrome

Variant	Frequency (% of Guillain–Barré syndrome cases)	Clinical features
Classic sensorimotor Guillain–Barré syndrome	30–85	Rapidly progressive symmetrical weakness and sensory signs with absent or reduced tendon reflexes, usually reaching nadir within two weeks
Pure motor	5–70	Motor weakness without sensory signs
Paraparetic	5–10	Paresis restricted to the legs
Pharyngeal-cervical-brachial	<5	Weakness of pharyngeal, cervical and brachial muscles without lower limb weakness
Bilateral facial palsy with paraesthesias*	<5	Bilateral facial weakness, paraesthesias and reduced reflexes
Pure sensory*	<1	Acute or subacute sensory neuropathy without other deficits
Miller Fisher syndrome	5–25	Ophthalmoplegia, ataxia and areflexia. Incomplete forms with isolated ataxia (acute ataxic neuropathy) or ophthalmoplegia (acute ophthalmoplegia) can occur. Overlaps with classical sensorimotor Guillain–Barré syndrome in an estimated 15% of patients
Bickerstaff brainstem encephalitis	<5	Ophthalmoplegia, ataxia, areflexia, pyramidal tract signs and impaired consciousness, often overlapping with sensorimotor Guillain–Barré syndrome

*Does not fulfil commonly used diagnostic criteria for Guillain–Barré syndrome (bilateral limb weakness) or criteria for Miller Fisher syndrome

Adapted with permission from Springer Nature from Leonhard et al. [2]. Copyright Springer Nature (2019).

and Schwann cell components or in the nerve axon (axolemma), respectively. An active area of research has been to tease out the role of T cell-mediated injury in a process that appears to be predominantly humorally mediated.

It is known that *Campylobacter jejuni* carries epitopes in the lipo-oligosaccharide of of its cell wall, which elicits anti-ganglioside responses such as GM1 or GD1a. It is estimated that 2–3 cases per 10,000 *Campylobacter* infections trigger Guillain–Barré syndrome.

Zika virus, which was discovered in 1947 and spread throughout the Americas in 2015, is well known for causing congenital defects in foetuses, but also causes Guillain–Barré syndrome at a similar infection rate to *Campylobacter* infection. Six pathogens have been temporally associated with Guillain–Barré syndrome (Table 25.4).

In 1976, there was a seven-fold increase in the incidence of Guillain–Barré syndrome in the USA following a swine influenza vaccination campaign. Subsequent studies of influenza vaccines have shown a marked reduction in this adverse effect – one additional Guillain–Barré syndrome case per one million vaccinations. Evidence for such an association has been looked for in France in the other direction; a self-controlled case series of 4,000 patients with Guillain–Barré syndrome. The risk of developing Guillain–Barré syndrome was no higher in the six weeks following vaccination than in other time periods. However, the risk of developing Guillain–Barré syndrome in the six weeks following an acute respiratory tract or gastrointestinal infection was increased almost four-fold. Other vaccines do not appear to increase the risk of Guillain–Barré syndrome in the paediatric or adult population [3].

Ten Steps in Managing Guillain–Barré Syndrome

In late 2019, the first globally applicable guidelines for the diagnosis and management of Guillain–Barré syndrome were published [2]. This was prompted by the recognition that outbreaks of infectious disease can trigger Guillain–Barré syndrome, such as the association with Zika virus infection. The international guidelines provide an important template in management.

One important guideline recommends monitoring of Guillain–Barré syndrome patients. As up to 22% of Guillain–Barré syndrome patients require mechanical ventilation [2], identifying evolving respiratory distress, autonomic cardiovascular dysfunction, severe swallowing dysfunction, diminished cough reflex and rapid progression of weakness may necessitate admission to an intensive care unit. It is good practice to anticipate deterioration and consider the following as signs of respiratory distress: breathlessness at rest/talking, inability to count to 15 in a single breath, use of accessory respiratory muscles, and increased respiratory rate or heart rate (documented in early warning charts). Monitoring vital capacity is helpful but facial weakness can impair technique; vital capacity should be above 20 ml/kg (1.5L for men and 1.0L for women). Pulse oximetry and arterial blood gas measurements can also be used.

Table 25.4 Recognised triggers of Guillain–Barré syndrome

Campylobacter jejuni
Cytomegalovirus
Hepatitis E virus
Mycoplasma pneumonia
Epstein–Barr virus
Zika virus

Treatment and Outcomes

Intravenous immunoglobulin (0.4 g/kg for five days) and plasma exchange (200–500 ml plasma/kg in five sessions) are equally effective treatments for Guillain–Barré syndrome.

Intravenous immunoglobulin is easier to administer and more widely available. Mortality in Guillain–Barré syndrome is 3–10%. A second course of intravenous immunoglobulin does not appear to improve outcome in patients with a poor prognosis, but consideration of nodo-paranodopathies is required.

References

1. Willison HJ, Jacobs BC, van Doorn PA. Guillain–Barré syndrome. *Lancet.* 2016;388(10045):717–27.
2. Leonhard SE, Mandarakas MR, Gondim FAA et al. Diagnosis and management of Guillain–Barré syndrome in ten steps. *Nat Rev Neurol* 2019;15(11):671–83.
3. Chen Y, Zhang J, Chu X, Xu Y, Ma F. Vaccines and the risk of Guillain–Barré syndrome. *Eur J Epidemiol.* 2020;35(4):363–70.

Learning Points

- Guillain–Barré syndrome is an immune-mediated disease of the peripheral nerves and nerve roots.
- Guillain–Barré syndrome most commonly follows an infection from *Campylobacter jejuni*, cytomegalovirus, hepatitis E, *M. pneumonia*, Epstein–Barr virus and Zika virus.
- Intravenous immunoglobulin and plasma exchange have similar evidence of efficacy in Guillain–Barré syndrome.
- Global guidelines provide a 10-step management plan for patients with Guillain–Barré syndrome.
- A poor response to therapy for Guillain–Barré syndrome should prompt consideration of nodo-paranodopathy as an alternative diagnosis.

Patient's Perspective

1. **What was the impact of the condition?**
    a. Physical (e.g. practical support, work, activities of daily living)
    I had fully recovered quite quickly but in recovery it was hard trying to re-learn something that is taken for granted when it used to be so easy and that is basic everyday things (walk, talk, eat, stand up, go to the toilet etc).
    b. Psychological (e.g. mood, emotional well-being)
    I'm a man of God. So, my courage and determination to get better after the treatment came from that and the support of my family.
    c. Social (meeting friends, home)
    When I came into hospital full time it was horrible. Not being able to physically take part in my social life. Although some people visited, it was not the same.

2. **What could you not do because of the condition?**
    Eventually walk, talk, swallow. I struggled breathing. I struggled with any muscular movement. Paralysis is traumatic and at a stage I couldn't even toilet myself, so dignity went out the window.

3. **Was there any other change for you due to your condition?**
    I haven't had any long-term side effects.

4. **What is/was the most difficult aspect of the condition for you?**
    When I was admitted to ICU, then I knew it was real. I was lying next to similar patients, people in a coma and very, very sick people; that was the scary part.

5. **Was any aspect of the experience good or useful? What was that?**

   Absolutely! It turned me into a better human being. I'm grateful every single day and thankful for the specialists working on me, God and my family for the love and support. I will never take anything for granted again.

6. **What do you hope for in the future for your condition?**

   I feel that my youth has been very much on my side. Because I was young and fit and healthy, it benefitted me a lot. I hope everyone is as lucky as what I have been.

When Speech and Swallow Fail

History

An 89-year-old left-handed man presented with a two-month history of difficulty swallowing after an operation for a left retinal detachment. He described choking. He had particular difficulty with crumbs. He had nasal regurgitation. A speech and language therapist confirmed problems with the pharyngeal phase of his swallowing, in that there was incomplete pharyngeal swallow, severe pharyngeal dysphagia and an aspiration risk. The patient had also noticed over the same two months that as he talked his speech became slurred. He had no breathing or walking difficulties and denied any diplopia, blackouts or dry mouth.

In his past medical history, he had metastatic prostatic cancer, type 2 diabetes mellitus, essential hypertension, chronic kidney disease stage 3, ischaemic heart disease and chronic obstructive pulmonary disease.

Medication included goserelin, lansoprazole, atorvastatin, ascorbic acid and lactulose.

He was single and neither smoked cigarettes nor drank alcohol.

Examination

He was alert and orientated but had mild dysarthria, which worsened with talking. Eye movements were normal. He had a nasogastric tube in situ. He had a pigmented left lower leg (due to radiotherapy for bony metastases). He had a right ptosis. Orbicularis oris was weak bilaterally. Neck flexion was weak at grade 4/5. Tongue movements were intact. He had no limb or tongue fasciculations. Limb tone was normal. He had mild bilateral shoulder abduction and hip flexion weakness (grade 4/5). His reflexes were symmetrically present and sensation was intact. Plantar responses were withdrawal.

Clinical Diagnosis

In view of the fatigable dysarthria, bulbar weakness, proximal limb weakness and right ptosis, myasthenia gravis was suspected.

Investigations

Myasthenic antibodies were measured. Acetylcholine receptor antibody was positive 553 (normal range $0–5 \times 10^{-10}$ M). An anti-skeletal muscle antibody was positive. Muscle-specific kinase and voltage-gated calcium channel antibodies were negative. Neuronal antibodies (Yo, Hu, and Ri) were negative.

A CT scan of the chest showed no evidence of a thymoma (despite positive anti-skeletal muscle antibody). Lumbar puncture was unremarkable.

Nerve conduction studies showed a mild right median nerve lesion at the wrist and a moderate right ulnar nerve lesion at the elbow.

Repetitive nerve stimulation of right abductor pollicis brevis, right abductor digiti minimi and right trapezius did not demonstrate any decrement at 3 Hz.

Single-fibre EMG of the right frontalis muscle was performed. Eighteen pairs of apparent single muscle fibre action potentials were recorded. The mean difference between consecutive discharges was 61 μs (normal range 10–50 μs). Two pairs of fibres had extensive jitter.

Diagnosis: Myasthenia Gravis (Acetylcholine receptor Antibody Positive)

Outcome

He was treated with pyridostigmine, prednisolone and intravenous immunoglobulin. A tapering dose of prednisolone was used. Within weeks, speech and swallowing had recovered. With the help of carers, independent living was achieved. At 12 months, prednisolone had been tapered down to 15 mg/day.

Comment

Diseases of the Neuromuscular Junction

There are four immune-mediated disorders of the neuromuscular junction. They are myasthenia gravis, Lambert–Eaton myasthenic syndrome (associated with a presynaptic voltage-gated calcium channel antibody), myasthenia gravis Lambert–Eaton overlap syndrome and neuromyotonia or Isaacs syndrome (hyperexcitability of peripheral nerve due to excess release of acetylcholine at the presynaptic membrane). Leucine-rich glioma-inactivated 1 (LGI1) antibody and contactin-associated protein-like 2 (CASPR2) antibodies have been found in neuromyotonia and Morvan's syndrome (peripheral nerve excitability plus autonomic instability and encephalopathy).

Epidemiology of Myasthenia Gravis

Myasthenia gravis is an autoimmune disorder causing weakness due to impaired neuromuscular transmission. There are paraneoplastic and non-paraneoplastic forms of myasthenia gravis. The disorder is immunologically heterogenous with recognised antibodies to acetylcholine receptor and muscle-specific receptor tyrosine kinase (MuSK), but not in the same patient. Myasthenia gravis occurs in all races and in both sexes. Incidence has a bimodal distribution and incidence rates of myasthenia gravis peak between 60 and 80 years, particularly among males [1]. While improved ascertainment is likely, it also appears that the real incidence (pooled estimate 5.3 per million population per year) is increasing. This combined with marked geographical variation suggests that other factors require further study [1].

Clinical Features of Myasthenia Gravis

Fatigable and rapidly fluctuating asymmetric, intermittent and even alternating ptosis is the hallmark of myasthenia gravis. Up to 65% of patients initially have ocular symptoms (double vision and ptosis). Bulbar weakness presentation, including pooling of food in the mouth after attempted swallowing and unintelligible speech after prolonged talking, occurs in about a quarter of patients. Thick tongue, garbled or nasal speech, swallowing difficulty and decreased facial expression all occur. A weak tongue with atrophy has been particularly noted in MuSK antibody-positive myasthenia gravis, which usually affects young females and requires more aggressive treatment in order to achieve remission. Limb weakness is an unusual complaint. Eyelid closure weakness, jaw closure and opening weakness, elevated palate and tongue weakness may occur. The peek sign occurs following complete initial voluntary apposition of the eyelid margins. After less than 30 seconds, the eyelid margins separate and the sclera starts to show (positive peek test). Quivering eye movements, an overactive frontalis to overcome ptosis and the curtain sign (lifting of eyelid worsens contralateral ptosis), the icepack test, sleep/rest test and the less frequently used, edrophonium test are other clinical features of myasthenia gravis.

In myasthenia gravis, there is loss of immunological self-tolerance. About 70% of cases are associated with thymic hyperplasia; 10–15% are associated with thymoma.

Differential Diagnosis of Myasthenia Gravis

The differential diagnosis of myasthenia gravis is listed in Table 26.1. As myasthenia gravis is very treatable even in frail elderly patients with multiple comorbidities (such as our patient), it is important to consider and look carefully for myasthenia gravis.

Ocular versus Generalised Myasthenia Gravis

Ocular myasthenia gravis is restricted to ptosis, extraocular muscle or eyelid closure weakness. Ten to sixteen per cent of patients have just ocular myasthenia gravis. Most patients with ocular myasthenia develop generalised myasthenia gravis within two years of onset.

Antibodies in Myasthenia Gravis

In 1976, a version of the modern acetylcholine receptor antibody was first described. More than 80% of patients with myasthenia gravis have antibodies to the acetylcholine receptor. The immunoglobulins G1 (IgG1) and G3 (IgG3) acetylcholine receptor antibodies are thought to be pathogenic for myasthenia gravis – increasing turnover of the acetylcholine receptor and activating a membrane-attack complex. Patients with only an ocular form of myasthenia gravis (15%) have a lower frequency of acetylcholine receptor antibodies, but even among these patients, seropositivity can reach 71%.

Arthrogryposis multiplex congenita has been diagnosed in children of mothers who were initially asymptomatic despite having acetylcholine receptor antibodies. Foetal acetylcholine receptors have a γ subunit in place of the adult ε subunit. The IgG1 acetylcholine receptor antibodies in foetal acetylcholine receptor inactivation syndrome (FARIS) cross the placenta and interact with the foetal γ subunit of the acetylcholine receptor. The offspring have been characterised to have a spectrum from arthrogryposis multiplex congenita to milder forms

Table 26.1 Differential diagnosis of myasthenia gravis

Congenital myasthenic syndromes

Dysthyroid ophthalmopathy

Lid levator muscle dehiscence (non-fatigable)

Motor neurone disease

Mitochondrial disorders – chronic progressive external ophthalmoplegia

Lambert–Eaton myasthenic syndrome

Guillain–Barré syndrome (variants with prominent cranial neuropathies)

Botulism (infant, food-borne, wound)

Acute organophosphate poisoning

Tick paralysis (western USA)

Diphtheria

of myopathic face, ptosis, hyper-nasal speech, hearing loss, extraocular restriction and dia-phragmatic paresis.

The MuSK antibody (predominantly immunoglobulin G4) was identified in 2001. This antibody inhibits agrin-induced acetylcholine receptor clustering in muscle myotubules. MuSK antibody-positive myasthenia gravis patients account for 1–10% of all cases of myasthenia gravis. These patients often have more bulbar weakness in contrast to the generalised weakness observed in seronegative cases of maysthenia gravis.

Another sensitive and specific antibody is the lipoprotein receptor-related protein 4 (LRP4) antibody. Many factors contribute to the pathogenicity of these antibodies including the epitope, binding capacity, IgG subclass, antibody-cross-linking capacity, antibody concentration and access of the antibody to the muscle endplate [2].

Titin and ryanodine receptor antibodies are associated with thymoma-associated myasthenia gravis and late-onset myasthenia gravis [2].

Drug-Exacerbating and Drug-Induced Myasthenia Gravis

More than 40 drugs can increase muscle relaxation and so aggravate myasthenia gravis. Beta blockers, antibiotics (gentamicin) and statins may all aggravate the condition. A list of such drugs can be found at www.myaware.org/drugs-to-avoid.

Other drugs are known to induce myasthenic syndromes. These are usually of slow onset, are associated with human leukocyte antigen DR1 and may have a slow and incomplete recovery after drug cessation. Anti-acetylcholine receptor antibodies may be present. Penicillamine, quinidine and anti-programmed cell death 1 (PD-1) antibodies such as pembrolizumab can induce myasthenia gravis.

Repetitive Nerve Stimulation and Single-Fibre EMG: Jitter and Blocking

Every action potential in a motor axon elicits an action potential in each muscle fibre of the motor unit. At high rates of stimulation, this relationship fails as some muscle fibres become refractory. The compound motor action potential amplitude then progressively declines, the so-called decremental response. In normal individuals, stimulation less than 20 Hz does not elicit a decremental response. At slow rates of repetitive nerve stimulation (e.g. 3 Hz), a decremental response greater than 10% is abnormal and can be seen in some muscles in myasthenia gravis. Spinal accessory nerve stimulation of the trapezius is more sensitive than ulnar nerve stimulation of the abductor digiti minimi because distal muscles are less often affected than proximal muscles (as shown in our patient) and distal muscles are more likely to be cool, which can reduce the decremental response to the normal range.

Single-fibre EMG is a time-consuming investigation predominantly used in the diagnosis of myasthenia gravis, particularly seronegative myasthenia gravis. It was described in the 1960s but became more popular in 1979 when Erik Stålberg and Joze Trontelj published a monograph – Single-Fibre Electromyography [3]. However, it is important to be aware that false positive results can occur. Single-fibre EMG can be used for jitter analysis and determination of fibre density.

Jitter analysis is a more sensitive test to detect disorders of neuromuscular transmission than repetitive nerve stimulation. Single muscle fibres do not discharge exactly synchronously in creating a motor unit potential. This variation increases when synaptic transmission is less secure as in myasthenia gravis. The endplate potential is smaller, which means the muscle action potential is higher on the hump of the endplate potential. The oscilloscope is set to be triggered by the first muscle fibre action potential. The second muscle fibre action potential occurs a few milliseconds after the first. Jitter refers to the appearance of the potentials on the oscilloscope. Mean consecutive differences of the interpotential intervals are usually less than 55 µs for extensor digiti minimi. Failure of conduction is called blocking. A normal muscle may have increased jitter in one of 20 muscle fibre pairs, but increased jitter or blocking in two or more of 20 pairs is abnormal.

Clinical weakness is required for blocking to be detected. Similarly, clinical weakness is required for detection of pathological decremental response on repetitive nerve stimulation tests. However, our patient was not weak in the muscles tested with repetitive nerve stimulation. In any disease of abnormal neuromuscular transmission, jitter may, however, be increased in muscles that are clinically normal.

Myasthenic Crisis

Up to 20% of patients with myasthenia gravis experience a crisis (life-threatening respiratory failure), and most present within the first year of the onset of myasthenia gravis. Patients with MuSK myasthenia gravis or thymoma-associated myasthenia gravis are more likely to have a crisis. Such deterioration can be triggered by infections, aspiration, surgery or trauma, rapid tapering of immunomodulation, first-pregnancy, contrast agents in radiology and importantly drugs such as ciprofloxacin, aminoglycosides, macrolides, fluoroquinolones, beta blockers, calcium channel blockers and magnesium.

Management of Myasthenia Gravis

The natural history of myasthenia gravis without immunosuppression was described by Hans Oosterhuis in 1989 [4]. Among 73 patients with myasthenia gravis between 1926 and 1965, 18 patients (29%) died, 2 patients had deteriorated, 12 patients (16%) had remained unchanged, 12 patients (16%) had some improvement, 13 patients (18%) markedly improved and 16 (22%) spontaneously went into remission [4].

The mortality rate is now around 2%, with most of the improvement in mortality due to managing lung infections. Treatment guidelines from the Association of British Neurologists and American Academy of Neurology have emerged. The American Academy of Neurology 2020 International Consensus Guidance recommended thymectomy early in the course of non-thymomatous generalised myasthenia gravis patients aged 18–50 years with acetylcholine receptor antibody. There was a lack of evidence for myasthenia gravis patients with MuSK or LRP4 antibody. Thymectomy is recommended for thymoma, although it may not improve myasthenic symptoms. Existing and some emerging therapies for myasthenia gravis are outlined in Table 26.2.

Table 26.2 Therapeutic interventions in myasthenia gravis

Intervention	Comment
Attempt to avoid drugs that exacerbate myasthenia gravis	Aminoglycosides, beta blockers, botulinum toxin, corticosteroids (transient worsening within two weeks), macrolide antibiotics and immune checkpoint inhibitors (which can exacerbate myasthenia gravis as well as induce myasthenia gravis)
Pyridostigmine	For symptomatic management
Corticosteroids	Required if pyridostigmine not controlling myasthenia gravis
Intravenous immunoglobulin or plasma exchange	Quick acting and useful for patients in a myasthenic crisis

Table 26.2 (cont.)

Intervention	Comment
Steroid-sparing immune-suppressant/modulation	Azathioprine/mycophenolate/ciclosporin/tacrolimus/eculizumab. Eculizumab is not used for MuSK antibody myasthenia gravis
Rituximab	Anti-CD20 monoclonal antibody depletes B cells
Thymectomy	Used for thymoma patients. Evidence in acetylcholine receptor antibody-positive myasthenia gravis patients under 50 years old
Some emerging drugs	Efgartigimod – a neonatal Fc receptor blocker – FDA approval for acetylcholine receptor antibody-positive myasthenia gravis Rozanolixizumab and nipocalimab – high-affinity neonatal Fc receptor blockers Zilucoplan – C5 inhibitor

Excess or Lack of Acetylcholine

Novichok (meaning 'newcomer' in Russian) is a group of fourth-generation chemical weapons devised in the 1970s and 1980s. These chemical compounds inhibit acetylcholinesterase, preventing normal breakdown of acetylcholine. As a result, acetylcholine concentrations increase at neuromuscular junctions to cause involuntary contraction of all skeletal muscles known as a cholinergic crisis. Respiratory and cardiac arrest may follow with death due to heart failure or drowning in excess fluid secretions. Atropine, a fast-acting anticholinergic drug, can block the acetylcholine receptors.

Botulinum Toxin

Botulinum toxin, one of the most poisonous biological substances known, is a neurotoxin produced by *Clostridium botulinum*. Botulinum blocks the release of acetylcholine at the neuromuscular junction, autonomic ganglia, postganglionic parasympathetic nerve endings and postganglionic sympathetic nerve endings. Medical use of botulinum is increasing and it is used in conditions such as focal dystonias, hemifacial spasm, spastic movement disorders, chronic migraine and hyperhidrosis.

References

1. Carr AS, Cardwell CR, McCarron P, McConville J. A systematic review of population based epidemiological studies in myasthenia gravis. *BMC Neurol*. 2010;10(46).
2. Gilhus NE. Myasthenia gravis. *N Engl J Med*. 2016;375(26):2570–81.
3. Ståhlberg E, Trontelj JV. *Single Fibre Electromyography*. Old Woking: Mirvalle Press, 1979.
4. Oosterhuis HJGH. The natural course of myasthenia gravis: a long term follow up study. *J Neurol Neurosurg Psychiatry*. 1989;52(10):1121–7.

Learning Points

- Myasthenia gravis is a treatable neuromuscular disease.
- Diagnostic clues to myasthenia gravis include intermittent or fluctuating ptosis, diplopia and fatigable dysarthria.
- Most patients have antibodies to acetylcholine receptor (80%), MuSK or LRP4 while the rest are labelled as seronegative.
- Repetitive nerve stimulation and single-fibre EMG jitter can help confirm neuromuscular junction pathology in the absence of myasthenic antibodies.

- Conventional myasthenic treatment involves pyridostigmine, corticosteroids and an emerging number of steroid-sparing agents with thymectomy recommended in acetylcholine receptor antibody-positive patients under 50 years of age or in patients who have a thymoma.

Patient's Perspective

1. **What impact did myasthenia gravis have on you?**
   I could not swallow or talk properly for two months. I could not push myself up from a seat.

2. **What was your mood like?**
   I was so ill I did not know what to think. I had no intention of dying.

3. **What do you hope for in the future for people with this condition?**
   Hope.

History

A 15-year-old female student developed upper leg pain and back discomfort. Five weeks later, she noticed weakness in her arms and particularly in her legs, with associated pins and needles and numbness. Her leg weakness was worse in the morning, but progressed over 10 days. She had had no flu or cold symptoms, diarrhoea, rash or joint pain. Two days prior to hospital admission, she required help from her mother to dress. She then had difficulty getting up from a chair and going upstairs.

In her past medical history, she had asthma. She was taking no medication. She neither smoked cigarettes nor drank alcohol. She had one older healthy brother. One year before presentation, her mother had presented with, and fully recovered from, Guillain–Barré syndrome.

Examination

Higher mental function was normal. There was no dysautonomia. Cranial nerves testing including facial strength was normal. There was no evidence of optic atrophy or retinitis pigmentosa. She had mild neck flexion weakness. Her limb tone was flaccid. She had four limb weakness (grade 4/5) but more so distally in her upper limbs – at elbow flexion and elbow extension as well as her hands. Similarly, she was weak in her legs, worse distally at ankle dorsiflexion (grade 3/5). She had a modified Gower's sign and had difficulty standing on her heels and toes bilaterally. She was areflexic. She had no sensory impairment to vibration or pinprick. Her unsteadiness was attributed to the weakness.

Investigations

Lumbar puncture revealed an opening pressure of 17 cm cerebrospinal fluid (CSF), 6 red cells/µL, no white cells/µL, CSF protein of 1 g/L, CSF glucose of 3.4 mmol/L, serum glucose of 4.7 mmol/L.

Campylobacter serology was negative. A viral screen, B12, folate, thyroid profile and nuclear autoantibody screen were all negative.

Nerve conduction studies demonstrated a patchy demyelinating motor predominant neuropathy at presentation. She had prolonged distal motor latencies, poorly formed and delayed F waves and delayed sensory nerve action potentials, supporting a primary demyelinating, sensory motor neuropathy.

Demyelinating Neuropathy Screen

PMP22 gene dosage was normal and no *PMP22* deletion or mutation was detected (i.e. no evidence of Charcot–Marie–Tooth – CMT1A – or hereditary liability to pressure palsies). A demyelinating neuropathy gene panel was negative. Plasma protein electrophoresis revealed no paraprotein. Vascular endothelial growth factor (VEGF) was 136 pg/mL (normal range<771 pg/mL). Very long chain fatty acids were normal and a porphyrin screen was negative.

A nerve biopsy (right sural nerve) showed mild axonal loss with very mild demyelinating/remyelinating changes.

Management

Forced vital capacity monitoring was organised for the initial presentation. Within five days of intravenous immunoglobulin (0.4 g/kg/day for five days), there was an improvement. She was better at rising from a chair and going upstairs. Examination confirmed power improvement with only residual shoulder abduction and less distal weakness. Upper limb reflexes had returned.

However, within 12 weeks of her hospital admission, weakness had returned in both arms and legs. She became wheelchair-bound. She was re-admitted to hospital and had another course of intravenous immunoglobulin (0.4 g/kg/day for five days). This was associated with a further but incomplete improvement in that she still had distal limb weakness. A third course of intravenous immunoglobulin was given.

Periods of weakness ensued. Steroid therapy was used with intravenous immunoglobulin, but because there was little evidence of benefit and low-impact fractures occurred, further management was restricted to intravenous immunoglobulin. She has continued to require immunoglobulin therapy for over 10 years. Dosing has been titrated to her strength. She has gone to university and has been working full time in health care.

Diagnosis: Chronic Inflammatory Demyelinating Polyradiculoneuropathy

Comment

Epidemiology and Classification

Peripheral neuropathy is common, occurring in 2% of the population but rising to 8% in those over 55 years of age. Reports of the prevalence of chronic inflammatory demyelinating polyradiculoneuropathy (CIDP) vary from 1 to 9 per 100,000 [1]; in the south-east of England CIDP has a prevalence of ~3 per 100,000, more frequent than multifocal motor neuropathy (MMN) (~0.5 per 100,000) and paraproteinaemic demyelinating neuropathy (~1 per 100,000). Chronic inflammatory demyelinating polyradiculoneuropathy is the most common form of autoimmune polyneuropathy.

Neuropathies can be classified into inherited or acquired (metabolic, immune, neoplastic and infectious). Further characteristics can help to identify the aetiology of a neuropathy (Table 27.1) [2].

In 1982, Peter Dyck described CIDP. However, reports of chronic and recurrent polyneuritis extend back to an 1890 description by Hermann Eichorst, a German neurologist working in Switzerland. The European Federation of Neurological Societies (EFNS)/Peripheral Nerve Society (PNS) diagnostic criteria for CIDP emerged in 2010 and subsequently in 2021 for use in clinical secondary and tertiary settings [3]. However, the diagnosis is challenging and misdiagnosis is common. In addition, 25% of patients may not respond to first-line therapy of steroids, plasma exchange or immunoglobulins [1]. Monitoring a treatment effect is also challenging.

Table 27.1 Classification of peripheral neuropathies

Inherited or acquired	Inherited	Acquired			
		Metabolic	Immune	Neoplastic	Infectious
What nerve	Motor or sensorimotor	Sensory>motor	Variable		
What symptom	Positive neuropathic sensory symptoms uncommon	Positive neuropathic sensory symptoms very common			
Where	Distal, symmetric		Not distal, symmetric		
When	Insidious, gradual onset, slow progression		Definite date of onset, more rapid progression		
What setting	Family history, foot deformities, foot ulcers	Risk factors, diseases or exposures	Symptoms of vasculitis or systemic illness	Symptoms of cancer Paraproteinaemia	Symptom or risk of infection

Table 27.1 (cont.)

Inherited or acquired	Inherited	Acquired			
		Metabolic	Immune	Neoplastic	Infectious
Differential diagnosis	Charcot Marie Tooth disease/ hereditary motor and sensory neuropathy, hereditary liability to pressure palsy	Diabetic Alcohol Ureamic B12 deficiency B1 deficiency Drugs	Non-vasculitic: GBS, CIDP, MMN, Sarcoid, Sjögren, Nodo-paranodopathy Vasculitic: Polyarteritis nodosa, Wegener's granulomatosis, Eosinophilic granulomatosis with polyangiitis, SLE	Paraneoplastic Paraproteinaemic (monoclonal gammopathies)	Hepatitis B and C Lyme HIV Syphilis West Nile Diphtheria Leprosy

Adapted from Mauermann and Burns [2] with permission from Wolters Kluwer Copyright 2009.

CIDP Consensus Criteria

Clinical and electrodiagnostic criteria from the EFNS have been widely accepted as they have high specificity, being able to distinguish CIDP from Lewis–Sumner syndrome, MMN and other chronic neuropathy types [3]. While most patients with CIDP have a chronic onset with a progressive or relapsing course over more than eight weeks, patients with CIDP can present with an acute onset resembling Guillain–Barré syndrome (similar to our patient). Acute-onset CIDP should be suspected if deterioration occurs for more than two months from onset or three treatment-related fluctuations occur (also demonstrated in our patient). It is recognised that 5% of patients initially diagnosed with Guillain–Barré syndrome are later re-classified as having acute-onset CIDP. Such patients are less likely to have facial weakness, respiratory or autonomic nervous system involvement but more likely to have sensory signs than patients with Guillain–Barré syndrome.

The 2021 European Academy of Neurology/PNS guideline on diagnosis of CIDP is itemised in Table 27.2.

Among the CIDP variants, distal CIDP is also known as distal acquired demyelinating symmetric (DADS) neuropathy.

Multifocal CIDP is synonymous with Lewis–Sumner syndrome, which is also known as multifocal acquired demyelinating sensory and motor neuropathy (MADSAM), multifocal demyelinating neuropathy with persistent conduction block or multifocal inflammatory demyelinating neuropathy. Multifocal CIDP usually affects the upper limbs first.

Immunoglobulin M (IgM) paraprotein and anti-myelin associated glycoprotein (MAG) antibodies make a diagnosis of anti-MAG neuropathy. This is not CIDP due to the presence of different electrodiagnostic features, pathology and lack of response to intravenous immunoglobulin and corticosteroids. Similarly, another neuropathy – POEMS or polyneuropathy, organomegaly, endocrinopathy, M-paraprotein and skin changes – can mimic CIDP. However, POEMS is a monoclonal plasma cell proliferative disorder, which is usually associated with monoclonal lambda light chain (95%) usually immunoglobulins A or G (IgA or IgG) and a markedly elevated serum VEGF.

Table 27.2 Clinical criteria for CIDP

Typical CIDP

All of the following

- Progressive or relapsing, symmetric, proximal and distal muscle weakness of upper and lower limbs, and sensory involvement of at least two limbs

- Developing over at least eight weeks

- Absent or reduced tendon reflexes in all limbs

CIDP variants

One of the following, but otherwise as in typical CIDP (tendon reflexes may be normal in unaffected limbs):

- Distal CIDP: distal sensory loss and muscle weakness predominantly in lower limbs

- Multifocal CIDP: sensory loss and muscle weakness in a multifocal pattern, usually asymmetric, upper limb predominant, in more than one limb

- Focal CIDP: sensory loss and muscle weakness in only one limb

- Motor CIDP: motor symptoms and signs without sensory involvement

- Sensory CIDP: sensory symptoms and signs without motor involvement

Adapted from van den Bergh et al. [3] with permission from John Wiley and sons.

Sensory symptoms in the presence of normal motor and sensory nerve conduction studies may be due to chronic immune sensory polyradiculopathy (CISP) because the affected sensory axons are proximal to the dorsal root ganglia. CISP has immune-mediated pathology but it is not clear if the pathology is demyelinating and so CISP is not regarded as a sensory CIDP.

Autoimmune nodopathies are also excluded from the 2021 CIDP diagnostic criteria. Antibodies to contactin-1 (CNTN1), neurofascin 155 (NF155), neurofascin 140/186 (NF140/186) and contactin-associated protein 1 (CASPR1) have been identified in patients fulfilling the 2010 EFNS/PNS criteria for CIDP. However, different pathology and treatments mean that these are now excluded from the CIDP definition.

Electrodiagnostic Investigation of CIDP

Electrodiagnostic investigation is strongly recommended. For typical CIDP sensory conduction abnormalities in two or more nerves can include prolonged distal latency or reduced sensory nerve action potential or slowed conduction velocity. At least one of the following motor conduction abnormalities must also be identified in two or more nerves in typical CIDP: motor distal latency prolongation $\geq$50% above upper limit of normal (except for median nerve); reduction of motor conduction velocity $\geq$30% below lower limit of normal; prolongation of F wave latency $\geq$20% above upper limit of normal ($\geq$50% if amplitude of distal negative peak compound motor action potential (CMAP) <80% of lower limit of normal); absence of F waves (if these nerves have distal negative peak CMAP amplitudes $\geq$20% of lower limit of normal) and one or more demyelinating parameters in one or more nerves. Motor conduction block, abnormal temporal dispersion (>30% duration increase between the proximal and distal negative peak CMAP) and distal CMAP duration prolongation (interval between onset of the first negative peak and return to baseline of the last negative peak) are other electrodiagnostic features strongly supportive of demyelination [3]. The 2021 EFNS/PNS CIDP guideline provides specific electrodiagnostic criteria for the CIDP variants.

The sensitivity of the electrodiagnostic criteria is improved by examining more than four peripheral nerves. Supportive criteria are also recognised. Cerebrospinal fluid with elevated protein and leucocyte count <10/mm^3, MR imaging showing enhancement and hypertrophy of the cauda equina, lumbosacral or cervical nerve roots, or the brachial or lumbosacral plexuses, objective clinical improvement with immunomodulatory treatment and nerve biopsy showing unequivocal evidence of demyelination and/or remyelination by electron microscopy or teased fibre analysis are all recognised supportive criteria for CIDP [3].

Differential Diagnosis of CIDP

Chronic inflammatory demyelinating polyradiculoneuropathy has a large differential diagnosis (Table 27.3). Conditions can mimic typical CIDP, distal CIDP, motor and sensory CIDP and focal or multifocal CIDP.

Table 27.3 Differential diagnosis of CIDP

Typical CIDP	Multifocal and focal CIDP
AL amyloidosis, ATTRv polyneuropathy	Diabetic radiculopathy/plexopathy
CANOMAD	Entrapment neuropathies
Guillain–Barré syndrome	Hereditary neuropathy with pressure palsies
Hepatic neuropathy	MMN
HIV-related neuropathy	Neuralgic amyotrophy
Multiple myeloma	Peripheral nerve tumours (e.g. lymphoma, perineurioma, schwannoma, neurofibroma)
Osteosclerotic myeloma	Vasculitic neuropathy (mononeuritis multiplex)
POEMS syndrome	
Uraemic neuropathy	**Motor CIDP**
Vitamin B12 deficiency (including functional)	Hereditary motor neuropathies (e.g. distal hereditary motor neuropathies, spinal muscular atrophy, porphyria)
Inflammatory myopathies	
Distal CIDP	Motor neurone disease
Anti-MAG IgM neuropathy	Neuromuscular junction disorders (e.g. myasthenia gravis, Lambert–Eaton myasthenic syndrome)
Diabetic neuropathy	
Hereditary neuropathies (CMT1, X1, 4, metachromatic leucodystrophy, Refsum disease, adrenomyeloneuropathy and ATTRv polyneuropathy)	**Sensory CIDP**
POEMS syndrome	Cerebellar ataxia, neuropathy, vestibular areflexia syndrome
Vasculitic neuropathy	CISP
	Dorsal column lesions (e.g. syphilis, paraneoplastic, copper deficiency, vitamin B12 deficiency)
	Hereditary sensory neuropathies
	Idiopathic sensory neuropathy
	Sensory neuronopathy
	Toxic neuropathies (e.g. chemotherapy and vitamin B6 toxicity)

ATTRv: hereditary amyloid transthyretin; CANOMAD: chronic ataxic neuropathy ophthalmoplegia IgM paraprotein cold agglutinins disialosyl antibodies

Adapted from van den Bergh et al. [3] with permission from John Wiley and sons.

Table 27.4 Treatment options for CIDP

Intervention	Comment
Immunoglobulins	Initial dosage 2 g/kg Maintenance 1 g/kg Dose reduction and subcutaneous administration advocated
Corticosteroids	Low evidence level (mostly observational) for treatment with oral or intravenous corticosteroids Prednisolone 1 mg/kg or high-dose 500–1,000 mg methylprednisolone for three to five days
Plasma exchange	Small trials have shown 33–66% of CIDP patients have significant short-term improvement
Other immunotherapies	CIDP patients who do not respond have been treated with cyclophosphamide, ciclosporin, mycophenolate, rituximab, bortezomab and blood stem cell transplantation

Management Options

The first-line treatment options for CIDP include immunoglobulins, corticosteroids and plasma exchange (Table 27.4) [1].

For our patient, regular intravenous immunoglobulin has maintained strength and prevented disability. However, there are no known predictors of disease activity. A treatment cessation trial with close clinical monitoring has been shown to be efficient, cost-effective and safe. Effective treatment of CIDP prevents disability, which is largely determined by axonal damage.

References

1. Fisse AL, Motte J, Grüter T, Sgodzai M, Pitarokoili K, Gold R. Comprehensive approaches for diagnosis, monitoring and treatment of chronic inflammatory demyelinating polyneuropathy. *Neurol Res Pract.* 2020;2(42).
2. Mauermann ML, Burns TM. Pearls and oy-sters: evaluation of peripheral neuropathies. *Neurology.* 2009;72(6):e28–31.
3. van den Bergh PYK, van Doorn PA, Hadden RDM et al. European Academy of Neurology/ Peripheral Nerve Society guideline on diagnosis and treatment of chronic inflammatory demyelinating polyradiculoneuropathy: report of a joint task force – second revision. *Eur J Neurol.* 2021;28(11):3556–83.

Learning Points

- Chronic inflammatory demyelinating polyradiculoneuropathy is the most common chronic inflammatory neuropathy.
- Chronic inflammatory demyelinating polyradiculoneuropathy is a clinical and electrophysiological diagnosis.
- Typical CIDP is a chronic, progressive, stepwise or recurrent symmetrical proximal and distal weakness and sensory dysfunction in all extremities, developing over at least two months.
- There is a wide differential diagnosis of CIDP; misdiagnosis of CIDP is frequent.
- Usual CIDP treatments involve immunoglobulins, corticosteroids and plasma exchange.

Patient's Perspective

1. **What is/was the impact of the condition?**

   a. **Physical (e.g. practical support)**

   At my worst I was unable to walk or use my hands and arms. I relied on my mother for all of my needs to be met and would spend most of the time in bed.

   b. **Psychological (e.g. mood, future, emotional well-being)**

   I was diagnosed at 15 years of age and found it very challenging to go from an independent active teenager to managing the physical impact and consequently the emotional impact of these changes.

   c. **Social (e.g. meeting friends, home)**

   I was very sociable and attended various activities, e.g. cross-country prior to diagnosis. I found the impact of not being able to be as sociable very difficult.

2. **What could you not do because of the condition?**

   I missed out on a lot of special events and 'teenage years'. It restricted me from attending school, and as a result I had to be home-schooled, which left me feeling more socially isolated.

3. **Was there any other change for you due to this medical condition?**

   The impact on my mental health was extremely negative and difficult to manage at times.

4. **What is/was the most difficult aspect of the condition for you?**

   Losing my independence throughout my teenage years and not having the opportunity to complete my education within my school setting.

5. **Was any aspect of the experience good or useful? What was that?**

   I felt that I matured quickly following the diagnosis and I became very aware and in tune with my body and how to care for it.

6. **What do you hope for in the future for your condition?**

   I would hope there would be more treatment options that will enable people with this condition to live as independently as possible.

Increasing Golfing Handicap

History

A 70-year-old right-handed man with a history of stable ocular myasthenia gravis presented with progressive pins and needles in his hands, progressing to numbness over a few months. He described an inability to hold a golf club. He said that if he put his hand into a bag, he would not be sure without visual help if he would take out the intended object. His legs had also started to feel weak. On moving in a certain way, he experienced a stinging electrical shock feeling throughout his body. In the few weeks before a neurological consultation, his right foot had become weak. He also developed bladder urgency but had no problem with his bowels.

Past medical history included acetylcholine receptor antibody-positive ocular myasthenia gravis, a corneal graft, resection of a lumbar schwannoma four years earlier, a right total hip replacement with revision, a left total knee replacement and hypertension.

His medication was ramipril 2.5 mg/day, indapamide slow release 1.5 mg/day, pyridostigmine 30 mg qid and paracetamol.

He was an ex-smoker and drank no alcohol.

Examination

Higher mental function was intact. Pulse was 80 bpm and blood pressure was 183/90 mmHg. He had normal cranial nerves with no ptosis. His walking was slightly unsteady. Tone in all four limbs was mildly increased. He had a proximal asymmetric weakness (weakest at right shoulder abduction grade 4/5, finger abduction grade 3/5, left hip flexion grade 4/5). He was hyper-reflexic in all his limbs and had extensor plantar responses. He had decreased vibration sensation in his right foot but no clear sensory level.

Working Clinical Diagnosis: Cervical Myelopathy

Investigations

An MRI of the spine revealed an extradural soft tissue mass at C2–C3 vertebral bodies extending into the neural exit foramina (Figure 28.1A). The mass extended beneath the posterior longitudinal ligament behind the C2 and C3 vertebral bodies. Although there was no signal change within the cord, the spinal cord was displaced posteriorly (Figure 28.1B).

Management

A C2/C3 decompression was performed. Pathologically, the lesion was identified as a conventional chordoma.

He was clinically and radiologically monitored. A multidisciplinary team suggested radiotherapy (54 Gray in 30 fractions). The extent of disease prevented radical radiotherapy.

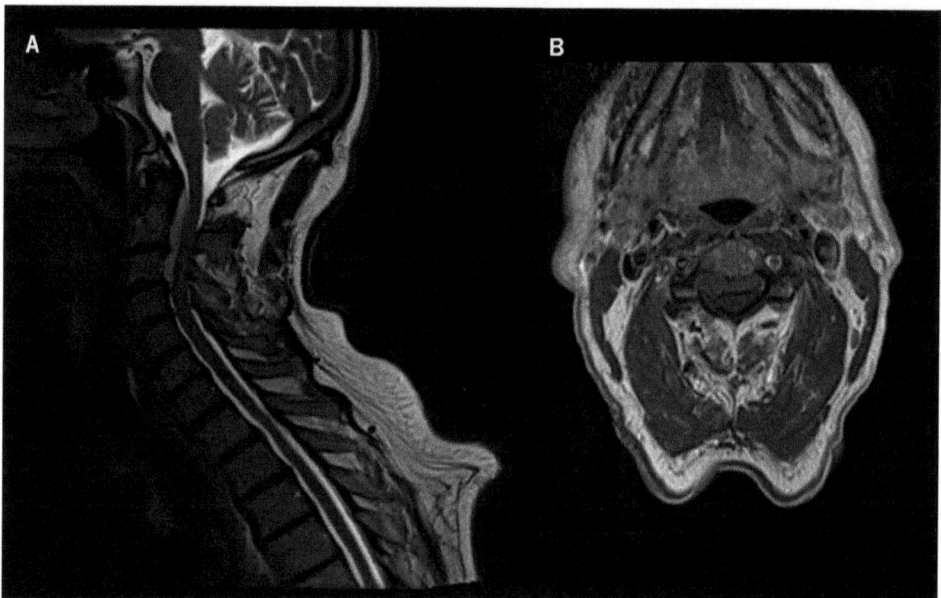

Figure 28.1 (A) A sagittal T2 MRI scan of cervical spine shows an extradural soft tissue mass extending down to C3 and displacing the spinal cord posteriorly. (B) An axial T1 with contrast MRI scan at the level of the upper cervical spine showing a mildly enhancing soft tissue mass displacing the spinal cord posteriorly.

Diagnosis: Cervical Myelopathy Secondary to Cervical Chordoma

Comment

Clinical Features of Myelopathy

Myelopathy is a neurological deficit related to the spinal cord. A simple classification of myelopathy involves compressive and non-compressive spinal cord lesions. The importance of the diagnosis lies in the need for early intervention for both compressive and non-compressive myelopathy in order to improve outcome. The essential clinical features include speed of symptom onset, disease course particularly for medical causes of myelopathy and the MRI appearance. Insidious onset or slowly progressive symptoms can be easily missed and result in diagnostic delay [1].

Clinical Features of Myelopathy

Weakness, spasticity, gait disturbance, clumsiness, hyper-reflexia and pathological reflexes (Hoffman and Babinski reflexes) accompanied by bowel, bladder and sexual dysfunction with a sensory level are the classical features of myelopathy. While the sensory level may not correspond precisely with the location of the vertebral body pathology, lower motor neurone signs (atrophy, hyporeflexia or inverted reflex and fasciculations) may provide a motor level.

Lhermitte's phenomenon is also known as the barber chair syndrome. This is either a tingling or (as in our patient) an electric shock feeling spreading down the arms and legs following neck flexion indicative of cervical spine pathology. However, Lhermitte's phenomenon (which is really a symptom rather than a sign) is not specific for any cervical spine disorder. It is most often reported in demyelination but can occur with vitamin B12 deficiency causing subacute combined deficiency of the cord with and without nitrous oxide exposure, tumour (as in our patient) and other inflammatory cord conditions including zoster myelitis. A reverse Lhermitte's phenomenon is defined by the tingling or electric shock feeling triggered by neck extension.

Functional hemisection of the spinal cord causing damage to one half of the spinal cord is called Brown-Séquard syndrome. Extramedullary (prolapsed cervical disc or tumour) and intramedullary lesions (demyelination and intrinsic spinal cord tumour) can produce this clinical picture. Involvement of the corticospinal tract causes ipsilateral spastic pyramidal weakness and root or anterior horn cell involvement causes segmental lower motor neurone signs at the level of the lesion. There is a dissociated sensory loss due to ipsilateral proprioceptive loss from the dorsal columns and contralateral pain and temperature loss due the early crossing of the spinothalamic tract (Figure 28.2). Brown-Séquard plus syndromes are also recognised. For example, a stab injury to the neck can cause Brown-Séquard plus bladder retention and bilateral extensor plantar responses [2].

Medullary Lesions

Intrinsic or intramedullary causes of myelopathy can be classified as ventral (motor neurone disease), central (trauma) and dorsal (multiple sclerosis, posterior spinal artery syndrome and some spinal epidural haematomas) pathologies.

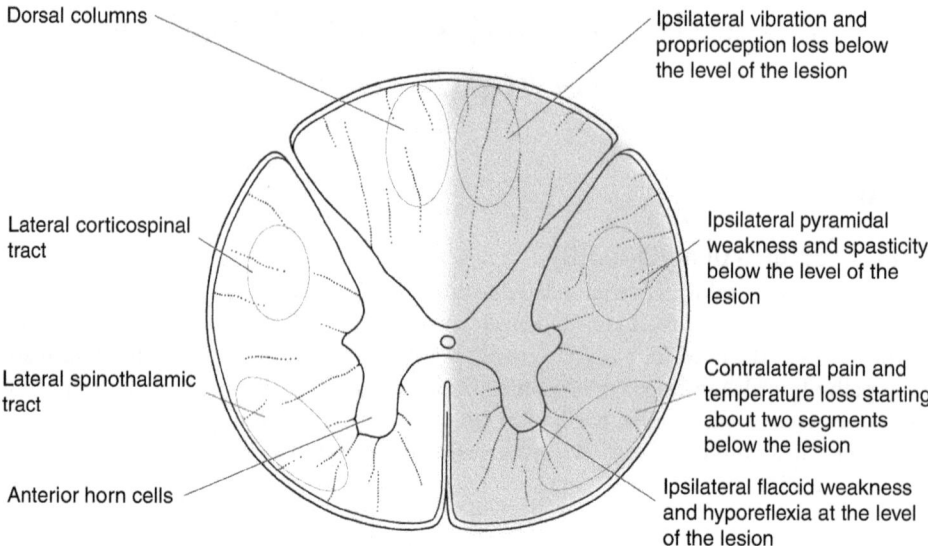

Figure 28.2 Schematic drawing of hemisection and injury to one half of the spinal cord causing Brown-Séquard syndrome.

Causes of Compressive Myelopathy

Degenerative disc disease, tumour and trauma are the major causes of compressive myelopathy. Degenerative disc disease or spondylosis is the most common cause of compressive myelopathy. Cervical spondylosis can present with neck pain (a common and non-specific symptom) and focal neurological symptoms such as numbness, poor co-ordination, poor balance and bladder problems. Cervical spondylosis usually occurs with age when disc herniation, ligament hypertrophy or ossification and osteophyte formation may occur. Worrying differential diagnosis includes tumour (particularly metastases from breast, prostate or lung cancer) and spinal abscess (often accompanied by severe local pain and fever) [3].

Surgical intervention for degenerative disc disease is performed when there is significant neurological dysfunction or progressive instability or deformity of the cervical spine.

Early recognition of metastatic spinal cord disease affects outcome whether treated with surgical decompression, radiotherapy or steroid therapy. Most metastatic cord compressions affect the thoracic cord (70%), next the lumbar spine (20%) and then the cervical spine (10%). Up to 20% of patients presenting de novo with metastatic spinal cord compression may not have had a cancer diagnosis. If ambulatory at presentation, intervention (steroids, radiotherapy or surgery) can preserve mobility in 80% of patients. As 30% of such patients live for a year, preserving ambulatory function can maintain quality of life.

Traumatic Spinal Cord Injury

Road traffic collisions, falls, gunshot or stab wounds and crushing industrial injuries are frequent causes of spinal cord injury. Some sports – diving, skiing, rugby and horseback riding – are implicated in traumatic spinal cord injuries.

Causes of Non-compressive Myelopathy

Myelopathy can occur without compression because of demyelinating, infectious, autoimmune, vascular and metabolic disorders (Table 28.1). The speed of onset can provide a diagnostic clue

[4]. Hyperacute presentation may suggest spinal cord infarction, with an abrupt onset within minutes and usually reaching nadir (maximum deficit) within an hour. An acute myelopathy can progress over days to weeks, but is defined as proceeding to its nadir within 21 days; transverse myelitis is the most common acute or even subacute presentation. Chronic progressive myelopathy may be due to progressive multiple sclerosis but is also seen with dural arteriovenous fistula, sarcoid, B12 deficiency, syphilis and human T cell lymphotropic virus myelitis.

Antibody-mediated disease and improved genetics of hereditary spastic paraplegia have improved specific diagnostic yield in non-compressive causes of myelopathy.

Chordoma

Chordoma is a rare bone tumour of notochordal origin with an estimated incidence of 8 per million per year. First recognised on the dorsum sellae in an autopsy by Rudolf Virchow in 1846, chordomas occur in the skull base (usually with a clival origin), at the centrum of the

Table 28.1 Some causes of non-compressive myelopathy and onset timeline

Cause of spinal cord lesion	Pathologies	Speed of onset	Features
Vascular	Infarction, haemorrhage	Hyperacute	Nadir usually one hour – initial areflexia with mute plantars. Often back pain and sensory level
Trauma		Hyperacute	Measured with American Spinal Injury Association (A–E) impairment scale
Decompression sickness/ Caisson disease		Hyperacute	Nitrogen bubbles in upper thoracic cord
Demyelinating	RRMS, NMOSD	Acute/subacute	
Inflammatory	Sarcoid	Acute/subacute	
Infectious	Syphilis, HTLV-1	Acute/subacute	
Metabolic/nutritional	B12 deficiency, copper deficiency	Subacute	B12 deficiency in Pernicious anaemia and nitrous oxide users Zinc excess from dental fixidents can cause copper deficiency
Vascular	Spinal dural arteriovenous fistula	Subacute/chronic	More common over 50 years and may be exacerbated by exercise or postural change
Neoplastic/ paraneoplastic	Ependymoma, metastases, lymphoma	Subacute/chronic	
Hereditary		Chronic	Hereditary spastic paraplegia panel
Progressive multiple sclerosis		Chronic	

NMOSD: neuromyelitis optica spectrum disorder; RRMS: relapsing-remitting multiple sclerosis mobile spine and in bones in the sacrococcygeal region. The median age of diagnosis is 58.5 years. Chordomas are classified into conventional (as in our patient), chondroid, dedifferentiated and poorly differentiated subtypes. In 1964, it was appreciated that higher doses of radiotherapy prolonged remission. Current management involves surgery and radiotherapy. Conventional chordoma is unresponsive to cytotoxic chemotherapy.

References

1. Davies BM, Mowforth OD, Smith EK, Kotter MRN. Degenerative cervical myelopathy. *BMJ.* 2018;360:8–11.
2. McCarron MO, Flynn PA, Pang KA, Hawkins SA. Traumatic Brown-Séquard-plus syndrome. *Arch Neurol.* 2001;58:1470–2.
3. Theodore N. Degenerative cervical spondylosis. *N Engl J Med.* 2020;383(2):159–68.
4. Mariano R, Flanagan EP, Weinshenker BG, Palace J. A practical approach to the diagnosis of spinal cord lesions. *Pract Neurol.* 2018;18(3):187–200.

Learning Points

*   Myelopathy symptoms include weakness, gait disturbance, clumsiness, sphincter disturbances and sexual dysfunction.
*   Myelopathy signs include weakness (with possible motor level), hyper-reflexia and pathological reflexes (Hoffman's reflex and extensor plantar or positive Babinski sign) accompanied by a sensory level. In the acute setting, reflexes may be absent.
*   Brown-Séquard syndrome causes a classical clinical picture of ipsilateral spastic pyramidal weakness, ipsilateral proprioceptive and vibration loss, and contralateral pain and temperature loss.
*   Common causes of cervical myelopathy include cervical spondylosis and demyelination.

Patient's Perspective

1. **What is/was the impact of the condition?**
    a. Physical (e.g. practical support, activities of daily living, golf)
    Golfing gradually became impossible. I needed to be accompanied on walks in case of tripping. I stopped going to the gym.
    b. Psychological (e.g. mood, emotional well-being)
    I was frustrated due to losing mobility and not knowing what was going on.
    c. Social (e.g. meeting friends, home)
    Family and friends were sympathetic. I avoided going far from home due to the urgency to urinate.
2. **What could you not do because of the condition?**
    *   *Zippers and buttons on clothing*
    *   *Hold/grip a cup of tea*
    *   *Use a knife and fork*
    *   *Get up from a chair*
    *   *Eventually I could not walk without crutches*
3. **Has there been any other change for you due to the condition?**
    Since surgery all symptoms disappeared except for pins and needles in my fingertips.
4. **What is/was the most difficult aspect of the condition?**
    Losing mobility and unable to do things on my own.
5. **Was any aspect of the experience of the condition good or useful? What was that?**
    No.
6. **What do you hope for in the future for people with this condition?**
    Early diagnosis.

History

A 41-year-old man described 'buckling' of his knees when he was laughing while attending a stock-car race. He recovered within seconds. He was sure that he did not lose consciousness. Over the next six months, he had multiple similar episodes, although not all of these seemed to have been associated with emotional change. He was admitted to hospital as he had three episodes in the same day. His partner explained that he could be eating and suddenly his head would drop, his mouth would open and his eyes close. His sister and partner confirmed that he was involuntarily falling asleep much more often during the day. His partner also reported that he was snoring more frequently. The patient described at least one episode of being unable to move while in bed.

Past medical history was unremarkable except for hypertension.

He was taking no medication. He smoked cigarettes and drank up to two litres of vodka per week.

Examination

While sitting in clinic providing the history, he had an event. His head flexed and his arms dropped by his side. His eyes were closed and were rolled up when opened. Cranial nerve and limb examinations following the event were normal.

Epworth sleepiness questionnaire score of 24 confirmed severe excessive symptoms (scores of 16–24 represent severe excessive daytime symptoms).

Two diagnostic tests were performed.

Investigations
Polysomnography

Poor quality of sleep was recorded; sleep was very fragmented with multiple arousals and very little N3 sleep (Figure 29.1).

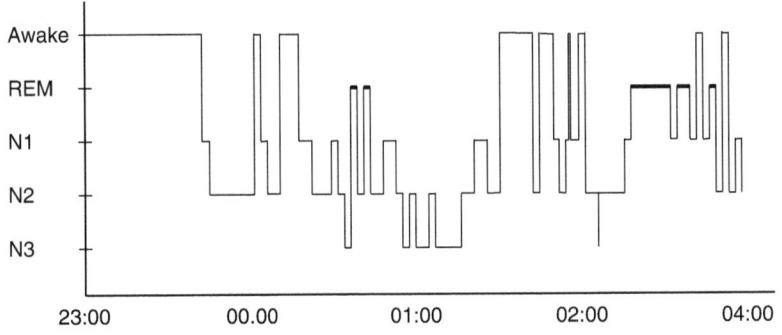

Figure 29.1 A hypnogram demonstrating poor-quality sleep with multiple arousals and very little N3 sleep.

His apnoea hypopnoea index or AHI was 6.6/hour, meaning that more than six episodes of apnoea and hypopnea occurred per hour during sleep These were associated with significant oxygen desaturations to as low as 86.9%, followed by arousals and re-saturation.

Multiple sleep latency testing (MSLT) was performed (Table 29.1).

Narcolepsy was confirmed based on the third edition of the International Sleep Disorder Classification.

Table 29.1 Multiple sleep latency and sleep onset rapid eye movement test results

Test	Result	Diagnostic of narcolepsy
Mean sleep latency	2 minutes 45 seconds	<8 minutes
Sleep onset rapid eye movement time (mean of 3)	3 minutes 20 seconds	<15 minutes

Diagnoses: 1. Type 1 Narcolepsy (i.e. Narcolepsy with Cataplexy)
2. Obstructive Sleep Apnoea

Management

Behavioural and pharmacological interventions were used. A short nap early in the afternoon helped. He was also treated for co-existent obstructive sleep apnoea with continuous positive airway pressure or CPAP until it was no longer required. He markedly reduced his alcohol intake.

Cataplexy was treated with sodium oxybate (the sodium salt of γ-hydroxybutyrate). This drug was obtained via an independent funding request. This highly sedating liquid taken at bedtime and 2.5–4 hours later was very helpful for the cataplexy. Venlafaxine has also helped his cataplexy.

Nine years later, he continued on both sodium oxybate 9 g per night in two divided doses and venlafaxine 150 mg per day. Cataplexy episodes had become much less frequent. His weight had reduced from 87 kg to 74 kg, and his quality of life had markedly improved.

Comment

Definition and Epidemiology of Obstructive Sleep Apnoea

Obstructive sleep apnoea causes recurrent collapse of the upper airway while sleeping, leading to recurrent episodes of hypoxia, hypercapnia and awakenings. Obstructive sleep apnoea is common, affecting nearly a billion adults globally. Prevalence of obstructive sleep apnoea is positively related to age and body mass index.

Apnoea is a cessation of airflow for at least 10 seconds. Hypopnoea is a 30% or more reduction in airflow or thoraco-abdominal excursion with at least 3% oxygen desaturation from baseline or an arousal. The AHI is the number of apnoeas plus hypopnoeas per hour of sleep time and defines the absence or presence and severity of obstructive sleep apnoea. AHI values ≥ 5 and <15 represent mild obstructive sleep apnoea, AHI ≥ 15 and <30 represent moderate obstructive sleep apnoea while AHI ≥ 30 is severe obstructive sleep apnoea.

Neurological Associations of Obstructive Sleep Apnoea

Obstructive sleep apnoea can remain undiagnosed for years, leading to increased risk of cardiovascular disease – hypertension, atrial fibrillation, pulmonary hypertension and ischaemic heart disease.

Neurological associations of obstructive sleep apnoea include headache, stroke, cluster headache (60–80% of patients compared to 15% in the general population), epilepsy and Parkinson's disease [1]. Apnoeas may cause an arousal from sleep and contribute to parasomnias. Treatment with CPAP can reduce morning headache, but no such evidence outside of case reports exists for cluster headache. Improved treatment of obstructive sleep apnoea can improve seizure control.

Definition and Epidemiology of Narcolepsy

Carl Westphal, Jean Baptiste Edouard Gélineau and Franz Fischer described narcolepsy between 1877 and 1880. Narcolepsy, which means 'to be seized by somnolence', is a common chronic sleepiness that affects 200–500 per million in Europe and North America [2]. It usually begins between the ages of 10 and 20 years, but there is often a 5–10-year delay from symptom onset until diagnosis. Narcolepsy is divided into type 1 narcolepsy, which is associated with cataplexy (sudden paralysis of most voluntary muscle usually in a rostral to caudal pattern) and low levels of hypocretin-1 (also known as orexin-A) in the cerebrospinal fluid (CSF). Type 2 narcolepsy, in which there is no cataplexy and normal CSF hypocretin-1 levels, is less well understood. Although remission is unlikely, age decreases the severity of excessive daytime sleepiness and cataplexy.

In narcolepsy, the regulation of rapid eye movement (REM) sleep is disturbed. The normal pattern of sleep stages is disrupted. REM sleep is characterised by saccadic or rapid eye movements, dreams and paralysis of most skeletal muscles. In narcolepsy, REM sleep can intrude at any time of the day. Our patient also had cataplexy, from the Greek 'kata' (down) and 'plak' (strike), reflecting brief episodes of voluntary muscle paralysis associated with REM sleep when the patient expects or experiences a positive emotion (such as enjoying stock-car racing for our patient). The other features of sleep paralysis (present in our patient) and hypnagogic hallucinations (occurring at night while falling asleep) can occur occasionally in the general population, but these features are less discriminating in making a clinical diagnosis than a history of cataplexy. Hypnopompic hallucinations occur in the morning on wakening up but are not as frequent in the general population as hypnagogic hallucinations.

The third edition of the International Classification of Sleep Disorders recognises narcolepsy if a subject has periods during daytime of an irrepressible need to sleep or actual lapses into sleep occurring for at least three months on a daily basis. Type 1 narcolepsy is diagnosed by either CSF hypocretin-1 deficiency (<110 pg/mL, or less than one-third of normative values on a standardised assay), or a mean sleep latency of <8 minutes and two sleep onset REM periods (SOREMPs) within 15 minutes of sleep onset on MSLT and/or overnight polysomnography, along with a clear history of cataplexy. Narcolepsy type 2 has the same MSLT and SOREMP criteria except cataplexy and/or CSF hypocretin-1 deficiency are not present.

Laughter and other happy or enjoyable emotions can trigger cataplexy; less often it is triggered by fear or anger emotions. Circuits from the medial frontal cortex and amygdala to the pons have been implicated in cataplexy.

The differential diagnosis of cataplexy includes: normal weakness when laughing, pseudocataplexy (negative emotion causing collapse but no head bobbing), laughter-induced syncope, gelastic seizures and hyperekplexia (increased startle and stiffness with sudden acoustic stimuli).

Pathology of Narcolepsy

In 1999, a mutation in a hypocretin receptor gene was implicated in familial canine narcolepsy. Despite the recognition of loss of hypocretin-1-producing neurones from the lateral hypothalamus in humans, no CSF or MRI markers of damage have been identified in narcolepsy. There are about 60,000 hypocretin-1-producing neurones; 90% of these neurones are lost in type 1 narcolepsy. Narcolepsy demonstrates seasonal variation; it most commonly occurs in late spring, possibly following a winter infection. The H1N1 influenza pandemic of 2009–10 suggested that narcolepsy has an immune-mediated basis. A vaccine (H1N1 Pandemrix) with a potent adjuvant was widely used in Scandinavia. One to two months after the vaccination, there was a dramatic increase (up to 12-fold) in the number of new cases of narcolepsy in young people with the human leukocyte antigen (HLA)-DQB1*06:02 allele (present in 98% of type 1 and 50% of type 2 narcolepsy patients but in only 12–30% of the general population). There was also a three-fold surge in new cases of narcolepsy in China, but not in Taiwan following the H1N1 infection of 2009–10 [3]. In summary, the HLA-DQB1*06:02 allele combined with young age and a particular immune stimulus seem to promote narcolepsy presentations. However, only 1 in 1,000 carriers of HLA-DQB1*06:02 develop narcolepsy. Narcolepsy has also been documented following traumatic brain injury [2].

Future research is directed at identifying the pathological process that destroys hypocretin-1-producing neurones.

Treatment

As in our patient, a short nap and good-quality nocturnal sleep can help many patients with narcolepsy. Drugs, which promote wakefulness, provide benefit. Modafinil reduces re-uptake of dopamine. Dextroamphetamine blocks re-uptake and increases the release of dopamine. Slow-release preparations can reduce drug abuse. Pitolisant, an inverse type 3 histamine receptor agonist can enhance wakefulness and is moderately effective for cataplexy. Venlafaxine and clomipramine are useful in treating cataplexy by increasing brainstem monoamines to suppress REM sleep. Sodium oxybate is effective at reducing cataplexy and daytime sleepiness. At full dose (as used by our patient – 4.5 g just before bedtime and then a second dose at 03:00), sodium oxybate can abolish 90% of cataplectic episodes. Activation of GABA-B receptors to enhance deep slow wave nocturnal sleep may explain how sodium oxybate produces very deep non-REM sleep.

Driving and Narcolepsy

Narcolepsy is another neurological disease that has driving implications. The UK Driver and Vehicle Licensing Agency (DVLA) guidelines for narcolepsy state that Group 1 car and motorcycle drivers 'must not drive and must notify the DVLA'. The guidelines go on to state '[a] licence may be reissued only when there has been satisfactory symptom control for at least three months before being considered for re-licensing. When an applicant or licence holder is not on appropriate treatment, relicensing may be considered after satisfactory objective assessment of maintained wakefulness, such as the OSLER [Oxford Sleep Resistance] test.' (Available at www.gov.uk/government/publications/assessing-fitness-to-drive-a-guide-for-medical-professionals.) The OSLER test assesses an individual's ability to maintain wakefulness and daytime vigilance.

Similar rules apply to Group 2 bus and lorry drivers with narcolepsy. However, in addition to the standards for group 1 licensing, 'relicensing may be considered subject to specialised assessment and a satisfactory objective assessment of maintained wakefulness, such as the OSLER test'.

Sleep Disorders and the Hypothalamus

While narcolepsy is the major sleep disorder due to hypothalamic pathology, other disorders may also involve hypothalamic damage. Kleine–Levin syndrome (hypersomnolence, compulsive hyperphagia and behavioural change such as an abnormally uninhibited sexual drive), ROHHAD (rapid-onset obesity with hypothalamic dysfunction, hypoventilation and autonomic dysregulation) and Prader–Willi syndrome (due to a genetic imprinting error causing a multisystem disorder with overeating, cognitive and behavioural problems) are other hypothalamic syndromes with sleep-related symptoms similar to narcolepsy.

Anti-IgLON5 Syndrome

Anti-IgLON5 syndrome is an important but rare differential diagnosis for sleep disturbance (non-REM and REM parasomnias) with a variety of neurological manifestations. Autoimmune and neurodegenerative pathophysiology have been implicated. Anti-IgLON5 syndrome, first recognised in 2014, causes sleep dysfunction, a progressive supranuclear palsy-like syndrome, a movement disorder such as chorea, brainstem and hypothalamic dysfunction causing dysphagia, dysarthria and autonomic dysfunction. Polysomnography shows abnormal sleep architecture, poorly differentiated non-REM sleep, REM sleep behaviour disorder, central hypoventilation, stridor and obstructive sleep apnoea. IgLON5 is a neuronal cell adhesion molecule widely expressed in the central nervous system. Neuronal loss, gliosis and accumulation of hyperphosphorylated neuronal tau (3-repeat and 4-repeat isoforms) have been found predominantly in the hypothalamus and tegmental brainstem nuclei. There is also a strong association with the HLA-DRB1*10:01 and DQB1*05:01 alleles.

References

1.   Cheng S, Stark CD, Stark RJ. Sleep apnoea and the neurologist. *Pract Neurol.* 2017;17(1):21–7.
2.   Bassetti CLA, Adamantidis A, Burdakov D et al. Narcolepsy – clinical spectrum, aetiopathophysiology, diagnosis and treatment. *Nat Rev Neurol.* 2019;15(9):519–39.
3.   Han F, Lin L, Warby SC et al. Narcolepsy onset is seasonal and increased following the 2009 H1N1 pandemic in China. *Ann Neurol.* 2011 Sep.;70(3):410–17.

Learning Points

- Obstructive sleep apnoea is a type of sleep-disordered breathing that causes hypopnoea and apnoea and has important neurological associations.
- Narcolepsy causes sleep dysregulation manifesting as excessive daytime sleepiness, cataplexy, hallucinations, sleep paralysis and disturbed sleep.
- Multiple hits from genetic and environmental factors as well as triggering events are implicated in the pathogenesis of narcolepsy.
- Cataplexy with narcolepsy constitutes type 1 narcolepsy and is associated with selective loss or dysfunction of hypocretin-1 neurones in the lateral hypothalamus causing profound deficiency of hypocretin-1 in the CSF.
- Sodium oxybate is the most effective treatment for cataplexy.
- Primary hypersomnias result in important driving restrictions.

Patient's Perspective

1.   **What is/was the impact of the condition?**

    a. Physical (e.g. practical support, looking after yourself)
    I have narcolepsy with cataplexy. It affected me physically by falling asleep randomly without warning. I was unable to walk and suffered a lot of falls, unable to walk upstairs, loss of control of my body by falling to the ground limp, unable to speak or move or express emotions.

    b. Psychological (e.g. mood, emotional well-being)
    It left me very depressed, as I was unable to do anything, including hobbies I once enjoyed, such as fishing. I was scared as no-one knew what was wrong with me and I felt worthless and a burden on my family.

c. Social (e.g. meeting friends or family, homelife)

I was unable to go out socially, as I would just fall. I was unable to talk or move. I was unable to go across to the shop, trapped in the house needing 24 hour supervision.

2. **What could you not do because of the condition?**

I could not walk, talk, eat, work. I couldn't make my own meals, I could no longer shower or bath unaccompanied. I couldn't hold a baby, couldn't hold a cup and had to have my food cut up.

3. **Was there any other change for you due to your medical condition?**

I put on a lot of weight, about three stone due to inactivity and unable to move. I suffered a lot of head injuries, bruises and cuts due to falls.

4. **What is/was the most difficult aspect of the condition for you?**

I was not able to do daily activities like walking, talking and laughing without having an attack. The fear of not knowing what was wrong, feeling I was dying. I lost all dignity, becoming dependent on others to wash, feed and monitor me.

5. **Was any aspect of the experience of the condition good or useful? What was that?**

No, it was the worst time of my life. I have never felt so low or worthless. The best thing was getting diagnosed and starting medication, giving me back some normality and quality of life.

6. **What do you hope for in the future for people with this condition?**

That people do not need to go so long without being diagnosed and receiving treatment. That better medication can be found as although a lot better, I still take attacks but not as frequent.

30 Covalent Cascade

History

A 71-year-old man was admitted to hospital with a five-week history of progressive unsteadiness and cognitive decline. He had worked as an electrician and often cycled 25 miles per day. Three weeks before admission he took three hours to change a washer on a water-tap, a procedure that he would have previously completed much more quickly. His wife and daughter had noticed increasing unsteadiness, slowness in using his mobile phone and decreasing communication. He had an unremarkable past medical history. He was a non-smoker and consumed no more than a glass of wine per week.

Examination

He was dyspraxic, having difficulty using his phone. He was orientated in year but not in day or month. He was mildly dysphasic but he was able to recount his history of unsteadiness. His visual acuity was 6/24 on the right and 6/12 on the left, both unaided. He had vertical gaze-evoked nystagmus and had impaired saccades. He had mild dysarthria and at times he had an occasional truncal jerk. He had left finger nose ataxia but no dysdiadochokinesia as his rapid alternate movements were intact. He had a broad-based gait and was unsteady on mobilising independently. He had bilateral heel shin ataxia. He had normal strength, reflexes and sensation. Plantar responses were flexor.

An investigation plan was devised.

Investigations

An MRI of the brain showed diffuse high signal (fluid-attenuated inversion recovery (FLAIR) and diffusion-weighted imaging (DWI)) in the cortex, more frontally with corresponding low signal on the apparent diffusion coefficient (ADC) map (Figure 30.1).

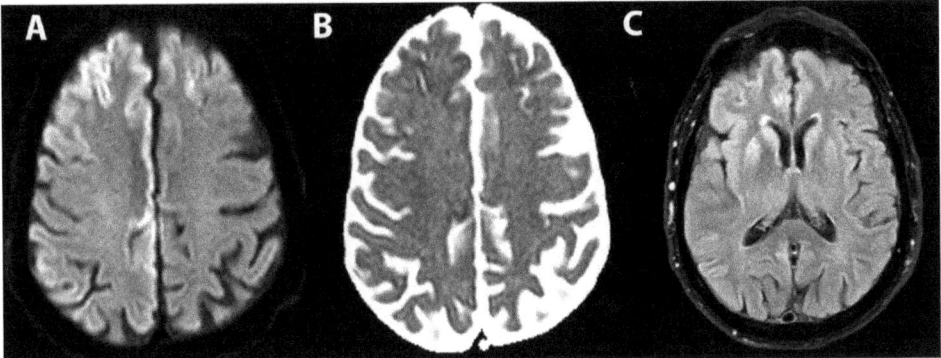

Figure 30.1 An axial MRI scan of the brain showing (A) high signal on diffusion-weighted imaging in the right cortex including parasagittal cortex, (B) restricted diffusion in the same cortical distribution and (C) high T2 signal in the caudate and putamen, particularly on the right.

EEG had a satisfactory background over the left hemisphere with an excess of slow waves, more notable over the right hemisphere (even numbered electrodes). Semi-periodic sharp waves were seen maximally over the right frontal region (Figure 30.2).

A lumbar puncture was carried out. Cerebrospinal fluid (CSF) had <1 white cell/µL and 525 red cells/µL. CSF protein was 0.46 g/L, CSF glucose was 3.7 mmol/L and plasma glucose was 5.4 mmol/L. PCR testing for herpes simplex viruses 1 and 2, varicella zoster virus, parechovirus, *Streptococcus pneumonia*, *Haemophilus influenzae* and *Neisseria meningitidis* was negative.

Among blood investigations, full blood count, CRP, electrolytes, liver function tests, thyroid profile, B12, folate and nuclear autoantibody screen were normal. A paraneoplastic screen (Hu, Yo and Ri), alpha-amino-3-hydroxy-5-methyl-4-isoxazolepropionic acide (AMPA) receptor, leucine-rich glioma-inactivated 1 (LGI1), contactin-associated protein-like 2 (CASPR2), n-methyl-D-aspartate receptor (NMDAR), glycine receptor and glutamic acid decarboxylases (GAD) antibodies were all negative. HIV and hepatitis screens were negative.

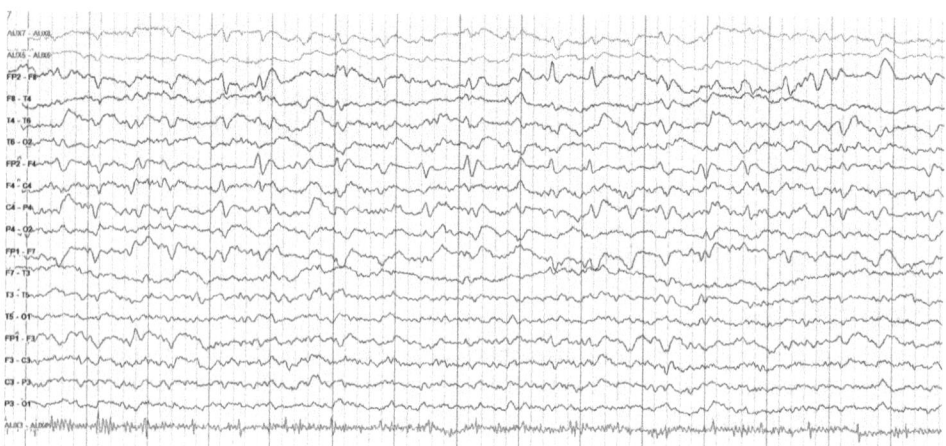

Figure 30.2 EEG shows an excess of slow waves over the left hemisphere and more so over the right hemisphere with some frontal periodicity.

Diagnosis: Probable Sporadic Creutzfeldt–Jakob Disease

Outcome and Investigation Results

Within a week he had become mute and was no longer mobile. He was referred to the national UK Creutzfeldt–Jakob Disease (CJD) surveillance unit. He had a remote telelink assessment.

Because of his rapid deterioration, he was transferred to a hospice and died there. No autopsy was performed.

Subsequent results from CSF obtained after death included a positive 14–3–3 protein and a positive real-time quaking-induced conversion (RT-QuIC) assay.

The complete open reading frame of the prion protein gene was sequenced and no mutations were identified. Prion protein codon 129 genotype was methionine valine (MV) heterozygous.

Comment

In 1920 in Leipzig, Alfons Maria Jakob (1884–1931) described three unrelated adults with spasticity and progressive dementia with cortical, striatal and spinal degeneration. Hans Gerhard Creutzfeldt (1885–1964) independently reported a similar disease in a 22-year-old woman in the same year. Creutzfeldt–Jakob disease is the most common form of prion disease (previously called spongiform encephalopathy). Brain tissue from patients with CJD contains aggregates of abnormal host-derived prion protein and a histopathological triad of spongiform changes, neuronal loss and gliosis [1].

Clinical Presentation

Rapidly progressive dementia (less than two years duration) is the hallmark of sporadic CJD. Other frequent symptoms include hallucinations, myoclonus, ataxia (all present in our patient from early on in hospital admission) and rigidity.

Epidemiology

The annual incidence of all human prion diseases is estimated at 1 per million per year. This figure is thought to be stable throughout the world. The peak age of onset of sporadic CJD is 65–74 years with almost equal sex distribution. There is a spectrum of human prion diseases recognised as idiopathic, familial and acquired prion diseases (Table 30.1) [2]. Prion disease, despite being rare, is a public health threat, as prions are resistant to inactivation and can transmit disease not only from one human to another but also, as vividly demonstrated in variant CJD, from animals to humans. Infection from animals to humans was identified in the UK as the cause of variant CJD by the CJD surveillance unit in 1995 in Edinburgh.

The differential diagnosis of CJD can include other neurodegenerative diseases, autoimmune/paraneoplastic encephalopathy, lymphoma and infections. Accurate diagnosis is crucial to avoid a misdiagnosis of a treatable disorder [3].

Pathology

Stanley Prusiner, an American neurologist, proposed in 1982 that all transmissible spongiform encephalopathies were due to proteinaceous infectious molecules free of nucleic acid and these are called prions. The discovery earned him the Nobel Prize for Medicine and Physiology in 1997.

Table 30.1 The spectrum of human prion disease

Group	Type of human prion disease
Idiopathic (85%)	Sporadic CJD Sporadic fatal insomnia Variably protease-sensitive prionopathy
Familial (15%)	Genetic CJD Fatal familial insomnia Gerstmann–Sträussler–Scheinker disease
Acquired	Kuru Variant CJD (ingestion of beef from cattle with prion disease) Iatrogenic CJD (dura mater, cornea and human pituitary gland-derived growth hormone)

Conformational conversion of the normal cellular prion protein (PrP^c (c denoting cellular)) into an extended misfolded β-pleated sheet pathological structure (scapie PrP or PrP^{sc}) results in a disease-associated PrP. The cause of sporadic disease remains speculative, but may result from a failure of a system known as the quality-control complex or proteostasis network. This may then result in release of misfolded PrP.

Sporadic prion disease has three distinct phenotypes: CJD, fatal insomnia and variable protease-sensitive prionopathy. The prion protein gene (*PRNP*) codon 129 polymorphism (MV) partially explains the different phenotypes. In addition, electrophoretic mobility of abnormally folded PrP after protease digestion yields two patterns – types 1 and 2 immunoblots. Ninety per cent of patients with sporadic CJD who are codon 129 methionine methionine (MM) have type 1 PrP^{sc} and more than 80% of patients with sporadic CJD who are 129 valine valine (VV) and 129MV have type 2 PrP^{sc}. The most common sporadic CJD sub-types are MM1, MV1, VV2 and MV2 [1].

Neuroimaging of CJD

High signal on DWI and FLAIR sequences in parts of the cerebral cortex (known as 'cortical ribboning'), basal ganglia and thalami are MRI features of CJD. The diffusion-weighted changes have a 91% sensitivity and 97% specificity for CJD. These MRI changes can occur at early stages of disease and can help in diagnosis. It is important however to bear in mind that immune-mediated encephalitides and focal seizures can show similar cortical changes.

Cerebrospinal Fluid in CJD

Real-time quaking-induced conversion of CSF is an in vitro prion amplification technique, which has a sensitivity of 95% and a specificity of 100%. Pathological PrP^{sc} acts as a seed for the propagation of more misfolded proteins derived from normal or recombinant protein. Repeated cycles of aggregate sonification or high-frequency shaking (RT-QuIC) amplify new seeds [1]. Cerebrospinal fluid 14–3–3 protein has a lower specificity (80%) for sporadic CJD. RT-QuIC can detect a minute amount of pathological prion protein in the CSF and has been added to the diagnostic criteria of CJD. Positive skin RT-QuIC assays suggest skin prion-seeding activity may be another diagnostic biomarker.

EEG in CJD

The progression of EEG abnormalities may be very rapid, as shown in another patient with sporadic CJD (Figure 30.3). The first EEG shows that the background was slower over the

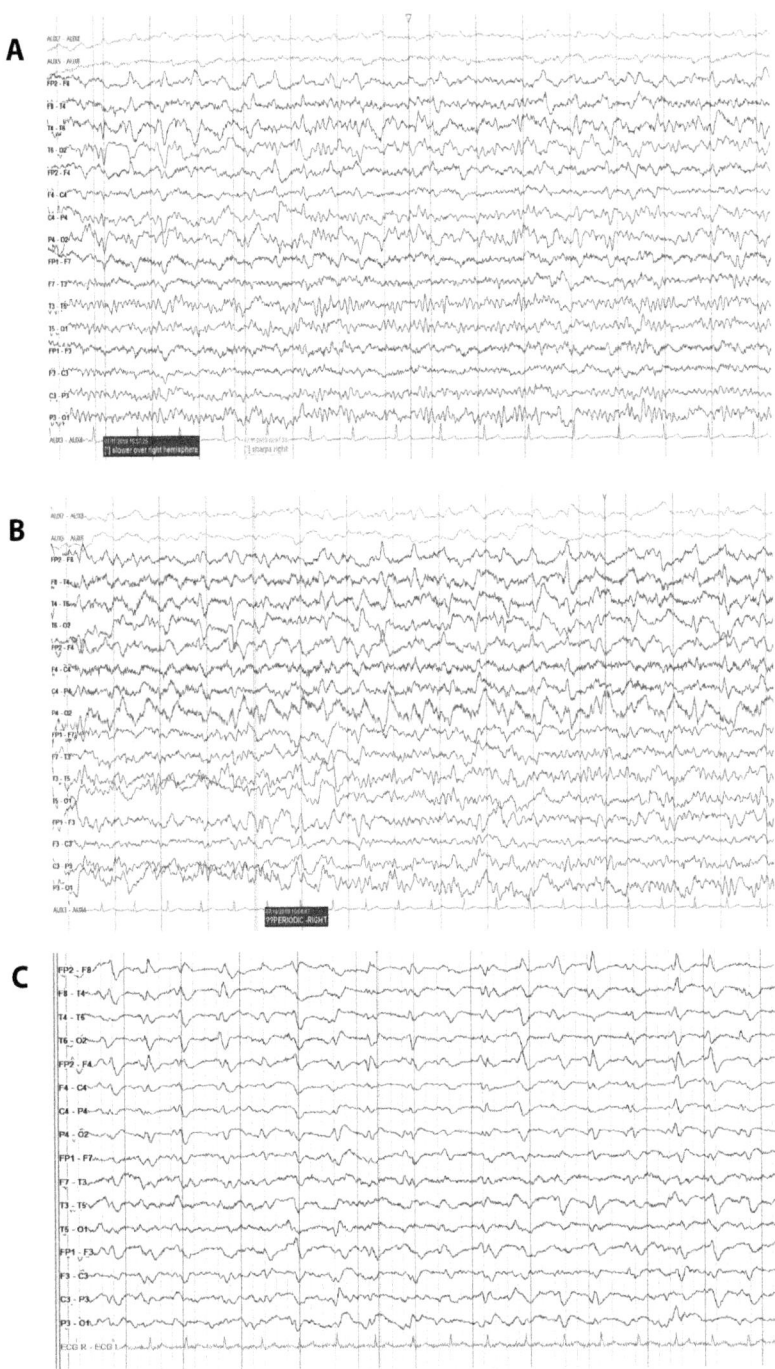

Figure 30.3 EEG progression over 15 days in another patient with (A) initial slowing on the right to (B) becoming more periodic on the right followed by (C) further bilateral slowing and marked periodicity.

right hemisphere with frequent sharp waves. The middle EEG was taken eight days later and shows that the slowing was more extensive involving the left hemisphere. The third EEG one week later shows marked slowing and periodicity.

Periodic sharp wave discharges have a reported sensitivity of just 67% and specificity of 86%. Periodic sharp wave complexes occur in the middle to late stages of disease. The periodic sharp wave complexes may be lateralised in earlier stages. Overall periodic sharp wave complexes are present in about two-thirds of patients with sporadic CJD; they are present in patients with codon 129MM and 129MV, but rarely in patients with 129VV homozygosity. Periodic sharp wave complexes tend to disappear in sleep and are attenuated with sedative medication and external stimulation. Typical periodic sharp wave complexes are uncommon in genetic CJD and do not occur in variant CJD.

Diagnostic Criteria

Criteria for sporadic CJD have been developed (www.cjd.ed.ac.uk/surveillance). A definite diagnosis requires a progressive neurological syndrome along with at least one of neuropathological, immunocytochemical or biochemical confirmation.

A probable diagnosis of CJD can be made in a patient with a rapidly progressive neurological syndrome and a positive RT-QuIC from CSF or other tissues. The typical EEG (generalised periodic complexes) or MRI brain findings (high DWI or FLAIR signal in caudate/putamen or at least two cortical regions) in the context of rapidly progressive cognitive impairment plus two clinical features from 1. myoclonus; 2. visual or cerebellar problems; 3. pyramidal or extrapyramidal features; and 4. akinetic mutism also make a diagnosis of probable CJD. Cerebrospinal fluid 14–3–3 analysis is no longer provided by the UK national CJD research and surveillance unit (NCJDRSU) since April 2022.

Treatment and Outcome

Creutzfeldt–Jakob disease is currently untreatable and invariably fatal. The NCJDRSU monitors the epidemiology of all forms of CJD and their experience contributes to an improving quality of care (www.cjd.ed.ac.uk).

References

1. Zerr I. Laboratory diagnosis of Creutzfeldt–Jakob disease. *N Engl J Med*. 2022.;386(14):1345–50.
2. Puoti G, Bizzi A, Forloni G et al. Sporadic human prion diseases: molecular insights and diagnosis. *Lancet Neurol*. 2012;11(7):618–28.
3. Chitravas N, Jung RS, Kofskey DM et al. Treatable neurological disorders misdiagnosed as Creutzfeldt–Jakob disease. *Ann Neurol*. 2011;70(3):437–44.

Learning Points

- Prion diseases are a group of rare, rapidly progressive, currently untreatable and fatal neurodegenerative diseases.
- Prion diseases occur as sporadic, genetic/familial, variant and iatrogenic forms.
- Diffusion-weighted MRI of the brain, EEG and CSF analyses can help make a probable diagnosis in the correct clinical setting.
- Real-time quaking-induced conversion of CSF has had a specificity of 100% for CJD in most series.

Perspective from the Patient's Daughter

1. **What was the impact of the condition on your father?**

   In the early stages – dizziness, forgetfulness, unsteady on his feet, unable to do simple things like use a phone or a TV remote control.

   Later stages – loss of speech, not able to walk, incontinence and difficulty breathing.

2. **What was the impact of the condition on your family?**

   A terrible shock to see such a healthy man deteriorate so rapidly. It was also difficult that so little is known about the disease and nothing could be done.

3. **What was the most difficult aspect of the condition for you and your family?**

   We couldn't say goodbye or discuss any last wishes because he wasn't able to speak or understand. [The initial COVID 19 pandemic surge prevented hospital visits.]

4. **Was any aspect of the experience good or useful? What was that?**

   My father became very carefree in the early stages. He showed no worry or concern throughout the illness. He never realised he was going to die and was very content.

5. **What do you hope for in the future for people with this condition?**

   That a cure can be found.

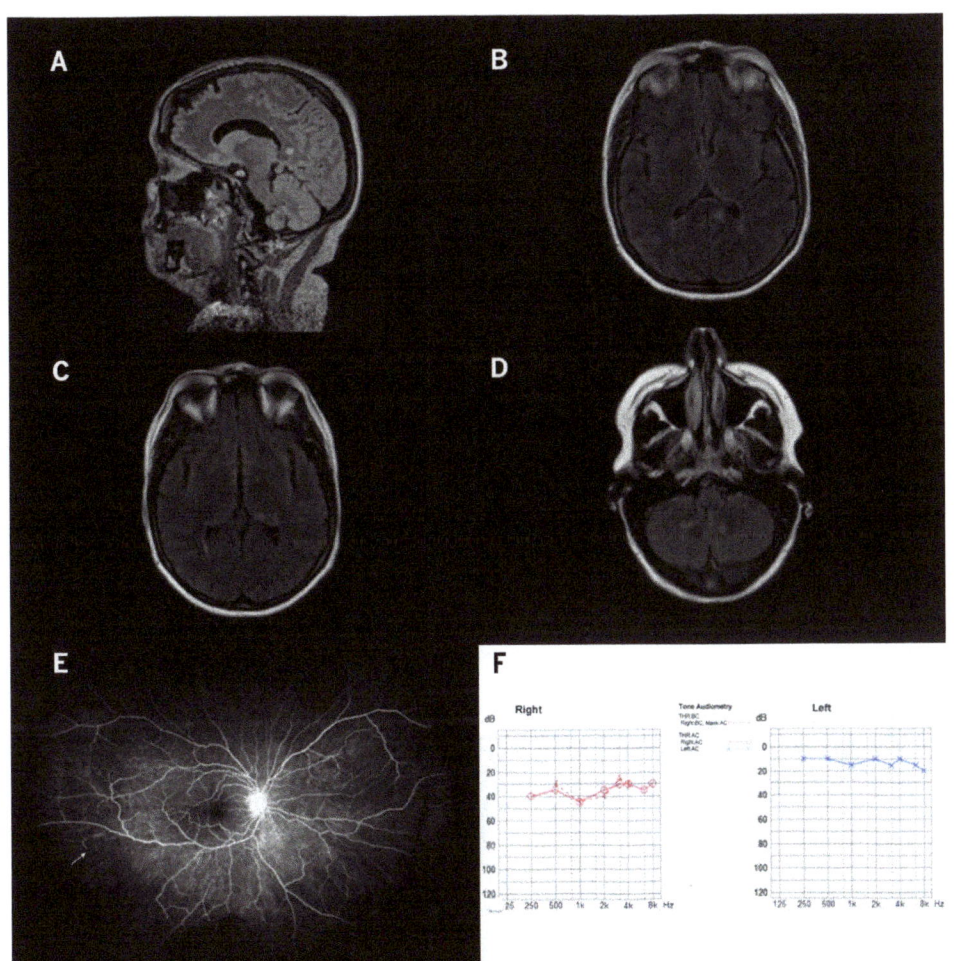

Figure 3.1 A (A) sagittal and (B) axial T2 FLAIR MRI scan of the brain, showing corpus callosal lesions. An axial MRI brain showing pulvinar lesion in (C) the left thalamus and (D) bilateral cerebellar lesions. Fluorescein angiography (E) shows a BRAO (arrow). (F) Audiometry demonstrates a right hearing deficit more prominent at lower frequencies.

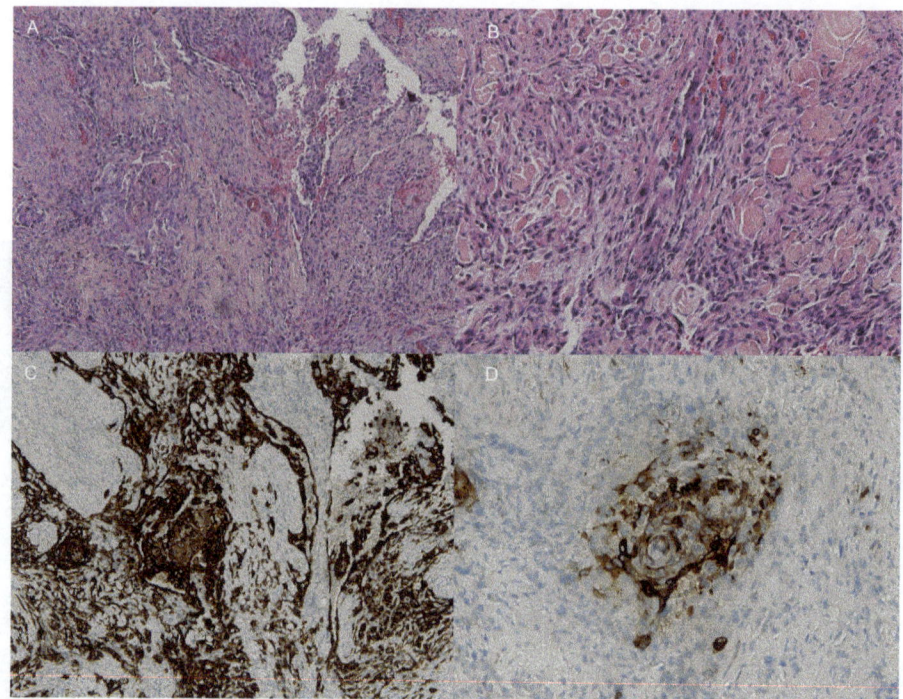

Figure 5.1 (A) Histology of the canthal tissue biopsy shows granulation tissue that is infiltrated by pleomorphic squamoid cells exhibiting dense eosinophilic cytoplasm, intercellular bridges and some keratinisation is seen focally. These atypical cells form nests and large groups with irregular contours as well as trabeculae and single cell forms. (B) Focally, sarcomatoid morphology with elongated spindle cell-like appearances and conspicuous mitotic figures are seen. There are also entrapped skeletal muscle bundles. (C) Cytokeratin 5/6 immunohistochemistry confirms the squamous phenotype of the lesional cells and highlights the tumour silhouette. (D) Epithelial membrane antigen immunohistochemistry shows patchy focal positivity that is consistent with squamous cell carcinoma.

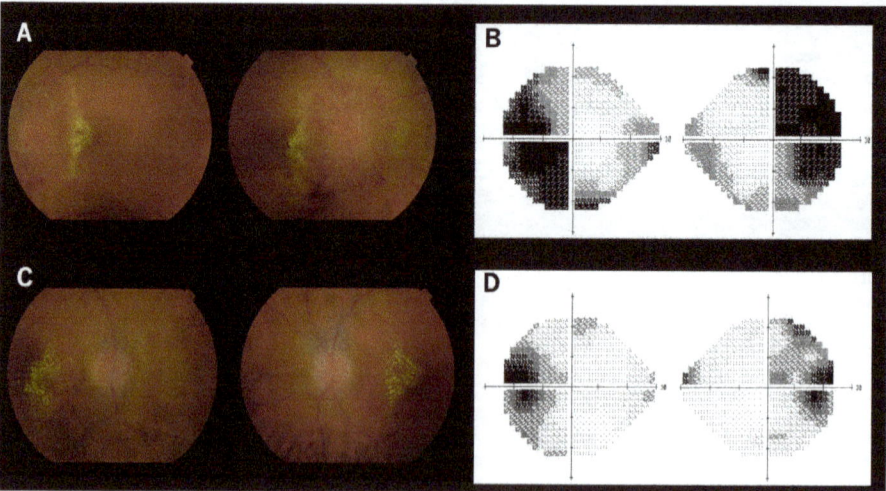

Figure 6.1 (A) Funduscopic photographs showing marked optic disc swelling alongside (B) perimetry showing predominantly bitemporal visual field constriction. Following shunt insertion, the (C) optic discs and (D) visual field appearances improved.

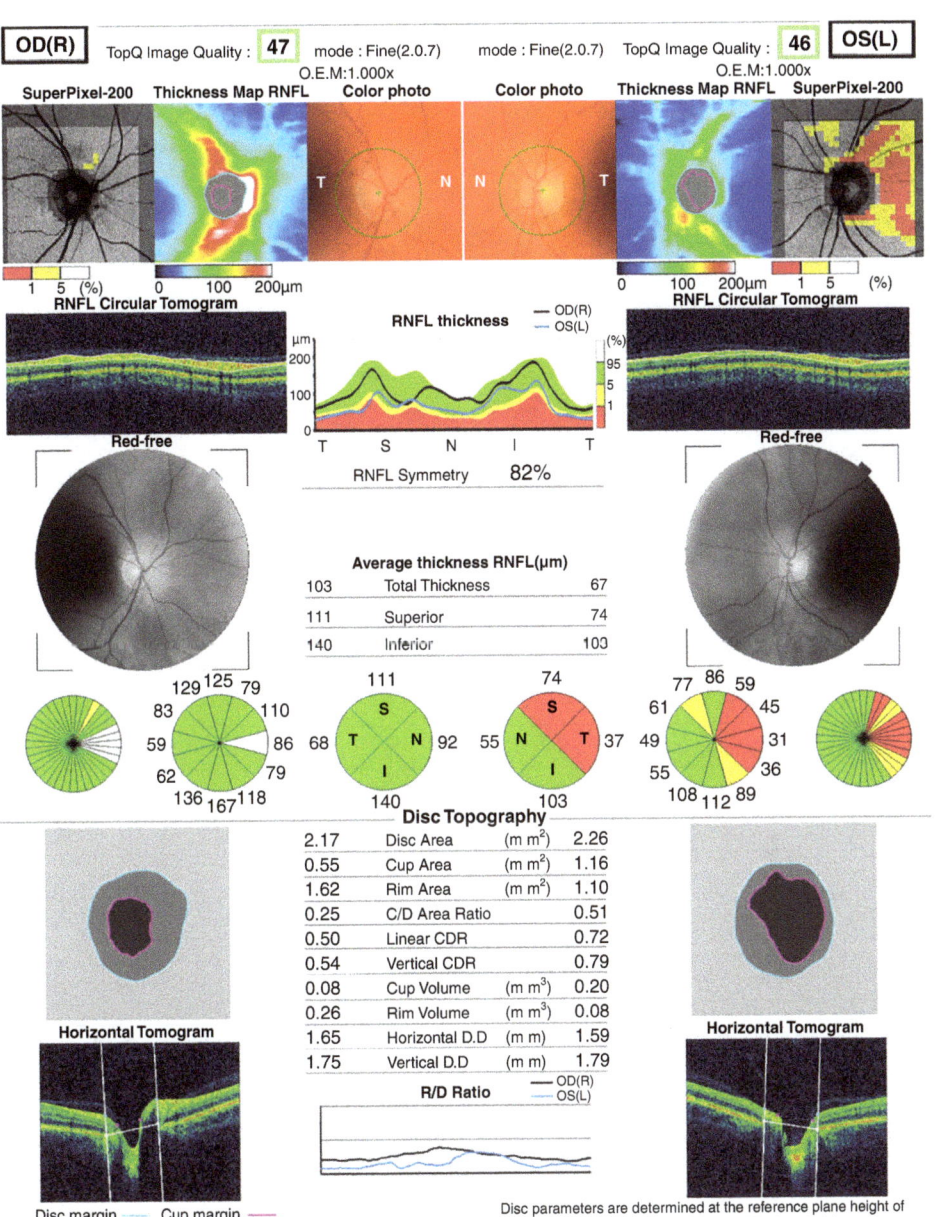

OD(R) TopQ Image Quality : **47** mode : Fine(2.0.7) mode : Fine(2.0.7) TopQ Image Quality : **46** **OS(L)**

O.E.M:1.000x   O.E.M:1.000x

SuperPixel-200 Thickness Map RNFL Color photo Color photo Thickness Map RNFL SuperPixel-200

RNFL Circular Tomogram   **RNFL Circular Tomogram**

RNFL thickness — OD(R) — OS(L)

RNFL Symmetry **82%**

Red-free   **Red-free**

Average thickness RNFL(µm)

103	Total Thickness	67
111	Superior	74
140	Inferior	103

Disc Topography

OD(R)		(m m²)	OS(L)
2.17	Disc Area	(m m²)	2.26
0.55	Cup Area	(m m²)	1.16
1.62	Rim Area	(m m²)	1.10
0.25	C/D Area Ratio		0.51
0.50	Linear CDR		0.72
0.54	Vertical CDR		0.79
0.08	Cup Volume	(m m³)	0.20
0.26	Rim Volume	(m m³)	0.08
1.65	Horizontal D.D	(m m)	1.59
1.75	Vertical D.D	(m m)	1.79

R/D Ratio — OD(R) — OS(L)

Horizontal Tomogram   **Horizontal Tomogram**

Disc margin — Cup margin —

Disc parameters are determined at the reference plane height of (OD(R):120/OS(L):120) um from the RPE plane in this version.

Figure 7.2 OCT demonstrating left retinal fibre layer thinning

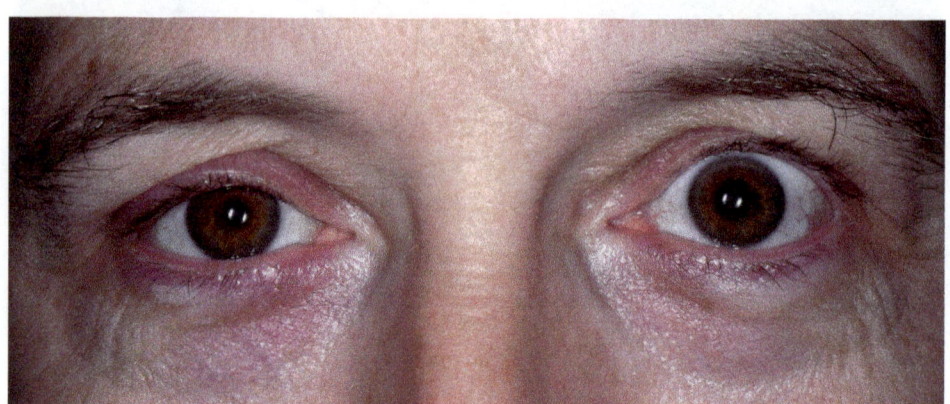

Figure 16.1 Right miosis and ptosis

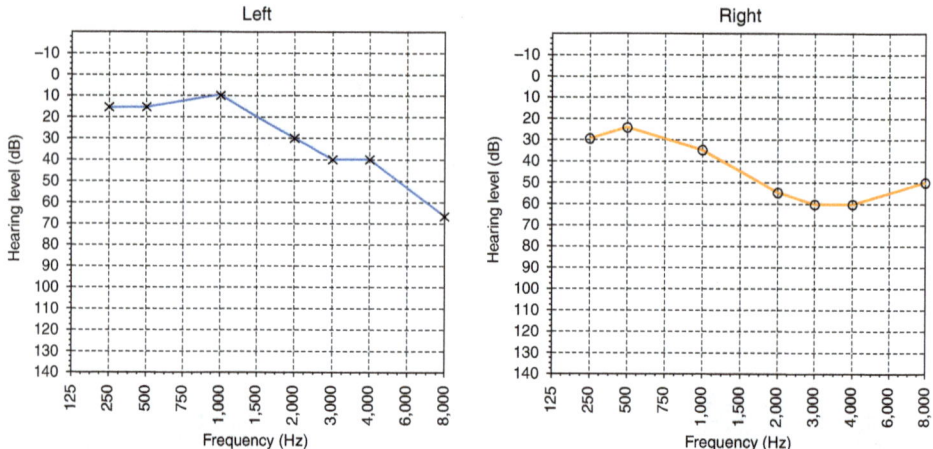

Figure 19.2 Audiometry showing bilateral deafness (i.e. hearing threshold beyond 25 dB). Hearing loss is worse on the left where it spans all hearing frequencies

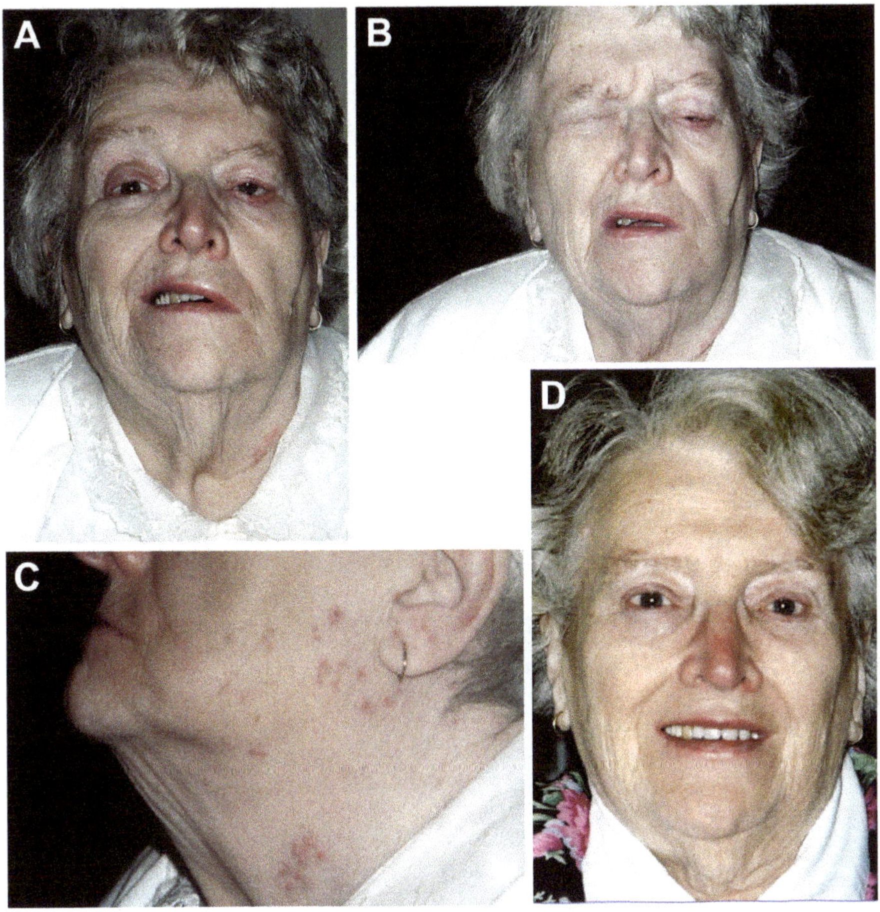

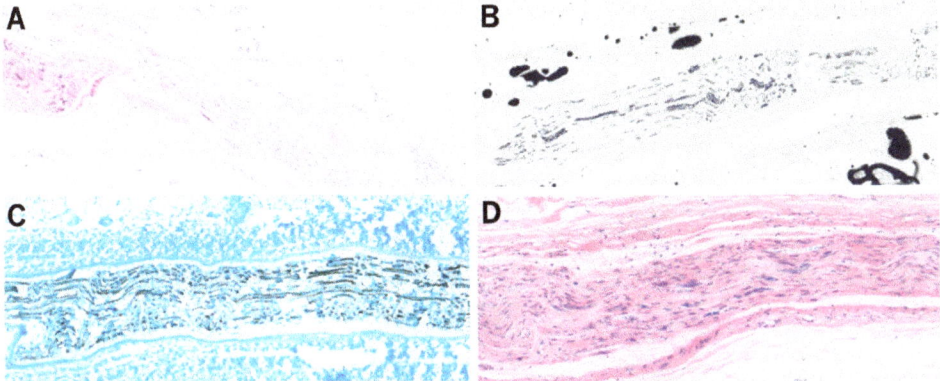

Figure 23.1 Features of Ramsay Hunt syndrome type 2. (A) An unfurrowed left forehead, widened left palpebral fissure due to sagging of left lower eyelid and drooping of the left mouth due to weakness of orbicularis oris. (B) Incomplete closure of the left eye. (C) Vesicular rash involving the left C2 dermatome (neck and pinna) as well as the left Vc dermatome. (D) Full recovery of facial nerve function after two months

Figure 24.4 Sural nerve biopsy. (A) A longitudinal section of the sural nerve showing axonal loss. (B) Myelin stain shows secondary myelin loss. (C) Immunohistochemistry for neurofilament protein shows axonal loss and fragmentation. (D) A histochemical stain, luxol fast blue, confirms little residual myelin

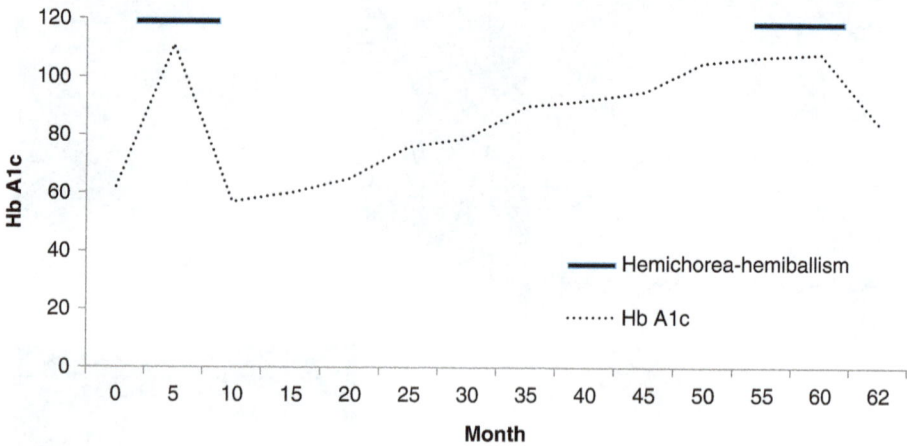

Figure 38.1 Haemoglobin A1c levels over five years with timeline for hyperglycaemia-induced hemichorea-hemiballism.

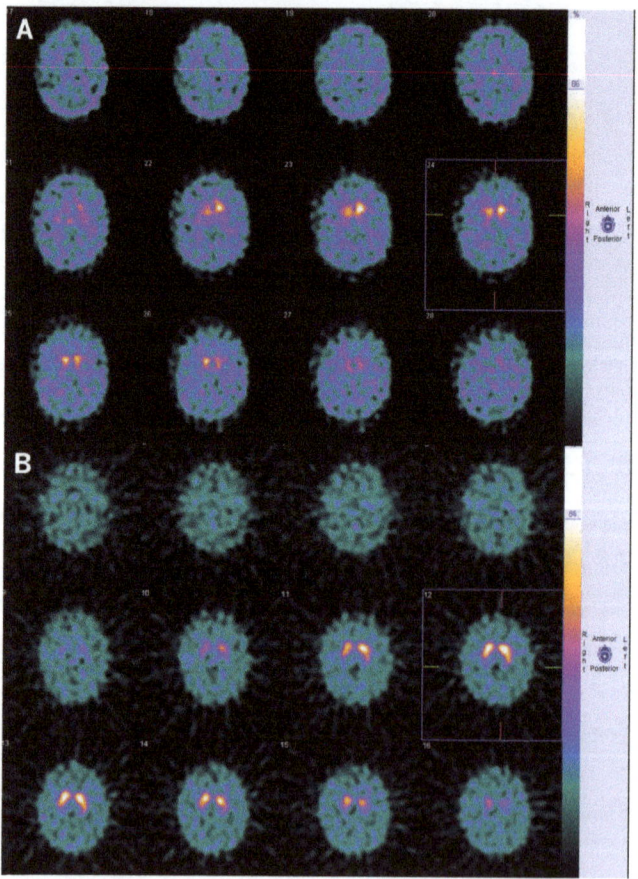

Figure 43.1 An I¹²³-ioflupane single-photon emission computerised tomography or DaT scan showing (A) decreased isotope in the putamen bilaterally of patient with Parkinson's disease and (B) a normal control in which the isotope shows up as two symmetrical crescent-shaped areas of equal intensity

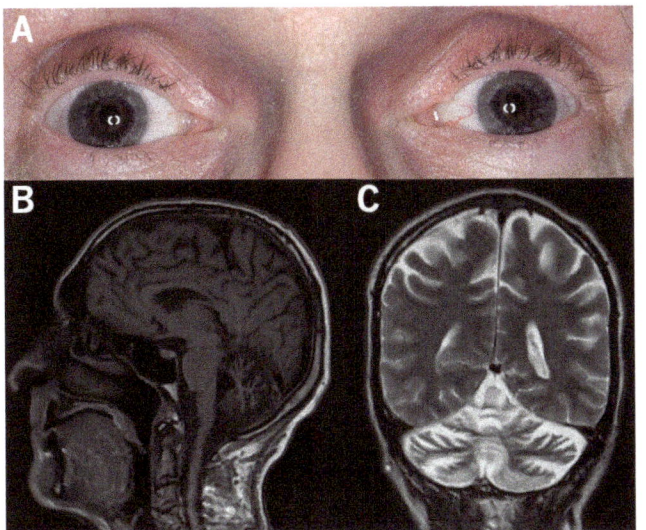

Figure 45.1 (A) Scleral telangiectasia. (B) Sagittal T1 and (C) coronal T2-weighted MRI scan of the brain showing diffuse cerebellar atrophy

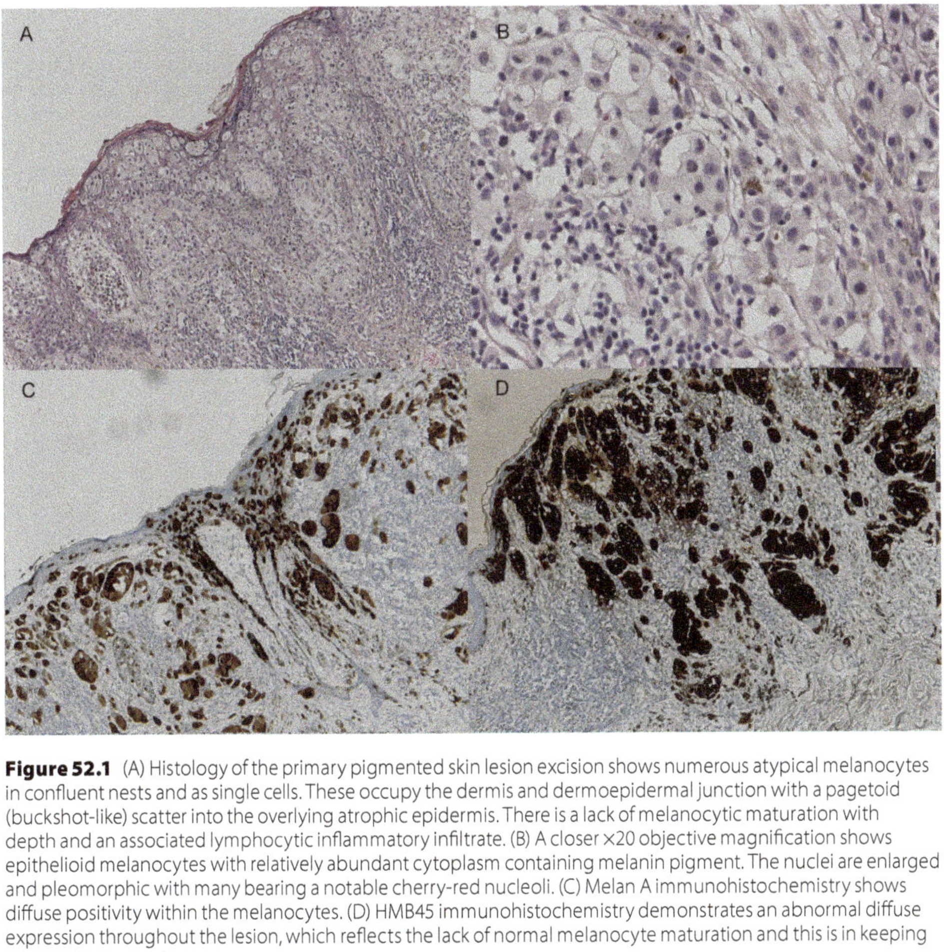

Figure 52.1 (A) Histology of the primary pigmented skin lesion excision shows numerous atypical melanocytes in confluent nests and as single cells. These occupy the dermis and dermoepidermal junction with a pagetoid (buckshot-like) scatter into the overlying atrophic epidermis. There is a lack of melanocytic maturation with depth and an associated lymphocytic inflammatory infiltrate. (B) A closer ×20 objective magnification shows epithelioid melanocytes with relatively abundant cytoplasm containing melanin pigment. The nuclei are enlarged and pleomorphic with many bearing a notable cherry-red nucleoli. (C) Melan A immunohistochemistry shows diffuse positivity within the melanocytes. (D) HMB45 immunohistochemistry demonstrates an abnormal diffuse expression throughout the lesion, which reflects the lack of normal melanocyte maturation and this is in keeping with malignant melanoma

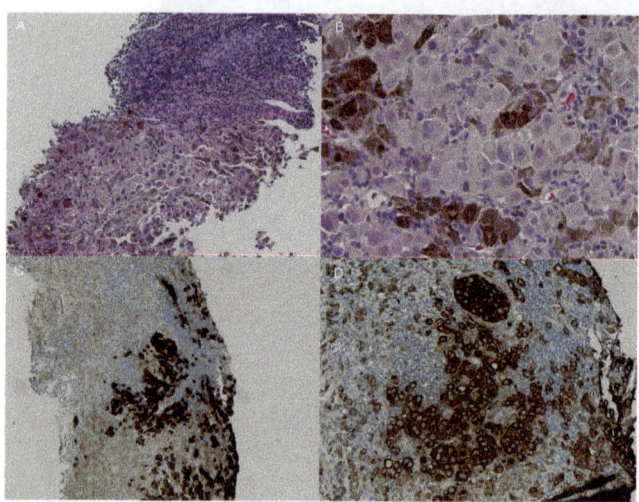

Figure 52.3 (A) Histology of the lymph node core shows infiltration by sheets, nests and single epithelioid cells with abundant eosinophilic cytoplasm and associated melanin pigment. (B) A closer ×20 magnification of the infiltrating cells shows them bearing large pleomorphic nuclei and notable cherry-red nucleoli. The diffuse and strong positivity for (C) melan A and (D) HMB45 immunohistochemistry are consistent with metastatic malignant melanoma

History

A 63-year-old right-handed female health care worker and driver developed a speech disturbance 12 months prior to assessment. A stammer progressed and word production diminished to single words. She could still understand commands, but sometimes these required repetition. Her family thought her memory was preserved but she was upset when she realised that she had put dog food into a freezer. Her handwriting remained clear. She had usually written in capitals. Although her spelling had never been perfect, she also started to leave out words. Short phrases could be repeated to her daughter but she lost that ability to speak over a few months. Her daughter had not witnessed grammatical errors or obvious omissions of small joining words in her spontaneous speech.

Self-care was preserved. She could still handle money and calculate change. There was no disinhibited behaviour but her mood became low. Despite supportive colleagues, she had to stop work. She stopped driving.

She smoked 20 cigarettes a day and drank one or two alcoholic drinks per week. She had four children.

Medication included mirtazapine for depression.

Examination

She had normal cranial nerves including saccades. In her limbs, tone, power, reflexes, co-ordination and sensation were normal. She needed verbal cues for the Luria hand sequence. She had effortful speech with a stammer and slurring of words. Speech was more affected than written communication. Folstein Mini-Mental State Examination score at initial assessment was 29/30 (dropped one point for recall). Montreal Cognitive Assessment score was 25/30 (dropping points on cube drawing: −1; language fluency: −1; abstraction: −1 and delayed recall: −2). Six months later, her mini-mental state examination was 23/30, Addenbrooke's Cognitive Examination 64/100 (attention and orientation 15/18; memory 12/26; fluency 4/14; language 19/26 and visuospatial score 14/16). The answers to these sections could be written down so as not to bias performance from the lack of verbal output. Recognition memory was better than spontaneous recall; her recognition of four faces from an array was perfect, suggesting preserved non-verbal memory.

Investigations

ESR, full blood count, electrolytes and thyroid profile were normal. A dopamine transporter scan showed no evidence of parkinsonism. A CT of the brain had been reported as normal but there was widening of the left Sylvian fissure. An MRI of the brain showed atrophy of the inferior frontal lobe and anterior insula (Figure 31.1).

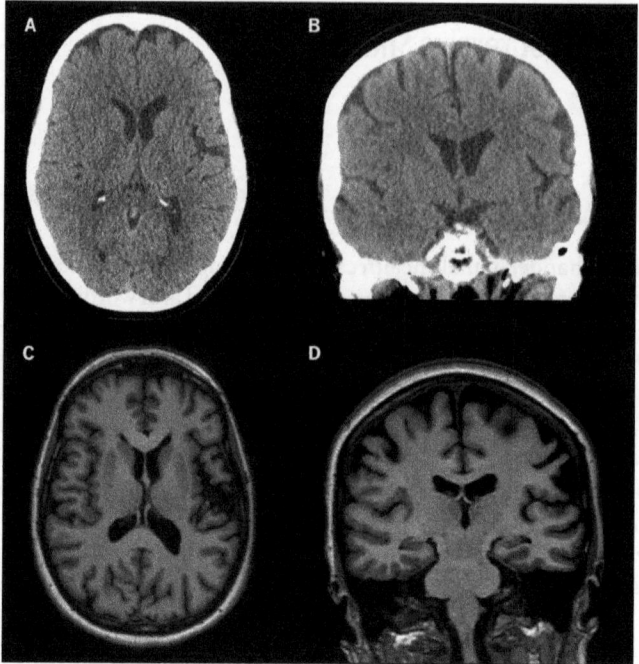

Figure 31.1 An (A) axial and (B) coronal CT scan of the brain showing widened left Sylvian fissure. An (C) axial and (D) coronal T1-weighted MRI scan of the brain demonstrating left inferior frontal atrophy.

Diagnosis: Progressive Non-fluent-agrammatic Primary Progressive Aphasia

Comment

What Are the Primary Progressive Aphasias?

Focal degeneration of language brain systems causes primary progressive aphasias. They are uncommon, with a conservative estimate of prevalence of 3 per 100,000 population. Accurate clinical diagnosis is challenging but important as the primary progressive aphasias have major adverse implications for family life, work and social functioning, all described by our patient. In 2011, a clinical classification was described of the three most commonly reported types of primary progressive aphasia and the classification was designed to be most applicable early in the presentation [1]. Patients are first diagnosed with primary progressive aphasia and are then divided into the clinical variants based on specific speech and language features of each sub-type. The classification facilitates 'imaging-supported' sub-type if the expected pattern of atrophy is identified. A 'definite pathology' classification is applied with pathological or genetic data.

Consensus Diagnostic Criteria of Primary Progressive Aphasia

Recognition of initial prominent difficulty with language as the main cause of impaired activities of daily living is the first step in the diagnosis (as was documented in our patient) [1]. A progressive language disorder ensues with 'gradual progressive impairment of language production, object naming, syntax or word comprehension' [1]. Exclusion criteria include episodic and non-verbal memory loss and visuospatial impairment at an early stage of the disease.

The next step in diagnosis requires analysis of speech and language features in order to characterise the specific variant of primary progressive aphasia (i.e. non-fluent-agrammatic variant, semantic variant or logopenic variant). This can be done clinically, supported by imaging and/or pathology. At least one core feature must be present for the non-fluent-agrammatic variant whereas two core features are required for both semantic and logopenic variants (Table 31.1).

Neuroimaging features of these three classical 'language-led dementias' are shown best with T1 coronal MR scanning.

Non-fluent-agrammatic Primary Progressive Aphasia

Agrammatism in language production or effortful speech are the core criteria of non-fluent-agrammatic variant of primary progressive aphasia. In agrammatism speech is usually limited to short, simple phrases along with omissions of morphemes (function words and inflections). Slow and laboured speech is effortful speech (as was present in our patient). Inconsistent speech sound errors can occur. Among the other features, our patient had mild impairment of sentence comprehension initially and difficulty with syntax but had preserved single-word comprehension and object knowledge. Clinical features may include a re-emergence of a childhood stutter preceding speech decline. Also, when requested to select between alternatives, the patient may consistently produce the wrong response, so-called binary reversal [2].

The imaging abnormalities of non-fluent-agrammatic primary progressive aphasia are confined to the left inferior frontal gyrus, insula, premotor and supplementary motor areas.

Table 31.1 Current consensus criteria for primary progressive aphasia

Level diagnosis	Non-fluent-agrammatic variant	Semantic variant	Logopenic variant
Clinical	*At least one of:*	*Both of:*	*Both of:*
Core features	Agrammatism in language production Effortful, halting speech with inconsistent speech sound errors and distortions (speech apraxia)	Impaired confrontation naming Impaired single-word comprehension	Impaired single word retrieval in spontaneous speech and naming Impaired repetition of sentences and phrases
Other features	*At least two of:* Impaired comprehension of syntactically complex sentences Spared single-word comprehension Spared object knowledge	*At least three of:* Impaired object knowledge, particularly for low-frequency or low-familiarity items Surface dyslexia or dysgraphia Spared repetition Spared speech production (grammar and motor speech)	*At least three of:* Speech (phonologic) errors in spontaneous speech and naming Spared single-word comprehension and object knowledge Spared motor speech Absence of frank agrammatism
Imaging-supported	*At least one of:* Predominant left posterior fronto-insular atrophy on MRI Predominant left posterior fronto-insular hypoperfusion/metabolism on SPECT/PET	*At least one of:* Predominant anterior temporal lobe atrophy on MRI Predominant anterior temporal hypoperfusion/metabolism on SPECT/PET	*At least one of:* Predominant left posterior perisylvian or parietal atrophy on MRI Predominant left posterior perisylvian or parietal hypoperfusion/metabolism on SPECT/PET
Pathologically definite	*At least one of:* Histological evidence of specific neurodegenerative pathology Known pathogenic mutation	*At least one of:* Histological evidence of specific neurodegenerative pathology Known pathogenic mutation	*At least one of:* Histological evidence of specific neurodegenerative pathology Known pathogenic mutation

Adapted from Gorno-Tempini et al. [1] with permission from Wolters Kluwer.

Frontotemporal lobar degeneration-tau is the most frequent pathological finding in non-fluent patients with agrammatism or motor speech disturbance.

Patients with the non-fluent-agrammatic variant may eventually develop motor features of corticobasal syndrome or progressive supranuclear palsy.

Semantic Variant of Primary Progressive Aphasia

Anomia and single-word comprehension deficits are the core criteria for the semantic variant. The naming problem is severe. There is an inability to comprehend low-frequency or low-familiarity words. This can involve impairment of object and person recognition even when presented in other modalities such as visual, tactile, olfactory and gustatory. There is impaired reading and writing of words that have an atypical relationship between spelling and pronunciation. In the early 1990s, Professor John Hodges and colleagues reported a comprehensive characterisation of semantic dementia.

Focal cerebral atrophy involves the dominant anteroinferior and mesial temporal lobe, including the amygdala and anterior hippocampus.

Logopenic Variant of Primary Progressive Aphasia

Sentence repetition deficits and word retrieval in spontaneous speech and confrontation naming are core features of the logopenic variant of primary progressive aphasia. Slow speech with word-finding problems but no agrammatism distinguishes this variant from the non-fluent-agrammatic variant. Maria Luisa Gorno-Tempini and colleagues described the logopenic variant of primary progressive aphasia in 2004. The confrontation naming is less severe in logopenic than in the semantic variant.

Imaging reveals atrophy of the temporo-parietal junction zone of the dominant hemisphere. This appears as widening of the left Sylvian fissure.

Clinical approaches to these suspected canonical primary progressive aphasias have been reported [2].

Pathology of Primary Progressive Aphasia

Patients with primary progressive aphasia have heterogenous neuropathology. Most patients have tau-positive, ubiquitin/transactive response DNA binding protein 43-positive fronto-temporal lobar degeneration pathology or Alzheimer pathology. Research continues into the core pathophysiological processes and how these contribute to the sub-types of primary progressive aphasia. One theory in non-fluent-agrammatic primary progressive aphasia describes impaired scaffolding of speech, impaired sequencing and scheduling of speech and interruption of predictive coding rules for other sensorimotor routines. This implies inflexible neural predictions from incoming sensory information [3].

Genetics of Primary Progressive Aphasia

The progranulin (*GRN*) gene can cause an autosomal dominant form of primary progressive aphasia. Hexanucleotide repeat expansions near the chromosome 9 open reading frame gene (*C9orf72*) and the microtubule-associated protein tau (*MAPT*) gene have also been implicated in primary progressive aphasia.

Management of Primary Progressive Aphasia

Management is challenging for a number of reasons. There are currently no known disease-modifying drugs for primary progressive aphasia and symptomatic treatments have limited evidence of efficacy. Supportive measures and education allow for social and financial planning. Non-pharmacological measures for enhancing communication can provide some support but these are often neither generalisable nor long-lasting. The rare dementia network is a source of support to family and caregivers (www.raredementiasupport.org/ppa).

References

1. Gorno-Tempini ML, Hillis AE, Weintraub S et al. Classification of primary progressive aphasia and its variants. *Neurology*. 2011;76(11):1006–14.
2. Marshall CR, Hardy CJD, Volkmer A et al. Primary progressive aphasia: a clinical approach. *J Neurol*. 2018;265(6):1474–90.
3. Ruksenaite J, Volkmer A, Jiang J et al. Primary progressive aphasia: toward a pathophysiological synthesis. *Curr Neurol Neurosci Rep*. 2021;21(3).

Learning Points

- Primary progressive aphasias are an uncommon, heterogenous and diagnostically challenging group of focal language-led dementias.
- Primary progressive aphasias are a selective brain network degeneration with devastating implications for family life, work and social functioning.
- Specific speech and language features can diagnose non-fluent-agrammatic, semantic and logopenic primary progressive aphasias supplemented by imaging and pathological (including genetic) findings.

Perspective from the Patient's Daughter

1. **What is the impact of the condition?**
   a. Physical (e.g. practical support, work, activities of daily)
   Needs assistance with some tasks. Decline in everything physically and mentally.
   b. Psychological (e.g. mood, emotional well-being)
   Low mood. Very little confidence.
   c. Social (e.g. meeting friends, home)
   Rare. Avoids.
2. **What can you not do because of the condition?**
   Speak. Difficulty reading and writing.
3. **Has there been any other change for you due to the condition?**
   Cannot eat certain foods. Difficulty swallowing. Persistent choking and coughing.
4. **What is/was the most difficult aspect of the condition for you?**
   (Very little) support outside of family, medical-GP. Little understanding and little knowledge.
5. **Was any aspect of the experience good or useful? What was that?**
   No.
6. **What do you hope for in the future for your condition?**
   Better support, knowledge and understanding of this condition, better services.

Patient's Own Writing

I CAN'T TALK NOW
HAVE TO SAY T CAN'T
MY CHILDREN I LOVE THEN
I CAN'T TALK TO MY GRAND CHILDREN

I CAN'T WORK AND CAN'T DRIVE AND IT
HARD TO WRITE AND CAN'T READ BOOKS

I WOULD BE LOST WITHOUT (name of daughter)
SHE IS MY ROCK

I FORGET THING I FEEL
IT GETTING WORSE

I DON'T UNDERSTAND SOMETIME
WELL THE HOUSE IS FULL
I FILL IT HARD TO EAT

32 Personality Change

History

A 65-year-old ex-mathematics and computer teacher had an apparent sudden change in behaviour. He stopped playing his weekly football, stopped tutoring (transfer test for primary-school students), went to bed at 18:30 and slept with the light on. His wife noticed that he had become more anxious and less adventurous. He was more easily irritated by noise. He had stopped driving for about a year prior to assessment, and his wife reported that before this he had become somewhat panicky when driving. His wife revealed that he had become disinhibited, became acerbic with people and had difficulty engaging in social conversations. He needed prompting to shave and change his clothes.

He had eight siblings. One brother had depression but there was no family history of dementia. His medication included bisoprolol 1.25 mg od, simvastatin 40 mg od and irbesartan 150 mg od.

Examination

His blood pressure was 180/97 mmHg. Pulse was 78 bpm and regular. Cranial nerves were normal. He was myopic. He had no bradykinesia. Tone, power, reflexes and sensation in his limbs were normal. He had no evidence of bradykinesia. Plantar responses were flexor.

On cognitive assessment, he scored 26 out of 30 on a Montreal Cognitive Assessment (dropping 4 points on delayed recall). He scored 91/100 in an Addenbrooke's cognitive examination (Table 32.1).

Table 32.1 Cognition

Addenbrooke's Cognitive Examination	91/100
Attention/orientation	18/18
Memory	24/26
Fluency	10/14
Language	25/26
Visuospatial	14/16

The repeatable battery for the assessment of neuropsychological status was developed to identify and characterise abnormal cognitive decline in older patients and as a neuropsychological screening battery for younger patients. Our patient's findings were summarised as:

- impaired immediate memory and delayed memory tasks
- borderline visuospatial and construction tasks
- low average language abilities and attention.

The Cambridge Behavioural Inventory is used to distinguish behavioural and psychiatric symptoms in Alzheimer's disease and behavioural variant of frontotemporal dementia. It assesses 81 items over 13 domains with a score from 0 (never) to 4 (constantly) based on the frequency of a behaviour). Our patient scored 94 within all 13 of the sub-sections. This demonstrated rigidity of thought, disturbed sleep, memory difficulties, problems with concentration and orientation, and reduced motivation.

Behavioural Assessment of the Dysexecutive Syndrome battery of tests assesses ability to plan an effective and efficient course of action. He had difficulty planning for unstructured activity.

Trail making test is a test of scanning, visuomotor tracking, divided attention and cognitive flexibility. This demonstrated slow processing and (part 4) difficulty in complex conceptual tracking.

Verbal fluency test performance was mixed. His letter fluency was average, but categorical switching was impaired, indicating difficulties in initiation and set shifting.

Section 1 of the Hayling sentence completion test was impaired. He could not complete section 2 (which is used to explore response inhibition). This reflected problems in the area of inhibition linked to frontal lobe functioning.

Function
Bristol Activity of Daily Living 5/60 (lower scores indicate greater independence.)

Mood
Geriatric Depression scale 9/15 in keeping with mild depression.

Behaviours

Neuropsychiatric Inventory Questionnaire
6/12 for behaviours

13/36 for severity (higher score = greater severity)

10/60 for distress (higher score = greater distress)

Carer Burden
Zarit Burden interview 38/88 (higher scores indicate greater burden)

Investigations
Blood tests revealed a normal ESR, full blood count, B12, folate and thyroid profile.

An MRI of the brain was performed over a two-year interval. There was progressive anterior lobe atrophy, more prominent on the right than left (Figures 32.1A and 32.1B). There was global atrophy, frontal more than posterior with temporal predominance. SPECT (Tc-99HMPAO-hexamethylpropyleneamine oxime) demonstrated bilateral frontal lobe hypoperfusion.

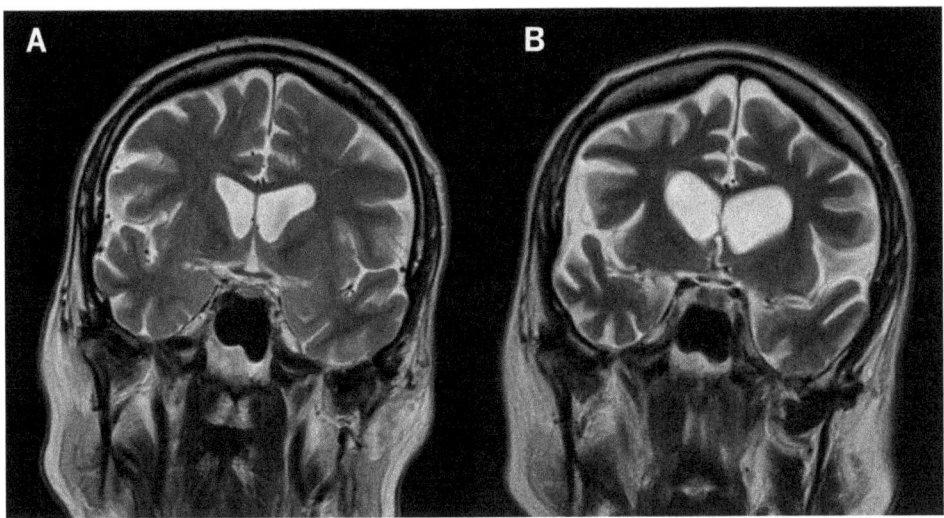

Figure 32.1 A (A) coronal T2 MRI scan of the brain showing frontal and temporal atrophy, which (B) progressed over two years with associated ventricular dilatation.

Diagnosis: Probable Behavioural Variant Frontotemporal Dementia

Management

At the age of 67 years, he had two tonic clonic seizures. He was treated with lamotrigine. He then developed a left hemiparkinsonian syndrome (hypomimic, resting left arm tremor, left pincer and left foot-tapping bradykinesia elicited with Fromment's manoeuvre). He continued to deteriorate and died aged 69 years.

Commentary

Dementias are usually denoted by a syndrome of failing memory and progressive impairment of other intellectual functions, but also include certain personality and behavioural changes. There are many causes of dementia. One classification includes dementia as the only evidence of disease (e.g. Alzheimer's disease, frontotemporal dementia), dementia associated with other neurological signs (cerebrovascular disease, Huntington's disease, Parkinson's disease, tauopathies such as progressive supranuclear palsy and white matter disease such as multiple sclerosis) and dementia associated with other medical disease (HIV and syphilis).

Frontotemporal Dementia

Frontotemporal dementia is a group of neurodegenerative disorders that cause not only cognitive impairments but also behavioural changes due to frontotemporal lobar degeneration (FTLD). Progressive behavioural change, executive dysfunction and language impairment make up the distinctive features of frontotemporal dementia. Behavioural variant frontotemporal dementia (bvFTD) and three distinct primary progressive aphasias (non-fluent-agrammatic, semantic and logopenic variants) all have recognised diagnostic criteria. Frontotemporal dementia can present with parkinsonism, atypical parkinsonism (akinetic-rigid syndrome, corticobasal syndrome and progressive supranuclear palsy-like phenotypes) or motor neurone disease.

Behavioural Variant Frontotemporal Dementia

Behavioural variant frontotemporal dementia occurs mostly sporadically, with 20% having an autosomal dominant mutation in three common mutations – hexanucleotide repeat expansions near the chromosome 9 open reading frame gene (*C9orf72*), progranulin (*GRN*) and microtubule associate protein-tau (*MAPT*).

There was a particular clue for bvFTD in this patient because of the marked frontal network dysfunction, which can cause significant changes in personality and behaviour. Disruptions in non-motor frontal-subcortical circuits (thalami to frontal lobes) are recognised causes of apathy, disinhibition and executive dysfunction.

The 2011 international consensus criteria for bvFTD require progressive deterioration of behaviour and/or cognition by observation or history from a knowledgeable informant [1]. The patient fulfilled criteria for probable bvFTD (Table 32.2).

The early profound changes in our patient's personality and behaviour favour this diagnosis, which is more frequent and severe than the frontal variant of Alzheimer's disease.

Table 32.2 International consensus criteria for bvFTD

I. Neurodegenerative disease
The following symptom must be present to meet criteria for bvFTD
A. Shows progressive deterioration of behaviour and/or cognition by observation or history (as provided by a knowledgeable informant)

II. Possible bvFTD
Three of the following behavioural/cognitive symptoms (A–F) must be present to meet criteria. Ascertainment requires that symptoms be persistent or recurrent, rather than single or rare events.

A. Early* behaviour disinhibition (one of the followings symptoms (A.1–A.3) must be present):
A.1. Socially inappropriate behaviour
A.2. Loss of manners or decorum
A.3. Impulsive, rash or careless actions

B. Early apathy or inertia (one of the following symptoms (B.1 or B.2) must be present):
B.1 Apathy
B.2 Inertia

C. Early loss of empathy or sympathy (one of the following symptoms (C.1 or C.2) must be present):
C.1 Diminished response to other people's needs and feelings
C.2 Diminished social interest, interrelatedness or personal warmth

D. Early preservative or stereotyped, compulsive/ritualistic behaviours (one of the following symptoms (D.1–D.3) must be present):
D.1 Simple repetitive movements
D.2 Complex, compulsive or ritualistic behaviours
D.3 Stereotypy of speech

E. Hyperorality and dietary changes (one of the following symptoms (E.1–E.3) must be present):
E.1 Altered food preferences
E.2 Binge eating, increased consumption of alcohol or cigarettes
E.3 Oral exploration or consumption of inedible objects

F. Neuropsychological profile: executive/generation deficits with relative sparing of memory and visuospatial functions (all of the following symptoms (F.1–F.3) must be present):
F.1 Deficits in executive tasks
F.2 Relative sparing of episodic memory
F.3 Relative sparing of visuospatial skills

III. Probable bvFTD
All of the following symptoms (A–C) must be present to meet criteria
A. Meets criteria for possible bvFTD
B. Exhibits significant functional decline (by caregiver report or as evidenced by Clinical Dementia Rating Scale or Functional Activities Questionnaire scores)
C. Imaging results consistent with bvFTD (one of the following (C.1–C.2) must be present):
C.1 Frontal and/or anterior temporal lobe atrophy on MRI or CT
C.2 Frontal and/or anterior temporal hypoperfusion or hypometabolism on PET or SPECT

IV. Behavioural variant FTD with definite FTLD pathology
Criterion A and either B or C must be present to meet criteria
A. Meets criteria for possible or probable bvFTD
B. Histopathological evidence of FTLD on biopsy or at post-mortem
C. Presence of a known pathogenic mutation

V. Exclusionary criteria for bvFTD
Criteria A and B must be answered negatively for any bvFTD diagnosis. Criterion C can be positive for possible bvFTD but must be negative for probable bvFTD
A. Pattern of deficits is better accounted for by other non-degenerative nervous system or medical disorders
B. Behavioural disturbance is better accounted for by a psychiatric diagnosis
C. Biomarkers strongly indicative of Alzheimer's disease or other neurodegenerative disorder

* As a general guideline 'early' refers to symptom presentation within the first three years

Reprinted with permission from Rascovsky et al. [1] with permission from Oxford University Press.

Distinguishing bvFTD from Primary Psychiatric Presentations

The diagnosis of bvFTD has some symptom overlap with non-degenerative primary psychiatric disorders. Indeed, a prior psychiatric diagnosis is observed in up to 50% of patients with bvFTD [2]. The standard neuropsychological battery of tests for bvFTD, 3D-T1 brain MRI with standard review protocol and ^{18}F-fluorodeoxyglucose PET scan improve the diagnostic accuracy of bvFTD. A strictly normal ^{18}F-fluorodeoxyglucose PET scan excludes bvFTD.

Other differential diagnosis includes cerebrovascular disease (multiple frontal infarctions), substance abuse and frontotemporal brain sagging syndrome due to intracranial hypotension. A behavioural variant phenocopy lacking clinical progression can be seen with personality disorders or high-functioning autism spectrum disorder. The majority of patients with bvFTD phenocopy remain stable over many years. However, a small minority of such patients may harbour the *C9orf72* expansion.

Pathology and Epidemiology of Frontotemporal Dementia

The pattern of frontotemporal atrophy suggests an underlying diagnosis of FTLD, which is characterised by ubiquitinated protein aggregates mostly in neurones. Frontotemporal lobar degeneration sub-types are recognised with different inclusions including tau, transactive response DNA-binding protein 43 (TDP-43), fused in sarcoma protein (FUS) and ubiquitin proteasome system (UPS) markers.

Frontotemporal dementia is a leading cause of early-onset dementia. Peak prevalence is 13 per 100,000 in the early sixties. Behavioural variant frontotemporal dementia accounts for about 50% of all frontotemporal dementia patients.

Right Temporal Variant of Frontotemporal Dementia

There has been debate that a predominantly right temporal variant of frontotemporal dementia may exist (i.e. a right hemisphere equivalent of semantic primary progressive aphasia). Prosopagnosia, episodic memory impairments and behavioural change such as disinhibition, apathy, compulsiveness and loss of empathy have been described as common initial symptoms. Core clinical features have been proposed to include at least two of prosopagnosia, memory deficit and behavioural changes (at least two of disinhibition, apathy-inertia, loss of empathy, compulsiveness). Although our patient had more right temporal atrophy than left temporal atrophy and sufficient behavioural change, he did not have prosopagnosia or memory impairment to diagnose right temporal variant of frontotemporal dementia [3].

References

1. Rascovsky K, Hodges JR, Knopman D et al. Sensitivity of revised diagnostic criteria for the behavioural variant of frontotemporal dementia. *Brain*. 2011;134(9):2456–77.
2. Ducharme S, Dols A, Laforce R et al. Recommendations to distinguish behavioural variant frontotemporal dementia from psychiatric disorders. *Brain*. 2020;143(6):1632–50.
3. Erkoyun HU, Groot C, Heilbron R et al. A clinical-radiological framework of the right temporal variant of frontotemporal dementia. *Brain*. 2020;143(9):2831–43.

Learning Points

- Frontotemporal dementia is a group of neurodegenerative disorders characterised by behavioural and cognitive impairments.
- Behavioural change with disinhibition, apathy, loss of empathy and executive dysfunctioning with relative preservation of memory and visuospatial abilities are characteristic of the behavioural variant of frontotemporal dementia, the most common variant of the condition.

- Psychiatric diagnoses are not unusual in the early stages of bvFTD.
- Advanced bvFTD exerts a heavy burden on relatives and carers.

Perspective from Patient's Wife

1. **What was the impact of the condition on your husband?**

   a. Physical (e.g. practical support)
   He lost all of his abilities of independence. Personality change.

   b. Psychological (e.g. mood, emotional well-being)
   Crabbit all of a sudden. Impatient. Couldn't care less about anything. Selfish. Unsettled. Imagination would seem real to him.

   c. Social (e.g. meeting friends, home)
   He couldn't cope with friends visiting. He would be anxious and even ask them to go. He got aggressive with some. He knocked a cup from the hand of one friend. He didn't want to visit people.

2. **What could he not do because of the condition?**
   Concentrate, play, turn the computer on, unlock the door, drive, read, watch a football match on TV, sit still, wait, understand what was being said to him, hold a conversation.

3. **Was there any other change for your husband due to his medical condition?**
   He thought that there were people upstairs a lot of the time. He would see them. He had three watches and he wore them all at the same time. He would take a dislike to someone and would be really mean to them, saying he didn't want them in the house.

4. **What is/was the most difficult aspect of the condition for you as his wife?**
   Losing my really independent husband who could do anything he wanted.
   Putting him into a nursing home – the worst thing.

5. **Was any aspect of the experience of the condition good or useful? What was that?**
   Meeting other people with similar experiences.

6. **What do you hope for in the future for people with this condition?**
   That they would never have it. More support.

History

A 29-year-old woman had a two-year history of intermittent burning in her feet, restless legs, back spasms and tremulousness on wakening. On occasions, her legs 'left' her, resulting in falls. She had pins and needles in her face, hands and legs. She had episodes of blurred vision. Her health deteriorated in the year before her first neurology inpatient assessment. Her symptoms continued with tremor, weakness in her legs, cold and burning feelings in her feet, pain in her eyes, blurred vision, pins and needles in her hands and feet, jerks and seizures. Sometimes she was conscious but unresponsive during 30-second seizure-like episodes.

She had four hospital admissions over two years. Ongoing visual disturbance, seizures and falling were persistent problems. An ophthalmologist diagnosed a right optic neuropathy at one stage but this was withdrawn after detailed assessment and the diagnosis was revised to right amblyopia and dry eyes. An MRI brain scan had shown mucosal oedema in a sphenoid sinus.

Past medical history included stress incontinence and tonsillectomy. Three years before her neurological symptoms began, she had a 10-day inpatient hospital stay including an ICU admission due to an extended spectrum beta-lactamase *Escherichia coli* pyelonephritis. This had been a very frightening experience.

She had two children. Her medication was amitriptyline 75 mg od, gabapentin 100 mg tid, co-codamol 30/500 and pizotifen 1.5 mg od. She did not smoke cigarettes. She drank alcohol once every six weeks.

Examination

She was alert and orientated. Visual acuity on the right was $6/9^{-2}$ and visual acuity on the left was 6/6 unaided. Ishihara plate test was 14/14 for both eyes. The remaining cranial nerves were normal. She was distressed at times due to spasm and jerks of her right leg. Power delivery was inconsistent with giveway strength but could reach 5/5. Reflexes were symmetrically present. Sensation (light touch, vibration and pin prick) was intact.

Investigations

MRIs of the brain, spine and orbits were reported as normal. During hyperventilation for an EEG, she had an episode of stopping hyperventilation, dropping her hands by her side, rolling her head backwards and briefly not responding. She complained of blurring of her vision. This was thought to be a typical episode of 'zoning out'. It was not associated with any EEG change. She also experienced spasms that were not associated with a change in her EEG. Visual perimetry was unreliable.

Diagnosis: Functional Neurological Disorder

Management
She had multi-disciplinary input from physiotherapy, occupational therapy and clinical psychology. She made good progress but has been prone to relapses and fluctuation in her symptoms, with seizures and mobility issues becoming more prominent, compromising her ability to remain independent.

Comment

Definition of Functional Neurological Disorder
Paralysis, tremor, seizures, gait disorder, blindness and other motor or sensory symptoms due to a functional rather than a structural disorder account for functional neurological disorder. The symptoms of functional neurological disorder cause a high level of physical disability, frequently equated to that experienced by patients with multiple sclerosis.

Epidemiology
The incidence of functional neurological disorder is at least 12 per 100,000 per year. Women are affected more frequently than men. Functional and psychological symptoms may make-up 16% of neurological outpatient attendances and up to a third of new outpatients may have 'symptoms unexplained by organic disease'. Once diagnosed, it is very unusual for the diagnosis to be reversed and symptoms subsequently attributed to neurological disease [1].

Functional overlay from neurological disease is not uncommon and is one important reason for appropriate investigation. Neurological co-morbidities are frequently present and appropriate management of co-morbidities can improve functional neurological disorder.

Diagnostic Criteria for Functional Neurological Disorders
The fifth edition of the Diagnostic and Statistical Manual of Mental Disorders (DSM-5) had three important changes for functional neurological disorder from the fourth edition. The fifth edition emphasised how to make the clinical diagnosis (positive physical signs of internal inconsistency or incongruity with recognised disease), recognised that a psychological stressor often is not present, and importantly that feigned symptoms are probably rare, are separately classified and should not be considered a functional disorder.

Nomenclature
The terms 'conversion' and 'psychogenic' are being used much less frequently. Patients find the term 'functional' more acceptable than other terms. Professor Jon Stone, a neurologist, and Professor Alan Carson, a psychiatrist, both working in Edinburgh, have advanced our diagnostic and management strategies for this group of patients.

Assessment and Clinical Findings
Sufficient consultation time is crucial for achieving an accurate diagnosis. A previous history of functional disorder (e.g. irritable bowel syndrome) may exist, but may not be disclosed. A thick file and multiple symptoms may be present while the primary complaint may not be clear. Time is also important as the assessment plays an important therapeutic or management role [2].

Signs in functional neurological disorder are incongruent with neurological disease; they may also be inconsistent over time. The level of complexity of the task and disability may be disproportionate to objective findings. There are also features or signs specific for each sub-type of functional neurological disorder.

Functional Movement Disorders

Functional movement disorders (tremor – most frequently, dystonia, myoclonus, gait and parkinsonism) were originally defined by Stanley Fahn and Daniel Williams in 1988 as show-ing remission with suggestion, physiotherapy, psychotherapy, placebos and while the patient is not being observed. A number of iterations ensued to allow for the absence or presence of other features and laboratory-supported criteria for functional tremor and functional myo-clonus. Alberto Espay and Anthony Lang have proposed phenotype-specific diagnostic fea-tures for functional movement disorders [3].

For tremor entrainment or full suppressibility, distractibility, tonic co-activation at tremor onset, pause of tremor during contralateral ballistic movements and variability in frequency, axis or distribution are phenotype-specific criteria.

Functional Weakness

The co-contraction sign is highly reliable but false positives can occur in spastic patients. Motor inconsistency can occur in a paralysed arm for dressing (because attention is distract-ed). Collapsing weakness from light touch and give-way weakness are general signs with high specificity. Hoover's sign (weakness of hip extension that resolves during contralateral hip flexion against resistance) is highly reliable but can be caused by cortical neglect. The abduct-or sign involves weakness of hip abduction, which resolves with contralateral hip abduction against resistance (highly sensitive and specific).

In the arm, the abduction finger test can be used in patients with severe hand weakness – finger abduction against resistance for two minutes causes a synkinetic abduction of the fifth finger of the contralateral (functionally paretic) hand. Also drift without pronation is a highly reliable sign of functional weakness.

Functional Sensory Loss

Sensory signs of functional sensory loss have been reported but some have been reported in organic disease (i.e. they have low specificity). Midline splitting and splitting of vibration sense (e.g. frontal bone vibration) have high specificity and reliability; midline splitting can occur with thalamic lesions. Non-anatomical sensory loss is poorly defined. Systematic fail-ure (i.e. below chance performance) occurring 100% of the time on a discrimination task is specific and reliable for functional sensory loss.

Dissociative Seizures

Dissociative seizures (previously called psychogenic non-epileptic seizures) are a sub-type of functional neurological disorder in which individuals exhibit paroxysmal convulsive events and/or alterations in behaviour and consciousness that resemble epileptic seizures but are not associated with changes in cortical activity. There is a gold standard diagnostic criterion – typical event on video-EEG with a lack of epileptiform activity in the peri-ictal period with semiologic and historical consistency with dissociative seizures, as demonstrat-ed in this patient.

More than one type of spell can exist. Up to 30% of these patients may also have a history of epilepsy. Features favouring a diagnosis of epileptic seizures include seizures occurring from sleep, postictal confusion and postictal stertorous breathing. There are some signs that help distinguish dissociative seizures from epileptic seizures (Table 33.1).

Putative Mechanisms

Interest in functional neurological disorders has prompted advances in a search for mechanisms or causes. There are theories for a brain network disorder, a disorder of predictive processing and psychological models (predisposing, precipitating and perpetuating factors). All of these theories have supportive evidence but no one theory applies to all patients. Mind (psychological) and brain (neural) functions are increasingly recognised as mutually important in brain, personal and societal functioning.

Management

Communication of the diagnosis should take place with key family members present in order to help sustain the diagnosis. The diagnosis is not based around normal tests. It is also important not to rely on the stress hypothesis. In functional dystonia, attention and response to injury can be triggers without stress. Not all patients have previous trauma or stress. Neurologists should explain the rationale for the diagnosis, that the symptoms are real and that the manifestations of functional neurological disorder are not under conscious control.

Subsequent discussions with the patient may include explaining how derealisation or depersonalisation in dissociation may avoid sensory overload. Patients may be told that our predictions from previous experience may not always be right. Explanations of activation of the autonomic nervous system and cycles of fear and avoidance can help a patient understand attacks. Explaining the protective physiological mechanism of dissociation and how this can become habitual may help patients understand their attacks. Other patients may need explanation of how attentional bias may exacerbate symptoms.

Table 33.1 Features helpful in distinguishing dissociative seizures from epileptic seizures

Favouring dissociative seizures	Favouring epileptic seizures
Longer than 10 minutes	Usually less than 2 minutes (but partial seizures can last longer)
Fluctuating course	Usually stereotyped
Asynchronous limb movements	Asynchronous limb movements unusual except for frontal lobe partial seizures
Pelvic thrusting	Pelvic thrusting unusual except for frontal lobe partial seizures
Occurrence from preictal pseudosleep	Occurrence from sleep
Side-to-side head or body movement	Postictal stertorous (generalised tonic clonic seizures only)
Forced eye closure	
Ictal crying	
Memory recall of being in a generalised seizure	
Vocalisation during or after seizure	Vocalisation at beginning, primitive, no emotional expression

Adapted from Xiang et al. [4] under Creative Commons Attribution 4.0 International License.

Treatment should be tailored to the patient. Distraction techniques can be used to break a cycle such as at the start of a seizure when attention to something else may prevent a seizure progressing. Physical therapies for motor problems can be helpful, but these need to start early.

Prognosis

The mean delay to diagnosis of dissociative seizures is seven years. Up to 75% of patients with dissociative seizures may be misdiagnosed with epilepsy in the first instance. While remission from epilepsy can be as high as 70%, remission from dissociative seizures may be only 30%. Up to 80% of patients with limb weakness have persistent symptoms. Patients may also develop different subtypes of functional neurological disorders.

Early diagnosis, young age, not being invested in medical diagnosis, not taking medication and being in work are all positive prognostic predictors. Poor prognosis occurs in individuals with a late diagnosis, and who have multiple functional system disorders, psychiatric co-morbidities and a personality disorder. Developing the appropriate services may be key to improve the prognosis.

Neurologists have slowly embraced their role in diagnosis and management of patients with functional neurological disorder. Overcoming myths in functional neurological disorder will be important for neurologists and their patients. Some myths that may obstruct management of functional neurological disorder include: 1. functional neurological disorder is feigned behaviour; 2. functional neurological disorder is a diagnosis of exclusion; 3. functional neurological disorder treatment is solely psychological or psychiatric therapy; 4. there is no role for investigation in a diagnosis of functional neurological disorder; and 5. bizarre behaviour denotes functional neurological disorder.

References

1. Walzl D, Carson AJ, Stone J. The misdiagnosis of functional disorders as other neurological conditions. *J Neurol.* 2019;266(8):2018–26.

2. Stone J. Functional neurological disorders: the neurological assessment as treatment. *Pract Neurol.* 2016;16:7–17.

3. Espay AJ, Lang AE. Phenotype-specific diagnosis of functional (psychogenic) movement disorders. *Curr Neurol Neurosci Reports.* 2015;15(32).

4. Xiang X, Fang J, Guo Y. Differential diagnosis between epileptic seizures and psychogenic non-epileptic seizures based on semiology. *Acta Epileptologica* 2019;1:6.

Learning Points

- Functional neurological disorder is a clinical diagnosis. Clear positive evidence of functional neurological disorder is derived from examination signs and/or seizure features.
- Explaining a functional neurological disorder can have a therapeutic role.
- The impact of functional neurological disorder is compounded by misunderstandings that the condition is voluntary or caused entirely by psychological factors.

Patient's Perspective

1. **What is the impact of the condition on you?**

    a. **Physical (e.g. practical support, activities of daily living)**
    The impact can change from day to day. On a bad day I go through periods of taking tremors, seizures, falls. My body physically does not work. My brain knows what it wants to do, but unfortunately parts of my body do not respond. Daily living can be very difficult. From being washed to dressed these have to be done by my husband. Depending on how I am, activities can change; nothing is ever set in stone anymore.

b. Psychological (e.g. mood, emotional well-being)

My mood will be very low when I am in a relapse but that is to be expected. No-one enjoys being sick or being unable to do things for themselves. I can get a lot of mixed emotions. I can get angry and frustrated. When I can't walk or talk I feel worthless as a person, a wife, a mother, a friend. I know now this is only temporary but sometimes I am scared these emotions will not leave.

c. Social (e.g. meeting friends, home)

My whole social life changes and has changed certain aspects of my life. I've become anxious in many ways. I may be worried that I would take a seizure in a public place. I get embarrassed if I am out with aids, i.e. rollator or wheelchair, or when people stop to talk, I just want to go home as this is where I feel safe. There will be times when I am unable to leave my home and that is down to me being physically unable to walk. I will be in bed until I am able to do things for myself. I've cancelled plans with friends because I just cannot commit to them. I also know that my friends can get scared in case I take sick and they don't know what to do. This puts me in a position where I don't want to put them in that situation where they have to look after me. I just feel it's unfair and scary for them.

2. **What can you not do because of the condition?**

   This is a good question. The things I have not been able to do due to FND have had a massive impact on my life. I have felt at stages that I was unable to be a mother to my two girls; they have both been in situations with me when they have had to ring for ambulances due to me taking seizures. For periods I have been unable to walk as my legs will just not carry me – they would shake and tremor or just leave me. I've had countless falls due to this. I've been unable to dress myself, wash myself, take myself to the toilet. My husband has to carry me in his arms upstairs and put me to bed. I've been unable to feed myself at times. Plans such as holidays have been cancelled, days out with friends cancelled. I've been unable to work, which has had a massive impact on my life, particularly my mental health and providing for my two girls. I was a carer for eight years and going from being a carer to being cared for was so hard. I felt I lost my life, my dignity. I felt like I lost myself. I was no longer that girl who worked, who was active and fit. My whole life changed over a period of time. I felt a part of me lost being a good wife as I became the sick wife. At times I cannot talk, so I've been rushed to hospital when I've been unable to talk to explain my situation.

3. **Has there been any other change for you due to your condition?**

   I lost myself along the way. I've tried to find myself again. It changed so much in my life. It has changed how I look at things in life. I am on medication, which I do not like.

4. **What is/was the most difficult aspect of the condition for you?**

   I think the last time I was in hospital was one of my worst and most difficult times. I had relapsed so bad I hadn't walked in 5 weeks, endless seizures, endless falls. As I was in hospital during COVID, I couldn't see people at normal visiting hours. Waiting for results of scans has also been very worrying. I felt alone and scared and thought that I was never going to get back to walking. I remember coming round from seizures being on oxygen, heart traces and a team of medical people around me. I was grateful for them and how they looked after me when I was in that state.

   Another difficult aspect has been seeing the fear in my children's faces when they see me in these states. It's hard for me to accept that I do have an illness, a lifelong chronic one- that has been very hard. It's such a hard illness to explain and in my opinion the only way I feel, is that it is similar to MS. Maybe I feel this due to my work background in caring.

   I know I mentioned walking a lot but that is massive for me. Losing my mobility nearly finished me mentally. I think we all in life take for granted putting one foot in front of the other. At time I've felt like I can't go on any longer. I can't keep putting my family through this as everyone of our lives change. I then hold onto hope that I will be ok with time and that I have time.

5. **Was any aspect of the experience good or useful? What was that?**

   When I was last in hospital my daughter, who is 16, phoned me to tell me that her friend took a seizure in the school toilets and she knew how to work with her and get her friend the help that was needed. My daughters have had to see and grow up that little bit faster due to me, but I hope and believe that they have learned lifelong skills by living a childhood with FND.

6. **What do you hope for in the future for people with this condition?**

I hope in the future for anyone living a life with FND is more understood. I hope for more awareness of FND and more funding for training days for staff. I hope one day there will be a neurology ward as during every stay in hospital I have met staff who had never heard of FND, which blows my mind. How are they to look after someone with this condition when they know nothing about it, not even doctors know about it!

I also hope one day we will have better answers why this happens. We know triggers that can set it off. I for one know my life before this was so different; I was a completely different person. I took sepsis seven years ago and I have never been the same.

I hope doctors do not put it down to a mental health problem. My reasoning for saying this is that one time in A and E a doctor tried to tell me that I was depressed, which made me very upset. I was then admitted to hospital for nearly two weeks. My question here is how can depression make you unable to walk, talk, get dressed and do your normal day-to-day physical things.

34 Clouding of Consciousness in Hospital

History

A 70-year-old woman, who had been mobilising at home with a Zimmer frame, went off her food. She developed vomiting and diarrhoea and ate less food than usual for three weeks. She was then admitted to a surgical ward in hospital with abdominal pain. While in hospital, she became less responsive. A neurology referral was made two weeks into her admission. By that stage, she had had little nutrition for five weeks. She had been treated for a presumed urinary tract infection with piperacillin with tazobactam (a beta-lactamase inhibitor).

She had co-morbidities including congestive cardiac failure, chronic kidney disease, hiatus hernia, gastric ulcer and left pedicle conjunctival flap for spontaneous corneal perforation. She did not drink alcohol.

Examination

At the time of the neurology assessment, she was encephalopathic. Her alertness varied, making co-operation for examination difficult. She could move her limbs and open her eyes spontaneously but her only verbal communication was groaning. She had conjugate eye movements. She had a flaccid areflexic quadriparesis (power of 2–3 out of 5). She had flexor plantar responses. Although difficult to assess, sensation appeared diminished.

Investigations

Blood investigations from early in her hospital admission showed pancytopenia (platelets 70 $\times 10^9$/L). This recovered prior to the encephalopathy.

Other investigations were normal or negative including thyroid profile, liver function tests, ammonia (12 µmol/L, normal range 22–88 µmol/L), NMDA receptor antibody and nuclear autoantibody screen. Creatine kinase was 46 U/L (normal range <70 U/L), anti-GM1 antibody was negative, anti-GQ1b antibody was negative and porphyrin screen was negative. Lead, thallium and mercury levels were all normal or negative. A search for faecal *Campylobacter jejuni* was negative.

A nutritional screen showed a low selenium level of 0.44 µmol/L (normal range 0.6–1.3 µmol/L), low zinc level of 7.5 µmol/L (normal range 8.0–15.0 µmol/L), normal copper level of 15.4 µmol/L (normal range 12.6–26.7 µmol/L), normal B12 level of 245 pmol/L (normal range 118–701 pmol/L) and low folate level of 2.0 µg/L (normal range 3.9–26.8 µg/L).

At lumbar puncture, there was an opening pressure of 8 cm of cerebrospinal fluid (CSF), no white cells/µL, 85 red cells/µL, an elevated CSF protein at 2.47 g/L (normal range <0.4 g/L) and CSF glucose of 3.7 mmol/L (serum glucose 5.2 mmol/L). An infective screen (PCR for herpes simplex virus, varicella zoster and enterovirus) was negative.

An MRI of the brain showed increased T2 signal in a symmetrical distribution in periventricular regions, medial thalamic nuclei, the floor of the third ventricle, mammillary bodies, periaqueductal grey matter, the midbrain reticular formation and the tectal plate (Figures 34.1A and 34.1B).

An MRI scan of the spine revealed degenerative disc changes but no cord compression.

An EEG was dominated by diffuse slow activity, which appeared slower on the right. There were also sharp waves over both cerebral hemispheres. The findings were in keeping with a moderate diffuse encephalopathy.

Nerve conduction studies demonstrated a severe length-dependent axonal loss peripheral neuropathy affecting both sensory and motor fibres.

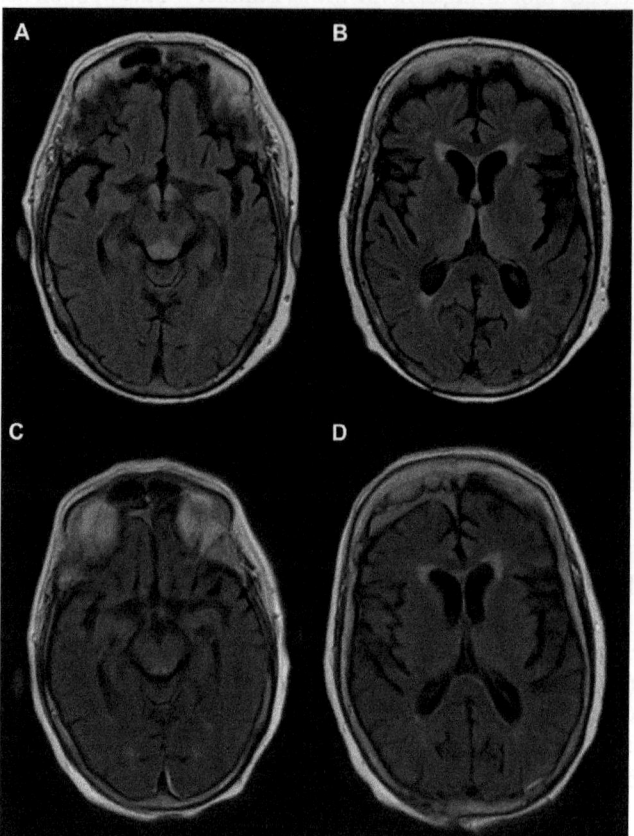

Figure 34.1 (A and B) An axial T2 FLAIR showing symmetrical abnormalities in periventricular regions, medial thalamic nuclei, the floor of the third ventricle, mammillary bodies, periaqueductal grey matter, the midbrain reticular formation and the tectal plate. (C and D) Two months later, the high signal changes had markedly improved.

Diagnosis: Dry Beriberi – Wernicke's Encephalopathy and Polyneuropathy

Management

The patient was treated with intravenous multivitamins (thiamine, riboflavin, pyridoxine, ascorbic acid and nicotinamide). She then had intravenous immunoglobulin at 2 g/kg over five days. A percutaneous enteral gastrostomy tube was inserted for nutrition.

A follow-up MRI of the brain at two months demonstrated a marked improvement (Figures 34.1C and 34.1D). There was a clinical improvement but she never reached her pre-hospital baseline. Mobility was limited, requiring a wheelchair, and feeding continued via a percutaneous enteral gastrostomy tube.

Comment

This patient demonstrated two manifestations of dry beriberi – Wernicke's encephalopathy and a polyneuropathy mimicking Guillain–Barré syndrome or acute inflammatory axonal neuropathy. There is considerable overlap in the clinical features of ascending polyneuropathy in dry beriberi and Guillain–Barré syndrome including an elevated CSF protein. The albuminocytological dissociation can occur in both diseases but there is typically a mild elevation in CSF protein in beriberi [1]. The markedly elevated CSF protein in our patient triggered empirical treatment with intravenous immunoglobulins. The clinical scenario may still have been explained in terms of 'Occam's or Ockham's razor' – two serious neurological manifestations of the one disease – dry beriberi neuropathy and Wernicke's encephalopathy due to thiamine deficiency. The differential diagnosis for the weakness includes acute, subacute and chronic demyelinating polyneuropathies, critical illness myopathy and critical illness neuropathy.

Dry beriberi patients present with a neuropathy, while wet beriberi patients have heart failure with or without neuropathy. The diagnostic features of Guillain–Barré–Strohl syndrome (often shortened to Guillain–Barré syndrome) include progressive limb weakness and areflexia.

Epidemiology and Clinical Presentation of Wernicke's Encephalopathy

Wernicke's encephalopathy has a well-recognised triad of encephalopathy, ataxia and eye movement abnormalities, but an affected patient may not have all three features [2], which can delay diagnosis. Although first described in 1881 by Carl Wernicke, thiamine deficiency was not recognised until the 1940s by Colin Campbell and Ritchie Russell as the cause of Wernicke's encephalopathy. Autopsy prevalence rates of Wernicke's encephalopathy (0.8–2.8%) exceed clinical diagnostic rates of Wernicke's encephalopathy [2]. The frequency of the clinical features of Wernicke's encephalopathy are:

- eye movement abnormalities including vertical nystagmus (29%)
- ataxia (23%)
- mental status changes (82%)
- all three features (16%)
- no features of the triad at presentation (19%)

Uncommon presentations are recognised, including stupor, hypothermia, hearing loss, hypotension and tachycardia, epileptic seizures and visual disturbances with papilloedema. Because of the under-recognition of Wernicke's encephalopathy, operational diagnostic criteria have been established particularly for alcoholic patients, and early parenteral thiamine treatment for any of the aforementioned presenting features [2].

Although red cell transketolase and thiamine levels had not been measured before treatment with high-dose thiamine in our patient, the MRI brain findings were characteristic of thiamine deficiency. Although folic acid, selenium and zinc were also deficient in our patient, the clinical and imaging features are best explained by thiamine deficiency.

Pathology of Wernicke's Encephalopathy

Thiamine is transported passively and actively across the blood–brain barrier. Body stores of thiamine can be depleted within 18 days. Thiamine is required for the production of thiamine pyrophosphate in glia and neurones to act as a coenzyme in intermediate carbohydrate metabolism, lipid metabolism, production of amino acids and generation of glucose-derived neurotransmitters (glutamic acid and gamma-aminobutyric acid). The importance of thiamine is further underlined as its other roles include synaptic transmission and axonal transmission.

Thiamine deficiency initially is associated with a decrease in α-ketoglutarate dehydrogenase, low intracellular glutamate, high extracellular glutamate and accumulation of lactate. Structural lesions ensue in particular parts of the brain including small haemorrhages in the periaqueductal grey matter, mammillary bodies and medial thalamus. A reversible component exists if prompt and sufficient thiamine therapy is provided, as shown in our patient. At neuropathology, chronically swollen astrocytes and proliferation of small blood vessels have been identified with relative neuronal and axonal sparing.

Adults require 1.4 mg/day of thiamine (recommendation 1.0–1.5 mg/day) but requirements of thiamine increase with caloric intake (0.33 mg of thiamine per 1,050 kcal consumed). Similarly, critically ill patients have higher requirements of thiamine.

Usually, Wernicke's encephalopathy is more likely in a patient with a history of excess alcohol and resulting malnutrition. However, Wernicke's encephalopathy can occur in any individual who is malnourished. In Asia, polished white rice, which is deficient in thiamine, has caused endemic beriberi. Recognised causes of Wernicke's encephalopathy are listed in Table 34.1, but genetic and epigenetic susceptibilities have also been identified.

As Wernicke's encephalopathy can cause death and can be difficult to recognise, intensive care and high dependency units often have a policy of high-dose thiamine infusions in all admitted patients. Wernicke's encephalopathy is an acute neuropsychiatric emergency. Without adequate thiamine replacement, progression to Korsakoff's syndrome or death can ensue. Korsakoff's syndrome manifests with irreversible cognitive and behavioural problems, including anterograde and retrograde amnesia, executive dysfunction, confabulation and apathy.

Management

There is understandably a lack of randomised controlled trials to inform evidence-based guidelines on management of patients with Wernicke's encephalopathy. However, a minimum of 500 mg of thiamine dissolved in 100 ml of normal saline is recommended three times a day for two to three days. In the UK, two ampoules of multivitamins are administered (250 mg of thiamine with 4 mg of riboflavin, 50 mg of pyridoxine in one ampoule and 160 mg nicotinamide and 500 mg of ascorbic acid or vitamin C in the second ampoule) for three to five days followed by one pair daily for a further three to five days.

Table 34.1 Causes of Wernicke encephalopathy

Clinical setting
Chronic alcohol abuse and malnutrition
Recurrent vomiting or chronic diarrhoea
Gastrointestinal surgical procedures including bariatric surgery
Cancer and chemotherapy (gastric carcinoma, large B-cell lymphoma and ifosfamide)
Systemic disease (renal disease, AIDS, chronic infectious febrile diseases)
Magnesium depletion (chronic diuretic, intestinal resection, Crohn's disease)
Drugs (intravenous high-dose nitroglycerin and tolazamide)
Nutritional imbalance (polished white rice is deficient in thiamine, absolute deficiency of food/thiamine)

Adapted from Sechi et al. [2] with permission from Elsevier.

Table 34.2 Reversible and easily overlooked encephalopathies

Encephalopathy	Useful pointers
Hepatic encephalopathy	Ammonia
Uraemic encephalopathy	Renal function
Hypoglycaemia	History, drugs, glucose, MRI of the brain
Electrolyte abnormalities	Sodium, calcium, magnesium
Pancreatic encephalopathy	Amylase
Wernicke's encephalopathy	Thiamine, red cell transketolase, MRI of the brain
Pellagra encephalopathy (dermatitis, diarrhoea and dementia)	Urinary N-methylnicotinamide and 2-pyridone Serum tryptophan and niacin
Medication-induced encephalopathy	Review of drug chart
• Cefepime	
• Ifosphamide	
Septic encephalopathy	Blood culture
Osmotic demyelination syndrome	Temporal electrolyte change and MRI of the brain
Fat embolism syndrome	CT of the brain
Overdose (e.g. barbiturate)	Prescription drug reserves

Adapted from Weathers et al. [3] with permission from Thieme.

An important clinical management issue is avoidance of intravenous glucose before treatment with thiamine in patients suspected of Wernicke's encephalopathy as glucose can precipitate Wernicke's encephalopathy.

This patient's journey highlights a cascade effect, which can ensue in an individual becoming deficient in thiamine.

Reversible Encephalopathies

In clinical practice, reversible encephalopathies are very important. Some such encephalopathies are listed in the Table 34.2 [3].

Haematologists are familiar with ifosphamide encephalopathy (drowsiness, confusion, hallucinations and seizures or severe coma) in patients receiving what was second-line treatment for diffuse large B-cell lymphoma. While Wernicke's encephalopathy and ifosphamide encephalopathy can co-exist, they appear to be separate entities despite use of thiamine in ifosphamide encephalopathy. Methylene blue is established as the main treatment and prevention of ifosphamide encephalopathy. Methylene blue shortens the duration of the encephalopathy by accepting electrons for the flavoprotein deficiency induced by ifosphamide and/or by inhibiting multiple amine oxidases, which prevent formation of the neurotoxic chloroacetaldehyde from ifosfamide-derived chloroethyl amine.

Fat embolism syndrome may be first identified by a radiologist reporting a CT brain scan on a 'confused patient'.

References

1. Shible AA, Ramadurai D, Gergen D, Reynolds PM. Dry beriberi due to thiamine deficiency associated with peripheral neuropathy and Wernicke's encephalopathy mimicking Guillain Barré syndrome: a case report and review of the literature. *Am J Case Rep.* 2019;20:330–4.
2. Sechi G, Serra A. Wernicke's encephalopathy: new clinical settings and recent advances in diagnosis and management. *Lancet Neurol.* 2007;6(5):442–55.
3. Weathers AL, Lewis SL. Rare and unusual … or are they? Less commonly diagnosed encephalopathies associated with systemic disease. *Semin Neurol.* 2009;29(2):136–53.

Learning Points

- Dry beriberi due to thiamine deficiency presents with encephalopathy and polyneuropathy.
- Wernicke's encephalopathy (eye movement abnormalities, ataxia and mental status change) can occur in any malnourished individuals, including patients without a history of excess alcohol consumption.
- Clinicians should have a low threshold for suspecting and treating Wernicke's encephalopathy with atypical presenting features such as unknown causes of coma or stupor, hypothermia or hyperthermia, or tachycardia or intractable hypotension.
- Avoid intravenous glucose before parenteral thiamine in patients suspected of Wernicke's encephalopathy as the glucose can precipitate more florid Wernicke's encephalopathy.

Perspective from Patient's Daughter

She never recovered. She needed help with all her activities of daily living. Her mood was low and social contacts were restricted to just family, who provided much of the help at home.

For others with this condition I hope they get the help they need before the condition worsens.

35 Leaky Effects of Rising Pressure

History

A 47-year-old man developed an altered mental state and right limb weakness while in hospital. He had been admitted to hospital with a blood pressure of 250/140 mmHg. A stroke thrombolysis call was made when he became confused with right-sided weakness. A CT scan of the brain and a CT angiogram from the arch of the aorta to the circle of Willis were performed. He was not treated with intravenous thrombolysis as he was improving.

Past medical history included hypertension and chronic kidney disease. He had no history of diabetes mellitus. He drank five beers per week and was a non-smoker.

Examination

He became increasingly alert during the examination, which had some variability. He had conjugate gaze. He had no facial weakness. He had right limb tactile inattention but no visual inattention. He was increasingly able to move his right arm and leg with power of at least grade 3–4/5. Reflexes were symmetrically present and his plantar responses were flexor.

Investigations

A CT of the brain showed a low-density left cerebellar lesion and general white matter disease. A CT angiogram from the arch of the aorta to the circle of Willis was normal.

An MRI scan of brain revealed a number of periventricular lesions and posterior confluent lesions. There was an extensive pontine lesion, a left cerebellar lesion and signal change in the splenium of the corpus callosum (Figures 35.1A and 35.1B). There was no restricted diffusion.

MRI brain scans five days later showed resolution of the pontine lesion and an improvement in the left cerebellar lesion (Figures 35.1C and 35.1D).

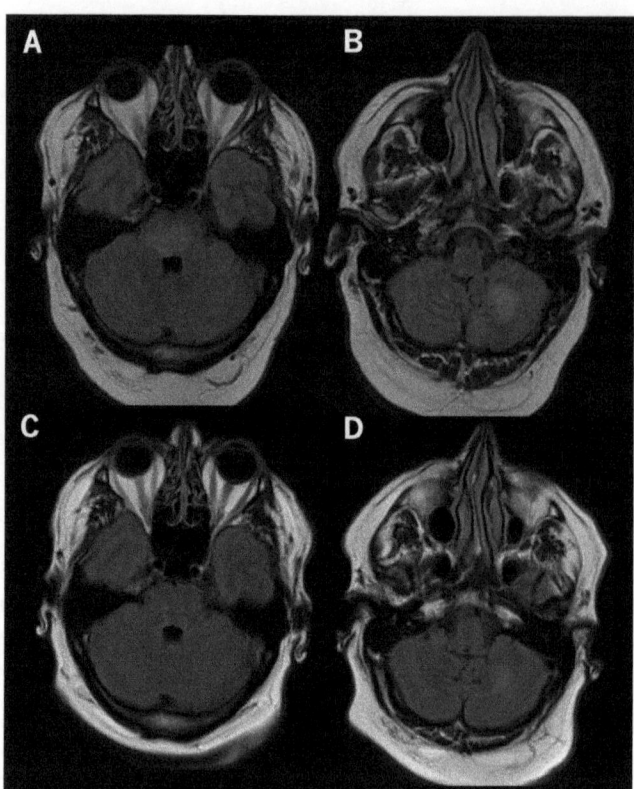

Figure 35.1 Axial FLAIR MRI brain scans showing (A) pontine and (B) left cerebellar high signal. Five days later, (C) the high signal in the pons had fully resolved while (D) the right cerebellar high signal had partially resolved.

Diagnosis: Posterior Reversible Encephalopathy Syndrome

Management

The patient's high blood pressure was treated with no further recurrences. The medication was adjusted to even out blood pressure control throughout the day.

Commentary

Definition of Posterior Reversible Encephalopathy

Posterior reversible encephalopathy syndrome (PRES) manifests with variable symptoms and signs including encephalopathy, disorders of consciousness, very high blood pressure, epileptic seizures, headache, visual disturbance and to a lesser extent focal neurological deficits [1]. Both clinical and radiological appearances are usually reversible; most patients show clinical and radiological recovery within a week. Although MRI of the brain can show vasogenic oedema and has increased the recognition of PRES, the condition lacks specific diagnostic criteria and so is almost certainly under-recognised.

Posterior reversible encephalopathy syndrome results from acute hypertension, severe fluctuations in blood pressure, direct endothelial injury from immunosuppressant drugs or autoimmune disorders or occurs in the setting of eclampsia. The prognosis is usually very good, although fatalities (from resulting ischaemic or haemorrhagic stroke) can occur in 3–6% [2]. The clinical symptoms of confusion, seizures, headache and visual symptoms are not specific for PRES.

Posterior reversible encephalopathy syndrome is in fact a misnomer; other parts of the brain as well as the brainstem [3] and even spinal cord can be affected. Imaging can be normal but the operational diagnostic framework relies on neuroimaging.

Pathophysiology

Elevated arterial blood pressure has been observed in the early stages of the majority of PRES patients. Cerebral perfusion pressure (mean arterial pressure – intracranial pressure) is maintained via autoregulation, which keeps cerebral bloodflow relatively constant over a range of blood pressure changes. One hypothesis (the hyperperfusion hypothesis) suggests that, once elevated, blood pressure exceeds the upper limit for autoregulation. Cerebral hyperperfusion follows from blood–brain barrier dysfunction with vascular leakage of plasma and macromolecules through tight junction proteins resulting in vasogenic oedema [1]. Relatively diminished sympathetic innervation of the posterior circulation has been postulated as the reason for posterior circulatory distribution prominence of the syndrome.

However, up to 30% of patients with PRES have normal or only modestly elevated blood pressure, suggesting, at least for these patients, that another mechanism may play a more prominent pathophysiological role. Another hypothesis involves circulating toxins (endogenous as in (pre-)eclampsia and sepsis or exogenous such as chemotherapeutic agents), which are thought to trigger endothelial dysfunction by interrupting the function of inter-endothelial adhesion molecules. Release of pro-inflammatory cytokines results in increased vascular permeability and vasogenic oedema [1]. A case series of 15 patients with PRES reported in the *New England Journal of Medicine* in 1996 included eclamptic patients and patients on immunosuppressive medication. However, the association between toxaemia of pregnancy and hypertension had been reported by 1897.

The pathophysiology involves loss of integrity of tight junctions, increased circulating cytokines, activation of endothelial cells, increased expression of adhesion molecules and increased circulating vascular endothelial growth factor (VEGF), which increases vascular permeability. Despite a number of theories of the pathophysiology of PRES, the final common pathway always involves endothelial dysfunction, disruption of the blood–brain barrier, local hyperperfusion and vasogenic oedema [1].

Imaging features have been studied in detail. Vasogenic oedema predominantly occurs in the parieto-occipital region, but lesions are common in the frontal lobe, cerebellum (as in our patient) and in the basal ganglia [4]. Restricted diffusion can occur in 15–30% and PRES is found in 17–38% of patients with reversible cerebral vasoconstrictor syndrome [2].

Suggested diagnostic criteria for PRES [1] have been proposed that consist of:

- acute onset of neurological symptoms
- focal vasogenic oedema on neuroimaging
- reversibility of clinical and/or radiological findings.

The differential diagnosis of PRES is large and includes vascular, neurodegenerative, auto-immune, paraneoplastic, infectious, metabolic and cancer-related conditions, as shown in Table 35.1 [4].

Table 35.1 Differential diagnosis of PRES

Category	Examples
Vascular	Cerebral ischaemia (posterior circulatory stroke) Cerebral venous sinus thrombosis Intracerebral haemorrhage Subcortical leukoaraiosis Central nervous system vasculitis Reversible cerebral vasoconstriction syndrome
Degenerative/autoimmune	Acute demyelinating encephalomyelitis Multiple sclerosis/acute disseminated encephalomyelitis Other autoimmune encephalitis (e.g. limbic encephalitis, Hashimoto's, Rasmussen, systemic lupus erythematosus, Behcet's disease) Cerebral autosomal dominant arteriopathy with subcortical infarcts and leukoencephalopathy (CADASIL) Mitochondrial encephalopathy, lactic acidosis, and stroke-like episodes (MELAS) Creutzfeldt–Jakob disease
Infectious	Herpes simplex encephalitis Other infectious encephalitis Progressive multifocal leucoencephalopathy
Cancer-related	Malignancy or tumour (lymphoma, gliomatosis cerebri, metastatic disease) Paraneoplastic encephalitis Chemotherapy-related demyelinating disorder Radiation necrosis
Metabolic	Metabolic encephalopathy Osmotic demyelination syndrome Toxic leucoencephalopathy

Adapted from Liman et al. [4] with permission from Wolters Kluwer.

A suggested diagnostic algorithm for PRES in the absence of an alternative diagnosis includes at least one acute neurological symptom (seizure, altered mental status, headache, visual disturbances), one or more risk factors (severe hypertension, renal failure, immunosuppressant drugs or chemotherapy, eclampsia, autoimmune disorder), and neuroimaging showing bilateral vasogenic oedema, cytotoxic oedema with PRES patterns or normal imaging [2].

The medulla oblongata regulates heart rate, stroke volume and vascular tone by responding to (carotid/aorta) baroreceptors and chemoreceptor signals. The rostral ventral medulla and upper cervical spinal cord, under influence from cerebral cortex, hypothalamus and the limbic system influence central blood pressure control. Cerebral autoregulation helps maintain relatively constant blood flow, although this shifts to the right in patients with chronic hypertension. This may at least partially explain how many patients tolerate hypertension without developing PRES more often.

Management of PRES

Posterior reversible encephalopathy syndrome in the brainstem and cerebellum can lead to hydrocephalus, requiring urgent neurosurgical intervention. Recommended management involves correcting the underlying pathology or removing the implicated medication. For hypertension, a reduction of blood pressure by 25% from baseline has been recommended, although there is no randomised prospective controlled trial evidence [1]. Other symptomatic treatments include anti-epileptic medication for seizures, but these can be withdrawn when recovery occurs.

References

1. Fischer M, Schmutzhard E. Posterior reversible encephalopathy syndrome. *J Neurol.* 2017;264:1608–16.

2. Fugate JE, Rabinstein AA. Posterior reversible encephalopathy syndrome: clinical and radiological manifestations, pathophysiology, and outstanding questions. *Lancet Neurol.* 2015;14(9):914–25.

3. McCarron MO, McKinstry CS. Vanishing brainstem edema. *J Stroke Cerebrovasc Dis.* 2008;17(3):156–7.

4. Liman TG, Siebert E, Endres M. Posterior reversible encephalopathy syndrome. *Curr Opin Neurol.* 2019 Feb.;32(1):25–35.

Learning Points

- Posterior reversible encephalopathy syndrome can present with a wide range of symptoms from mild encephalopathy to coma, epileptic seizures, headache and visual disturbance.
- Elevated blood pressure is a common feature of the early stages of PRES. Eclampsia and immunosuppressant drugs are recognised triggers of PRES.
- Different theories for the pathophysiology of PRES all involve endothelial dysfunction, breakdown of the blood–brain barrier, local hyperperfusion and vasogenic oedema.
- Despite the name, the pathology of PRES is not restricted to the posterior brain.
- Lesion reversibility on MRI of the brain can confirm a diagnosis of PRES.

Patient's Perspective

1. **What was the impact of the condition on you?**

    a. **Physical (e.g. practical support, washing, dressing activity)**
    I had no interest in washing or my appearance. I had no interest in getting my hair cut, in cooking, cleaning and day-to-day life.

b. **Psychological (e.g. mood, emotional well-being)**
I was moody and very argumentative. I was angry, fed-up and low.

c. **Social (e.g. meeting friends, interacting with family at home)**
I had no interest in meeting anyone or going anywhere. I was interacting with family in an argumentative way at home.

2. **What could you no longer do because of the condition?**
Activities such as walking a long distance caused tiredness.

3. **Was there any other change for you due to your medical condition?**
Besides the mood swings and tiredness, I had weakness in my arms and legs. I didn't always understand and sometimes I was confused.

4. **What is/was the most difficult aspect of the condition for you?**
Not knowing what was happening and now knowing it could happen at anytime, that I could have a stroke or heart attack because my blood pressure can't be controlled.

5. **Was any aspect of the experience good or useful? What was that?**
None as I always have that fear that it could happen anytime.

6. **What do you hope for in the future for your condition?**
I hope that this will help other people with my condition. I am always monitoring my blood pressure but fear the worst.

History

A 66-year-old woman was admitted to hospital with confusion. For three months, her son had noticed a deterioration in her memory. He also noticed new confusion but she retained her awareness of day and night. She had no falls but had lost over 10 kg in weight over four months. She experienced no hallucinations.

Past medical history included chronic obstructive pulmonary disease, hypothyroidism (previous subtotal thyroidectomy and radio-iodine treatment), anxiety and depression, diverticular disease, gastro-oesophageal reflux, osteopenia and coeliac disease.

Medication included multivitamins, levothyroxine 75 µg/day, fluticasone/umeclidinium/vianterol inhaler, calcium with vitamin D3, beclometasone/formoterol inhaler and fluoxetine 20 mg.

She smoked cigarettes (35 pack year history), but alcohol consumption was no more than two pints of Guinness in eight weeks. She had 11 siblings. One sister had died from ovarian cancer at the age of 56 years.

Examination

She knew her age and the day of the week but did not know where she was. Her Folstein mini mental score was 15 out of 30. She was not dysphasic. She had normal tone and power but was unsteady on heel-toe walking. Sensation was intact. She had absent ankle jerks.

Investigations

Electrolytes showed that sodium was reduced at 115 mmol/L, which was slowly corrected. Serum osmolality was 270 mOsm/kg, B12 was normal. Her folate level was low at 3.7 µg/L (normal range 3.9–26.8 µg/L).

An MRI scan of the brain showed increased signal in the medial temporal lobes (Figure 36.1).

At lumbar puncture, there was an opening pressure of 9 cm of cerebrospinal fluid (CSF), 1 white cell/µL, 7 red cells/µL, CSF glucose of 5.4 mmol/L (serum glucose of 5.0 mmol/L) and CSF protein of 0.34 g/L. PCR for herpes simplex virus 1 and 2, varicella zoster, enterovirus and parechovirus were negative. Cerebrospinal fluid cytology was negative.

A CT scan of the chest abdomen and pelvis as well as mammography revealed no evidence of malignancy.

HIV and syphilis tests were negative. N-methyl-D-aspartate (NMDA) receptor, leucine-rich glioma-inactivated 1 (LGI-1), contactin-associated protein-like 2 (CASPR2), α-amino-3-hydroxy-5-methyl-4-isoxazoleproprionic acid (AMPA) 1 receptor, AMPA2 receptor, γ-aminobutyric acid-B (GABA-B) receptor and glutamic acid decarboxylase (GAD) antibodies were all negative. Voltage-gated calcium channel antibody was negative.

An EEG had low amplitude and an excess of slow waves, at times maximal over the left temporal area and spreading to the left fronto-temporal area.

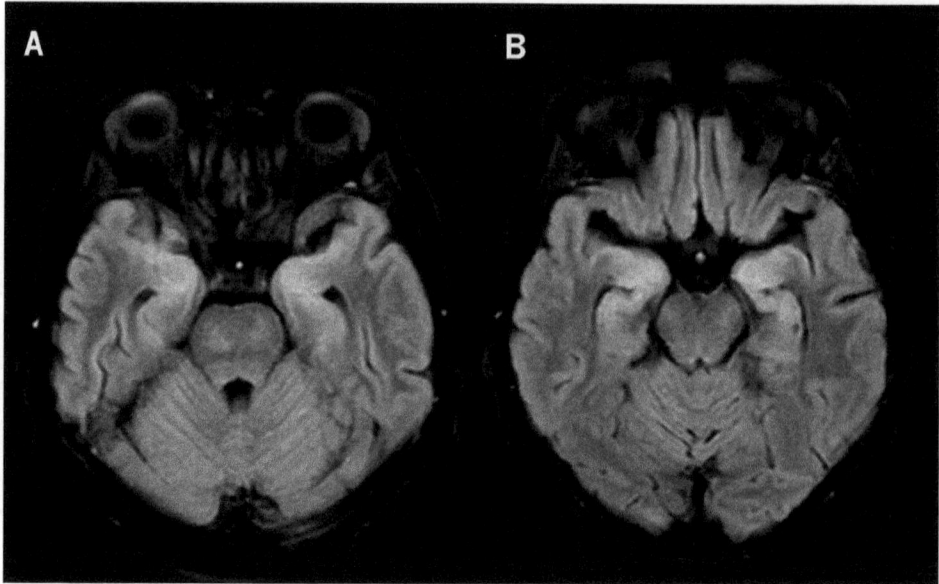

Figure 36.1 An axial T2-FLAIR MRI scan of the brain showing high signal in medial temporal structures consistent with encephalitis.

Differential Diagnosis

At the time of clinical assessment, infective and autoimmune/paraneoplastic encephalitides were considered.

Management

Despite correcting hyponatraemia and folate, the confusion did not resolve. Respiratory problems accumulated before stabilising. She was treated with intravenous aciclovir (10 mg/kg tid) for two weeks.

A paraneoplastic screen was negative for anti-Yo and anti-Ri antibodies but demonstrated a positive anti-Hu antibody in blood and CSF. Follow-up CSF analyses were otherwise normal or negative.

She was transferred to a nursing home and remained stable. Six months after her presentation, she developed a tonic-clonic seizure. A further seizure occurred two months later. No further seizures occurred when she was established on levetiracetam.

A search for malignancy included repeat CT of the chest abdomen and pelvis, PET scanning and mammography, which had remained negative after two years of follow-up. Serial MRI scans of the brain showed some fluctuation in the extent of the increased signal in the medial temporal lobes but no resolution.

Diagnosis: Anti–Hu Syndrome Limbic Encephalitis

Comment

Differential Diagnosis of Limbic Encephalitis

Limbic encephalitis has a number of causes, as outlined in Table 36.1 [1].

Definition of Paraneoplastic Neurological Syndrome

Paraneoplastic neurological syndromes are non-metastatic or remote neurological compli-cations of systemic malignancy due to immune-mediated neuronal dysfunction or death [2]. The high-risk phenotypes are encephalomyelitis, limbic encephalitis, rapidly progres-sive cerebellar syndrome, opsoclonus-myoclonus, sensory neuronopathy, gastrointestinal pseudo-obstruction (enteric neuropathy) and Lambert–Eaton myasthenic syndromes. The syndromes can precede detection of cancer by up to five years and occur when the underlying neoplasm expresses proteins, which are cross-reactive with neuronal proteins. The presence of a classical syndrome and the presence of the Hu antibody was previously considered a def-inite paraneoplastic syndrome, but revised criteria now categorise this as a high-risk pheno-type [1]. However, as explained later, the definite category should really have a co-existent cancer diagnosis. This was a particular issue for our patient. One in 300 people with cancer develop a paraneoplastic neurological syndrome, which may increase with the expanding use of immune checkpoint inhibitors.

In the 1960s, Peter Wilkinson and Jan Zeromski established that paraneoplastic neuro-logical disease could have an autoimmune basis. Tumours were thought to harbour antigens that cross-react with neuronal proteins but some antigens are not expressed in the associated tumour (e.g. Tr and Hodgkin's lymphoma). Two groups of antibodies have been detected in paraneoplastic neurological syndromes. Antibodies directed against neuronal cell-surface proteins such as NMDA receptor and LGI-1 protein cause non-lethal neuronal dysfunction. The associated conditions facio-brachial dystonic seizures and limbic encephalitis are often

Table 36.1 Differential diagnosis of limbic encephalitis

Disease
Herpes simplex encephalitis 1 and 2
Autoimmune/paraneoplastic encephalitis
Glioma
Status epilepticus
Lymphoma
Posterior reversible encephalopathy syndrome
Human herpes virus 6 and varicella zoster virus
Autoimmune systemic diseases (e.g. systemic lupus erythematosus, Behçet's disease)
Neurosyphilis
Chronic temporal lobe epilepsy
Wernicke's encephalopathy
Whipple disease

amenable to immune modulation treatment. A second group of antibodies, which include anti-Hu and anti-Yo, binds to intracellular proteins and ultimately leads to cell death, although the mechanisms are poorly understood.

Anti-Hu Syndromes

The anti-Hu (or ANNA-1) syndrome can manifest as a dorsal sensory neuronopathy (54%), cerebellar ataxia (10%), limbic encephalitis (9%), and encephalomyelitis or multifocal involvement. The presence of the anti-Hu antibody (often in serum and CSF) in the context of one of these high-risk phenotypes is almost invariably due to an underlying malignancy, most often small-cell lung cancer, neuroendocrine tumours and in children neuroblastoma [2]. However, in children, a non-paraneoplastic or autoimmune limbic encephalopathy presentation with an anti-Hu syndrome is recognised.

Role of Anti-Hu Antibodies

Hu (like Ma2, Yo and amphiphysin) is an intranuclear antigen. The anti-Hu antibodies are not thought to be pathogenic, but rather may be a marker of T-cell cytotoxicity against neurones. Importantly, paraneoplastic syndromes with antibodies to cell-surface antigens appear to have a better prognosis with immunosuppressive treatment combined with cancer treatment [2]. Vigorous treatment with immunoglobulins, cyclophosphamide and methylprednisolone has in general not been useful for paraneoplastic anti-Hu syndrome.

Paraneoplastic antineuronal antibodies with intracellular antigen targets that have a greater than 70% association with cancer are shown in Table 36.2. Anti-Hu, Ma1, Ma2, Ri, Tr and Yo are almost invariably associated with underlying malignancy. High-risk antibodies are defined as a greater than 70% cancer association [1].

Table 36.2 High-risk paraneoplastic neuronal antibodies against intracellular antigens

Antibody	Neurological phenotype	Frequency of cancer (%)	Associated malignancy
Hu	Sensory neuronopathy, chronic gastrointestinal pseudo-obstruction, encephalomyelitis, limbic encephalitis	85	Small-cell lung cancer, neuroendocrine tumours, retinoblastoma (infants)
CV2/CRMP5	Encephalomyelitis, sensory neuronopathy	>80	Small-cell lung cancer and thymoma
SOX1	Lambert–Eaton myasthenic syndrome with and without rapidly progressive cerebellar syndrome	>90	Small-cell lung cancer
Purkinje cell cytoplasmic antibody 2	Sensorimotor neuropathy, rapidly progressive cerebellar syndrome and encephalomyelitis	80	Non- and small-cell lung cancer and breast cancer
Amphiphysin	Polyradiculoneuropathy, sensory neuronopathy, encephalomyelitis and stiff person syndrome	80	Small-cell lung cancer and breast cancer
Ri	Brainstem/cerebellar syndrome, opsoclonus myoclonus syndrome	>70	Breast and lung (small and non-small-cell lung cancer)
Yo	Rapidly progressive cerebellar syndrome	>90	Ovary and breast cancer

Table 36.2 (Cont.)

Antibody	Neurological phenotype	Frequency of cancer (%)	Associated malignancy
Ma2 and/or Ma	Limbic encephalitis, diencephalitis and brainstem encephalitis	>75	Testicular cancer and non-small-cell lung cancer
Tr (DNER)	Rapidly progressive cerebellar syndrome	90	Hodgkin's lymphoma
Kelch-like protein 11 (KLHL11)	Brainstem/cerebellar syndrome	80	Testicular cancer

Adapted from Graus et al. [1] with permission from Wolters Kluwer.

Diagnostic Workup for Adults with Anti-Hu Syndrome

The diagnostic workup for a patient testing positive for anti-Hu antibody should include a thorough search for malignancy. Guidelines have been developed to screen for paraneoplastic tumours [3]. Cancers have been identified predominantly as small-cell lung carcinoma but non-small-cell lung cancer and extra-throacic neoplasms have also been identified in patients with anti-Hu syndromes (Table 36.3) [2].

The new diagnostic criteria for paraneoplastic neurological syndromes suggest that cancer screening should be guided by the phenotype and antibody [1]. High-risk phenotypes with high-risk antibodies require six monthly screening for two years as most tumours are diagnosed within two years.

In the updated 2021 diagnostic criteria for paraneoplastic neurological syndromes, a scoring system (PNS Care score) was devised based on the clinical phenotype association risk with cancer, antibody risk stratification and whether a cancer has been found or excluded after two years of appropriate cancer screening [1]. In this way, scores were assigned to identify definite, probable, possible and non-paraneoplastic syndrome categories. Our patient had a PNS Care score of 7 (high risk phenotype –3, high-risk antibody –3 and no cancer found within two years –1), which is a probable diagnostic level.

Immune-mediated adverse effects of immune checkpoint inhibitors have increasingly been recognised in oncology management. The diagnostic criteria for paraneoplastic neurological

Table 36.3 Neoplasms identified in anti-Hu syndrome patients

Tissue/histology
Lung/small-cell lung cancer
Lung/non-small-cell lung cancer
Prostate
Gastrointestinal
Breast
Bladder
Pancreas
Ovary
Neuroendocrine tumours
Neuroblastoma

syndromes will probably have to be applied more often in these scenarios including neuronal antibody testing when patients develop immune-related adverse effects of immune checkpoint inhibitors.

References

1. Graus F, Vogrig A, Muñiz-Castrillo S et al. Updated diagnostic criteria for paraneoplastic neurologic syndromes. *Neurol Neuroimmunol Neuroinflammation*. 2021;8(4):e1014.

2. Galli J, Greenlee J. Paraneoplastic diseases of the central nervous system. *F1000Research*. 2020;9:167.

3. Titulaer MJ, Soffietti R, Dalmau J et al. Screening for tumours in paraneoplastic syndromes: report of an EFNS Task Force. *Eur J Neurol*. 2011;18(1):19–e3.

Learning Points

- Paraneoplastic neurological syndromes are remote and immune-mediated neurological effects of cancer.
- Six high-risk clinical phenotypes include encephalomyelitis, limbic encephalitis, rapidly progressive cerebellar syndrome, opsoclonus-myoclonus, sensory neuronopathy, gastrointestinal pseudo-obstruction and Lambert–Eaton myasthenic syndrome.
- Paraneoplastic neuronal antibodies are either antibodies to neuronal cell surface proteins or antibodies directed at intracellular antigens.
- Antibody risk stratification along with clinical phenotype and cancer screening yield are required to measure the diagnostic certainty of a suspected paraneoplastic neurological syndrome

Perspective from Patient's Son

1. **What was the impact of the condition on your mother?**
   a. Physical (e.g. practical support)
   Support required with all aspects of daily living, cooking, cleaning, personal care, medication management and financial management.
   b. Psychological (e.g. mood, emotional well-being)
   Fluctuating moods, experiencing more frequent episodes of depression and agitation.
   c. Social (e.g. meeting friends, home)
   Initially required domiciliary care package, now resides in a nursing home. She does not engage socially with friends and outings. She maintains contact only with me.

2. **What could your mother not do because of the condition?**
   She can no longer do many tasks she previously could do independently. She requires support for all aspects of daily living.

3. **What is/was the change for your mother due to her medical condition?**
   She developed epilepsy, memory impairment. At present she is in receipt of nursing care due to the issues of living independently.

4. **What is/was the most difficult aspect of the condition for your mother?**
   Changing issues with memory have had a profound effect on mental health and well-being, relationships and ability to manage independently.

5. **Was any aspect of the experience good or useful? What was that?**
   Unfortunately there have been no positives.

6. **What do you hope for in the future for people with this condition?**
   Quicker diagnosis, input from multidisciplinary team at earlier stage, and assess needs on a holistic level.

History

A 20-year-old female university engineering student presented with a three-year history of 'déjà vu' events and impaired awareness episodes. The déjà vu phenomena were 'like dreams about which I cannot remember what happened'. She ran daily and estimated that about half of all her events occurred while running. At the onset of an event, she would often pause her watch and then not recall that she had paused her watch when she started running again. On one occasion, a more prolonged episode occurred. She had been running when she was next found sitting on a road as cars drove around her. Sometimes she could have multiple events in the one day. In a diary, she recorded multiple amnesic periods. At her part-time work, she could forget what she was doing or what she was supposed to be doing. Sometimes the déjà vu phenomenon would occur prior to the amnestic episodes but not always.

On another occasion, a running partner noticed that the patient suddenly was no longer running alongside her. The running partner found her sitting up against a wall complaining of nausea. The event lasted a few minutes and she wanted to run on afterwards. Her running partner noted that she had stopped her watch and forgot that she had done this. The running partner also reported that the patient was confused for 10–15 minutes in total.

During an EEG recording (see later) she reported not knowing where she was or who was carrying out the EEG.

Past medical history included childhood chickenpox and more recent COVID-19 disease. She was on no medication. She was a non-smoker and drank no more than two or three beers a month. There was no family history of epilepsy.

Examination

General and neurological examinations were normal.

Working Diagnosis: Focal Onset Seizures – Awareness Impaired and Behaviour Arrest – Possibly Triggered by Running

Investigations

ECG showed normal sinus rhythm with QTc of 398 ms.

An EEG captured a typical focal-onset seizure (Figure 37.1). Twenty minutes into the recording, her eyes glazed over and she became disorientated as she started to look around the room, initially to the right. She occasionally responded with one-word answers but her answers were not appropriate and she seemed very confused. At one point, her head and eyes were briefly fixed to the left side. The EEG showed an initial build-up of irregular slow activity at 2.5 Hz over the left hemisphere. This gave way to a long run of higher voltage rhythmical notched slow activity at 3–4 Hz mixed with frequent sharp discharges over the left hemisphere. This had an anterior and temporal emphasis and spread across the midline to involve, less impressively, the right anterior and temporal area. Irregular delta activity at 1.2–3 Hz was then seen over both hemispheres with a left-sided emphasis. The EEG started to improve after 1.5 minutes but she remained confused for another two minutes.

An MRI scan of the brain showed a 15 × 12 × 9 mm ovoid cortico-subcortical parafalcine mass in the right fronto-parietal region, which enhanced following contrast and was felt to represent a dysembryoplastic neuroepithelial tumour (Figure 37.2).

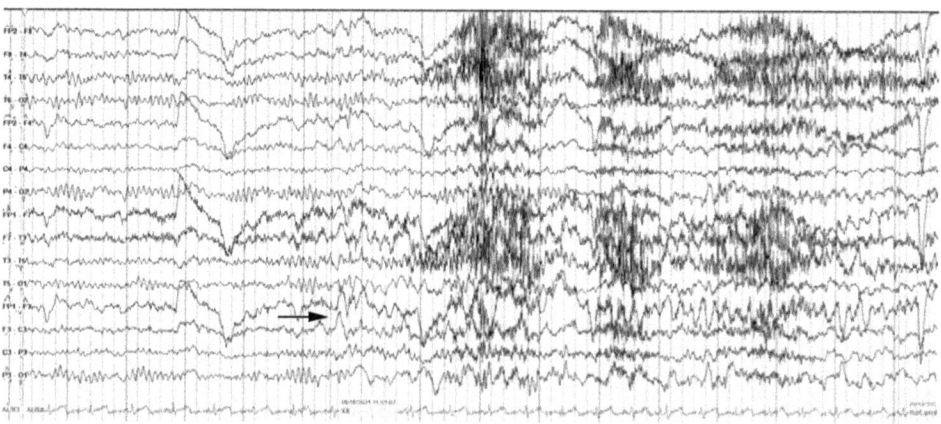

Figure 37.1 An EEG shows the build-up of slow activity over the left hemisphere (black arrow).

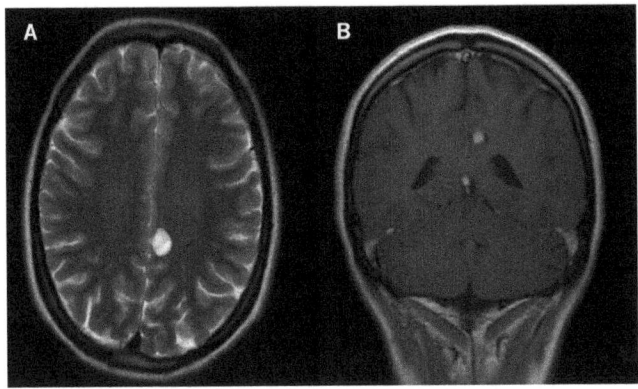

Figure 37.2 (A) Axial T2-weighted MRI scan of the brain showing ovoid high-signal lesion in left parafalcine fronto-parietal cortico-subcortical region. (B) Coronal T1 scan MRI scan shows contrast enhancement of the lesion.

Diagnosis: Focal Onset Awareness Impaired and Behaviour Arrest Seizures (or Posterior Cingulate Gyrus Seizures)

Commentary

Definition and Epidemiology of Epilepsy

A seizure is a transient occurrence of symptoms and/or signs due to abnormal excessive or synchronous neuronal activity in the brain. Epileptic seizures are classified into 1. focal onset seizures; 2. generalised onset seizures and 3. seizures of unknown onset.

Epilepsy is a disease with an enduring predisposition to generate epileptic seizures in an individual. It gives rise to neurobiological, cognitive, psychological and social consequences. In 2014, the International League Against Epilepsy (ILEA) updated its operational definition of epilepsy to reflect this. Previously, epilepsy was diagnosed when two or more unprovoked seizures more than 24 hours apart occurred in an individual. However, this may not be the most accurate definition, as individuals can grow out of epilepsy (i.e. lose the enduring predisposition to epileptic seizures) and other patients may have predisposing risk factors present after one seizure (e.g. a brain tumour), which make subsequent epileptic seizures very likely. The ILEA 2014 operational definition of epilepsy therefore includes one unprovoked (or reflex) seizure and a probability of further seizures similar to the general recurrence risk (at least 60%) after two unprovoked seizures, occurring over the next 10 years.

The ILAE 2017 classification of epilepsy attempts to define epilepsy with descriptions of the type of seizure(s), type of epilepsy and epilepsy syndrome as well as the aetiology of an individual's epilepsy. An operational classification of seizures is set out in Table 37.1 [1].

Table 37.1 2017 ILAE classification of seizures

Focal onset	Generalised onset	Unknown onset
Aware or impaired awareness	**Motor**	**Motor**
Motor onset	• Tonic-clonic	• Tonic-clonic
• Automatisms	• Clonic	• Epileptic spasms
• Atonic	• Tonic	**Non-motor**
• Clonic	• Myoclonic	• Behaviour arrest
• Epileptic spasms	• Myoclonic-tonic-clonic	
• Hyperkinetic	• Myoclonic-atonic	
• Myoclonic	• Atonic	
• Tonic	• Epileptic spasms	
Non-motor onset	**Non-motor (absence)**	
• Autonomic	• Typical	
• Behaviour arrest	• Atypical	
• Cognitive	• Myoclonic	
• Emotional	• Eyelid myoclonia	
• Sensory		
Focal to bilateral tonic-clonic		
		Unclassified

Adapted from Fisher et al. [1] with permission from Wiley.

There is a similar if not slightly higher incidence of epilepsy in males compared to females. Incident rates vary with the ILAE definition of epilepsy. One study adopting the more recent 2014 ILAE definition of epilepsy reported an age-adjusted incidence rate of epilepsy of 74 per 100,000 per year. Worldwide, there is an estimated 50–70 million people with epilepsy and 30% of those are medically refractory. Peaks in epilepsy incidence occur in infancy and old age.

Epilepsy is a symptom complex with multiple risk factors including genetic predisposition. A reliable eyewitness account in the clinical history can be crucial in making a diagnosis. Our patient is unusual in having a seizure captured during an EEG recording.

Management usually involves medication, which achieves remission in about two-thirds of patients. For drug-resistant seizures in appropriately selected patients, epilepsy surgery can achieve long-term seizure remission from focal-onset seizures.

Focal Epilepsy

The clinical signs or semiology of epilepsy are the motor, behavioural or subjective phenomena with or without loss of consciousness. History and video-telemetry can help localise seizure onset. Symptoms and clinical signs reveal the symptomatogenic zone, which can evolve as a seizure propagates (seizure semiology). The symptomatogenic zone is usually but not always close to the epileptogenic zone (area of the cortex required to generate seizures). The epileptogenic zone must be removed or disconnected for successful epilepsy surgery [2].

Some recognised focal seizure semiologies are summarised in Table 37.2 [2]. The temporal lobe is the most frequent site for the onset of focal seizures. The seizure semiologies are not always very specific. For example, whereas epigastric auras implicate the temporal lobe with 83% probability, autonomic auras implicate the temporal lobe in 58%, but the frontal lobe in 13% and hypothalamus in 15%. Olfactory auras are even less specific – 21% frontal, 28% parietal and 40% temporal in origin.

Clinically distinguishing absences (in idiopathic or genetic generalised epilepsies) from focal impaired awareness seizures is important. Absences are shorter, motor arrest lasting a matter of seconds, without preceding aura or postictal confusion.

Auras are common in temporal lobe seizures, and include an abdominal aura or rising epigastric sensation, gustatory and olfactory hallucinations and somatosensory tingling.

Ictal foreign language has been observed and can be a localising feature (non-dominant temporal lobe) in focal epilepsy.

Cingulate Seizures

Cingulate gyrus epilepsy is rare and a wide range of clinical manifestations can make the diagnosis challenging. The cingulate (name derived from a 'belt' or 'girdle') gyrus has extensive brain connections and is part of the limbic system. The anteroposterior sub-divisions of the cingulate cortex have different functional roles, which can explain the semiology of cingulate seizures alongside the seizure spread patterns. The posterior cingulate cortex, the location of the presumed dysembryoplastic neuroepithelial tumour in our patient, plays an important role in memory as it receives input from the hippocampus. It is recognised that, like our patient, the electroclinical findings can suggest temporal lobe epilepsy, although it is often difficult to localise ictal onset with scalp EEG [3]. Posterior cingulate epilepsy can cause what used to be called dyscognitive or dialeptic seizures – with impairments in perception, attention, emotion, memory or executive function. This may have contributed to the delay in referral for our patient.

Table 37.2 Focal seizure semiologies

Location	Semiology
Frontal	Brief (usually 30 seconds), prominent vocalisation, often occur from sleep, cycling, rocking, grimacing, bilateral motor with retained awareness, ictal scalp EEG may not show changes. Focal atonic seizures due to involvement of negative motor areas
Frontal – primary motor cortex	Contralateral, unilateral Jacksonian march along the homunculus
Frontal – supplementary motor cortex	Asymmetric bilateral tonic posturing with or without impaired awareness
Frontal –orbitofrontal cortex	Impaired awareness and automatisms, which may evolve to more complex motor seizures
Frontal -dorsolateral frontal cortex	Early head and eye version
Temporal	Most frequent site of onset of focal seizures Behavioural arrest, manual and oral automatisms in two-thirds and variable loss of awareness with postictal confusion. Duration 2–3 minutes
Mesial temporal	Abdominal aura – rising epigastric sensation and experiential phenomena – fear, déjà vu and jamais vu. Early flushing or tachycardia, which may progress to behavioural arrest, automatisms and impaired awareness
Lateral temporal lobe	Auditory (humming, ringing and buzzing) or vertiginous features. Dominant hemisphere ictal dysphasia
Parietal	5% of epilepsies Frequent auras. Diverse and subjective nature including contralateral somatosensory aura. Proprioceptive-induced seizures are rare but unique to parietal lobe epilepsy
Occipital	Usually a visual aura or eye deviation, blinking or nystagmus. Primary visual cortex produces an elementary visual aura usually less than 2 minutes (longer in migraine) – pulsating and usually lateralised (contralateral to hemisphere where seizure onset occurs. Complex visual hallucination less frequent

Seizures from the anterior cingulate gyrus can cause intense fear, screaming, aggressive vocalisation, complex gestural automatisms and even ill-formed visual hallucinations. Anterior cingulate seizures have more features in common with frontal lobe seizures. Gelastic (laughing or giggling) seizures, which are usually due to a hypothalamic hamartoma, may also arise from the anterior cingulate gyrus.

Exercise-Induced Seizures

Seizures triggered by exercise have been reported for both idiopathic generalised epilepsies and more often symptomatic focal epilepsies of frontal and temporal lobe origin. However, exercise-induced seizures are rarely reported in the literature and, in general exercise may protect against seizures.

There is some evidence that exercise may be an under-recognised form of reflex epilepsy. Exercise-associated seizures usually have temporal lobe abnormalities and in most patients seizures are lateralised (as in our patient) to the left hemisphere. However, it is important to bear in mind that exercise brings physiological and psychological benefit. Where exercise-associated seizures occur, social support is encouraged to increase confidence and safety.

References

1. Fisher RS, Cross JH, D'Souza C et al. Instruction manual for the ILAE 2017 operational classification of seizure types. *Epilepsia*. 2017;58(4):531–42.

2. Chowdhury FA, Silva R, Whatley B, Walker MC. Localisation in focal epilepsy: a practical guide. *Pract Neurol*. 2021;21:481–91.

3. Enatsu R, Bulacio J, Nair DR et al. Posterior cingulate epilepsy: clinical and neurophysiological analysis. *J Neurol Neurosurg Psychiatry*. 2014;85(1):44–50.

Learning Points

*   Epileptic seizures are usually diagnosed from a detailed eye-witnessed account and occasionally are picked up on a video-electroencephalogram recording.

*   Seizure semiology can help localise the symptomatogenic zone of a seizure.

*   Cingulate seizures are rare and have a wide range of manifestations.

*   The posterior cingulate receives input from the hippocampus and so seizures can impair perception, attention, emotion, memory or executive functioning.

Patient's Perspective

1. **What is the impact of the condition on you?**

    a. Physical (e.g. practical support, study, travel)
    I'm a third year at uni and have to miss a lot of class travelling to and from appointments and scans. I had to suddenly stop running which has ruined my fitness as I have been running for 13 years.

    b. Psychological (e.g. mood, emotional well-being)
    It's been very stressful and hard to explain my condition to people. My meds make me very tired and a bit anxious. My friends don't understand and I feel like they are always baby-sitting me.

    c. Social (e.g. meeting friends, home)
    On nights out with friends or at family gatherings I can always feel everyone watching me. I feel like my friends are babysitting me on nights.

2. **What can you not do because of the condition?**
    I'm not allowed to run alone or drive until my seizures stop completely. My diabetic friend went skydiving and it took her a long time to get a doctor's permission, and I realised I'll never be allowed to do anything like that.

3. **Has there been any other change for you due to the medical condition?**
    I have to get an MRI scan every three months and regular blood tests, but I have a fear of needles in veins. I faint nearly every time a needle goes in my arm so now I regularly feel dizzy and pass out at appointments.

4. **What is/was the most difficult aspect of the condition for you?**
    I was training six days per week before I found out I had epilepsy. I really miss long solo runs and competing in races. I can't train alone until my seizures stop and now I'm slower than I was before.

5. **Was any aspect of the experience good or useful? What was that?**
    Luckily my medication has started working quickly and I feel like my short term memory is improving.

6. **What do you hope for in the future for people with this condition?**
    I wish there would be more information about the different types of seizures because I went three years undiagnosed since I didn't know my seizures were seizures.

38 Involuntary Arm Movement

History

A 71-year-old woman with a history of type 2 diabetes mellitus developed involuntary move-ments of her left arm and left leg. These were predominantly proximal, irregular, unpredict-able, purposeless and at times had a ballistic or explosive and large amplitude pattern. The movements stopped during sleep. She associated the involuntary movements with the onset of pain in her first carpo-metacarpal joint. A local anaesthetic-steroid injection had helped ease the pain. Her diabetic control had recently deteriorated.

She had a past medical history of chronic kidney disease, hypothyroidism and hypertension.

Medication included amitriptyline 25 mg nocte, omeprazole 10 mg/day, gliclazide mr 300 mg mane, rosuvastatin 10 mg nocte, bisoprolol 5 mg/day, hydralazine 50 mg bd, irbe-sartan 300 mg/hydrochlorothiazide 35 mg, levothyroxine 150 µg/day and aspirin 75 mg/day.

Examination

Higher mental function was normal. Cranial nerves were intact. Hemichoreic and hemibal-listic movements of the left arm and to lesser extent the left leg were present. Her only other limb abnormality was bilaterally absent ankle jerks.

Investigations

Serial haemoglobin A1c (HbA1c) measurements had shown a recent deterioration in diabetic control (Figure 38.1). CT brain and MRI brain scans demonstrated predominantly right basal ganglia calcification (Figure 38.2).

Management

Her diabetic management was changed and improved. The involuntary movements stopped after three months.

Four years later the involuntary movements returned to her left arm and leg, but were less prominent compared to the original presentation. Again, there had been a record of increas-ing HbA1c levels (Figure 38.1). A follow-up CT scan of the brain was unchanged. She declined further MR imaging due to claustrophobia.

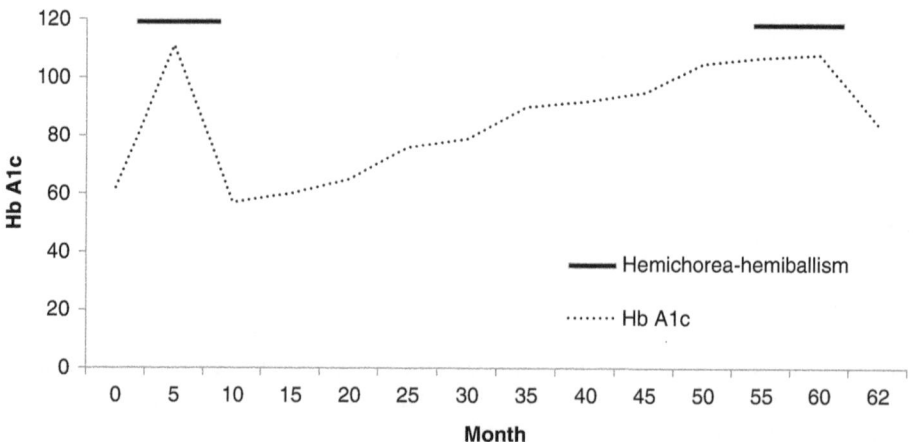

Figure 38.1 Haemoglobin A1c levels over five years with timeline for hyperglycaemia-induced hemichorea-hemiballism.

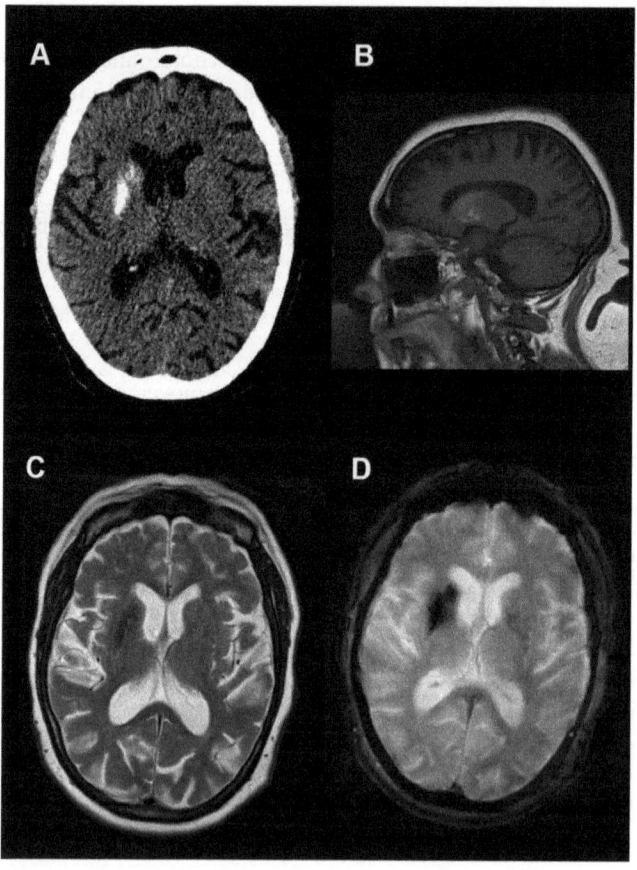

Figure 38.2 (A) A CT brain scan showing high signal in the right basal ganglia – caudate and putamen. (B) A sagittal T1-weighted MRI brain scan showing high signal in the right basal ganglia. (C) Axial T2-weighted and (D) gradient-echo MRI brain scan showing low signal in the right basal ganglia.

Diagnosis: Left Hemichorea-Hemiballism Secondary to Hyperglycaemia

Comment

Hyperkinetic Movements

Movement disorders are classified as hyperkinetic or hypokinetic. The hyperkinetic movements are tremor, dystonia, tics, chorea, myoclonus, stereotypies and paroxysmal dyskinesias.

Chorea

Chorea comes from the Ancient Greek verb for 'dance' and is defined as involuntary, arrhythmic movements of a forcible, rapid, jerky type. In contrast, ballism, from the Greek for 'throw' refers to explosive involuntary movements involving proximal limb muscles and are of a wide range and flinging [1]. Ballism often merges into chorea. Hemiballism (unilateral ballism) can result from cerebral infarction, haemorrhage, tumour or other focal lesions such as arteriovenous malformation, infections and immune-mediated conditions such as Behçet's disease, head injury and drugs (dopamine antagonists) as well as hyperglycaemia (Table 38.1). Hemiballism is thought to result from lesions in the contralateral subthalamic nucleus or striatum. Lesions in the subthalamic nucleus reduce excitatory innervation to the internal globus pallidus (GPi), which then results in reduced inhibitory signals to the thalamus. This causes increased excitation of the primary motor cortex. Where subthalamic lesions are not apparent, it is suggested that subthalamic innervation is altered, leading to chorea-ballism. In a review of clinicopathological cases of hemichorea-hemiballism, Professor Alastair Compston reported how James Purdon Martin and colleagues demonstrated that subthalamic lesions alone were not necessary for a patient to have hemichorea-hemiballism but that the condition could occur whenever irregular impulses came from an intact globus pallidus [2]. More recent research with lesion network mapping has shown that strokes in different anatomical locations associated with hemichorea-hemiballism have a common functional single network connected to the contralateral posterolateral putamen.

Table 38.1 Causes of hemichorea-hemiballism

Non-ketotic hyperglycaemia
Stroke (functionally connected to the contralateral posterolateral putamen)
Tumour
Vascular malformation
Demyelination
Vasculitis (e.g. systemic lupus erythematosus)
Trauma
Infection (tuberculoma and toxoplasmosis)
Wilson's disease
Thyrotoxicosis
Autoimmune encephalitis (anti-LGI-1 and anti-CASPR2)

CASPR2: contactin-associated protein-like 2; LGI-1: leucine-rich glioma inactivated-1

Athetosis is derived from a Greek word meaning 'unfixed' or 'changeable' and is an inability to sustain any part of the body in one position. The maintained posture is interrupted by relatively slow, sinuous, purposeless movements, which have a tendency to flow into each other. Finally, dystonia is a persistent posture in one or other of the extremes of athetoid movement.

Hyperglycaemia-induced hemichorea-hemiballism was first described in 1960 by Stephen Bedwell. By 2003, there were more than 60 reported cases of hyperglycaemia-induced hemichorea-hemiballism (making it the second commonest cause of hemiballism after stroke). A systematic review published in 2020 identified 176 patients with diabetic striatopathy, 17% newly diagnosed with diabetes mellitus and 88% presenting with hemichorea-hemiballism [3]. An example of hemichorea-hemiballism is available on youtube at: www .youtube.com/watch?v=GzRV5HCyVl4.

Risk factors for hyperglycaemia-induced hemichorea-hemiballism include advanced age, being female and being of East Asian origin. Hemichorea-hemiballism emerges with hyperglycaemia and resolves in 25% with normoglycaemia [3], as demonstrated twice by our patient. However, over 70% of published cases had also received anti-chorea medication, usually haloperidol [3]. Bedwell reported recurrence of the movement disorder with further hyperglycaemia, as was observed in our patient. Twenty per cent of patients have hemichorea-hemiballism for more than three months [1].

Patients reported with hyperglycaemia-induced hemichorea-hemiballism have high T1 signal in the putamen on MRI brain imaging; similar changes are variably found in the globus pallidus and caudate nuclei. Two-thirds have signal abnormalities on T2-weighted MR imaging. Some have diffusion-weighted imaging abnormalities but findings from blood-sensitive sequences such as gradient echo imaging have been varied [1]. Software for MR quantitative susceptibility mapping can help distinguish intracranial calcification from haemorrhage.

There has been little pathological investigation of hyperglycaemia-induced hemichorea-hemiballism. In the putamen, necrotic foci have been found surrounded by gliosis with prominent infiltration by gemistocytic astrocytes. Macrophage infiltration and evidence of haemorrhage in the form of focal microhaemorrhages and haemosiderin deposits have been reported along with confluent infarction, small foci of tissue necrosis, arterial lumen narrowing with fibrosis and punctate calcification [3]. Some have speculated that reactive astrocytes may be a reaction to microinfarction but no occluded blood vessels were found. The pathophysiology remains to be clarified but a two-hit hypothesis seems likely.

Untreated so-called striatopathy with persistent hyperglycaemia can result in persistent symptoms and caudate atrophy.

References

1. Postuma RB, Lang AE. Hemiballism: revisiting a classic disorder. *Lancet Neurol.* 2003;2(11):661–8.

2. Compston A. Hemichorea resulting from a local lesion of the brain. (The syndrome of the body of Luys.) By James Purdon Martin, MD (London). *Brain* 1927:50; 637–651; Hemichorea associated with a lesion of the corpus Luysii. By James Purdon Martin and N.S. Alcock. *Brain.* 1934:57; 504–516; and Hemichorea (hemiballismus) without lesions in the corpus Luysii. By J. Purdon Martin (From the National Hospital, Queen Square, W.C.1) *Brain.* 1957:80; 1–10. *Brain.* 2006;129(7):1633–6.

3. Chua CB, Sun CK, Hsu CW et al. 'Diabetic striatopathy': clinical presentations, controversy, pathogenesis, treatments, and outcomes. *Sci Rep.* 2020;10(1):1–11.

Learning Points

- Chorea consists of involuntary, arrhythmic movements of a forcible, rapid and jerky nature.
- Hyperglycaemia can trigger hemichorea-hemiballism (diabetic striatopathy), particularly in elderly women.
- A common functional network involving the posterolateral putamen has been implicated in stroke causes of hemichorea-hemiballism.
- Correction of hyperglycaemia usually helps resolve hyperglycaemia-induced hemichorea-hemiballism.

Perspective from Patient's Daughter

1. **What was the impact of the condition on your mother?**

    a. **Physical (e.g. practical support, mobility, activities of daily living)**
    Mom experienced difficulty with the following daily activities:
    - *Dressing*
    - *Bathing/personal hygiene*
    - *Cooking*
    - *Eating*

    b. **Psychological (e.g. mood, emotional well-being)**
    Her mood was affected by the constant arm movement. It also made her very tired.

    c. **Social (e.g. meeting friends, family, home)**
    We are/were only a small family, so this was not really relevant.

2. **What could she not do when she had the movements?**
    She used to have a lot of trouble resting/sleeping due to the arm movements.
    She experienced difficulty with eating with a knife and fork, often having to have things cut up so she could just use a fork to eat with.
    Driving a vehicle was not possible.

3. **What was the most difficult aspect of the condition for your mother?**
    From what I observed, it was the constant uncontrollable arm movements, that affected her daily and the fact that she did not know what was causing it or how to stop it. She also suffered from a painful thumb joint in the same arm and did have one or two injections to ease that. She felt that the two were related (i.e. the pain and the arm movements).

4. **What do you hope for in the future for people with this condition?**
    I never knew, until researching what I now know is the condition my mother had, that this was caused by her diabetes. I don't think my mother was very good at managing her diabetes, and had I been more aware of this being the cause, then I would have been able to step in and try to help and guide her with better health choices (as I believe that her diabetes was largely down to poor diet choices). So, I think it would be a good goal to do as much as possible to inform and educate both patients and their families, on what, if anything they can do themselves to either prevent or treat this condition.

39 Salt Control

History

A 38-year-old woman had a long history of an eating disorder and laxative abuse. She smoked 10 cigarettes per day. She was admitted to hospital with abdominal pain and 'constipation'. Prior to admission, she had been observed to be drinking a lot of water. She had returned from Rome a day before her hospital admission. In hospital, she was agitated. Her admission serum sodium was 102 mmol/L. She was admitted to the High Dependency Unit. The hyponatraemia was corrected (Figure 39.1) initially with normal saline and three-times normal saline but a large diuresis ensued.

Following recovery of her serum sodium level, she was discharged. Because of slurred speech and poor balance, she was re-admitted to hospital three days later.

Examination

Neurological assessment requested following re-admission found her to be alert and orientated. Heart rate, blood pressure and respiratory rate were all normal. Strength and sensation were intact. She had impaired rapid alternate movements, horizontal nystagmus and brisk reflexes. Plantar responses were flexor.

Investigations

MRI scan of the brain demonstrated T2 high signal changes in the central pons (Figure 39.2A). There were also T2 hyperintense changes within the lentiform nuclei and caudate nuclei bilaterally (Figure 39.2B).

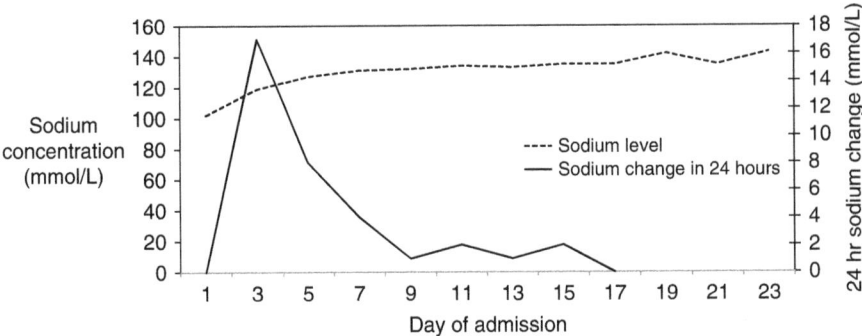

Figure 39.1 Daily plasma sodium levels and 24-hour changes in plasma sodium following hospital admission.

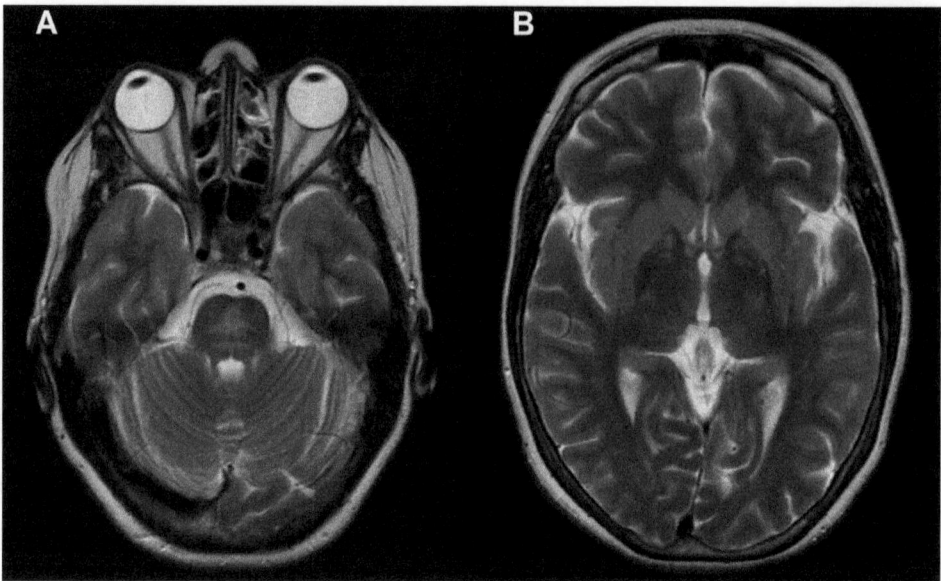

Figure 39.2 An axial T2-weighted MRI scan of the brain showing (A) high signal within the pons and (B) bilateral high signal within the basal ganglia and thalami.

Diagnosis: Osmotic Demyelination Syndrome (Previously Known as Central Pontine Myelinolysis)

Outcome

She never really improved. Slurring of speech and unsteadiness have remained as a major disability.

Comment

Hyponatraemia

Hyponatraemia is categorised as mild (130–4 mmol/L), moderate (125–9 mmol/L) or severe (<125 mmol/L). Assessing the volaemic state of a patient helps classify hyponatraemia as hypovolaemic (diarrhoea, vomiting, burns, Addison's disease, renal loses from diuretics), euvolaemic (syndrome of inappropriate antidiuretic hormone (SIADH), drugs, hypothyroidism, adrenal glucocorticoid insufficiency) or hypervolaemic hyponatraemia (cardiac failure, cirrhosis, chronic kidney disease and nephrotic syndrome). However, assessment of volaemic status is not very reliable.

The commonest cause of hyponatraemia is SIADH, although many other causes (listed earlier) exist. The essential criteria for SIADH are itemised in Table 39.1 [1].

Our patient was hyponatraemic at the time of her first admission to hospital. She had not consumed sufficient solutes in her diet to maintain renal ionic gradients for water excretion. Water overload ensued [2], and explained the low serum sodium levels on admission to hospital. When this occurs in the context of excess beer consumption, it is called beer potomania from the Latin 'poto' meaning 'I drink'.

Osmotic Demyelination Syndrome

Osmotic demyelination syndrome was first described in 1959 by Raymond D. Adams and colleagues [3], and was associated with chronic alcoholism, malnutrition and severe liver failure. The clinical spectrum varies from locked-in syndrome to isolated ataxia (the latter demonstrated in our patient). There have been few published cases with isolated ataxia and dysarthria due to osmotic demyelination syndrome. Sudden shifts in serum sodium can trigger osmotic demyelination syndrome but this is not a prerequisite for development of the condition.

Table 39.1 Essential criteria for diagnosis of SIADH

Essential criteria
Effective serum osmolality <275 mOsm/kg
Urine osmolality >100 mOsm/kg at some level of decreased effective osmolality
Clinical euvolaemia
Urinary Na concentration >30 mmol/L with normal dietary salt and water intake
Absence of adrenal, thyroid, pituitary or renal insufficiency
No recent use of diuretics

Adapted from Spasovski et al. [1] with permission from Oxford University Press.

Sepsis, renal impairment and a history of excess alcohol are recognised triggers of osmotic demyelination syndrome (previously known as central pontine myelinolysis).

More than half of all patients make a good recovery but death has been reported in up to a quarter of patients with osmotic demyelination syndrome. Imaging may reveal asymptomatic findings. The pathological process has not been clearly identified. The syndrome is now described as osmotic demyelination syndrome in order to emphasise that extrapontine demyelination can occur (as occurred in our patient).

For our patient, the admission serum sodium was 102 mmol/L. Osmolality was 218 mOsm/kg. Urinary sodium was <20 mmol/L. The serum sodium had risen by 8 mmol/L in eight hours and by 17 mmol/L within the first 24 hours. A diuresis occurred because solute (previously lacking in the diet) was now available to the kidney, increasing serum sodium and predisposing to osmotic demyelination syndrome. This type of low-solute hyponatraemia is recognised in the non-alcoholic patient. Guidelines exist for diagnosis and management of hyponatraemia [1]. Osmotic demyelination syndrome is less likely to occur if the rise in serum sodium concentration is less than 10 mmol/L in the first 24 hours and less than 8 mmol/L in each following 24 hours.

References

1. Spasovski G, Vanholder R, Allolio B et al. Clinical practice guideline on diagnosis and treatment of hyponatraemia. *Eur J Endocrinol*. 2014;170(3):G1–47.
2. Fox B. Crash diet potomania. *Lancet*. 2002;359:942.
3. Adams RD, Victor M, Mancall EL. Central pontine myelinolysis: a hitherto undescribed disease occurring in alcoholic and malnourished patients. *AMA Arch Neurol Psychiatry*. 1959;81(2): 154–72.

Learning Points

- Osmotic demyelination syndrome can present with a wide spectrum of neurological findings from isolated ataxia to a locked-in syndrome.
- There is little correlation between clinical findings and MRI brain appearance in osmotic demyelination syndrome.
- Guidelines for diagnosing and treating hyponatraemia are important measures to reduce the incidence of osmotic demyelination syndrome.
- A favourable recovery from osmotic demyelination syndrome can occur in about half of patients.

Patient's Perspective

1. **What was the impact of the condition?**
   a. **Physical (e.g. job, driving, practical support)**
   They put the sodium in too quickly. I thought I was in hell, I didn't know where I was. I fell out of bed. I couldn't walk in a straight line. Because I couldn't walk upstairs, I slept downstairs.
   b. **Psychological (e.g. mood, future, emotional well-being)**
   Terrible. I had an eating disorder. I had been drinking loads of water and taking laxatives.
   c. **Social (e.g. meeting friends, home)**
   Nobody wanted to speak to me. They didn't know how to handle me. I rarely go out.
2. **What could you not do when you left hospital?**
   I had difficulty coping at home. I lived with my mother initially after discharge but now I live alone.
3. **Was there any change for you due to your medical condition?**
   My co-ordination is off. I fell and fractured ribs three years ago.

4. **What is most difficult aspect of the condition?**

   I have no social interaction. I live in a bungalow and I live alone. In the last three to four years I have lost my motivation probably because my co-ordination problem.

5. **Was any aspect of the experience good or useful? What was that?**

   Nothing.

6. **What do you hope for in the future for your condition?**

   I hope there is more awareness about CPM [central pontine myelinolysis] to prevent people developing this condition.

A Young Man with More Than Dizziness

History

A 45-year-old man, who was a non-smoker and rarely drank alcohol, was admitted to hospital with new and sudden onset of headache, dizziness and vomiting. He described the floor and walls moving towards him. He also felt a spinning sensation. He was unsteady. Movement seemed to exacerbate the dizziness and vomiting. He remained unsteady in hospital but the dizziness improved. Past medical history was unremarkable. He was on no medication.

Examination

He was apyrexic, alert and orientated. His heart rate was 72 beats per minute, and his blood pressure was 119/76 mmHg. He had no heart murmur and no evidence of hypermobility. Neurological examination revealed horizontal gaze-evoked nystagmus, normal head impulse test and mild right arm and leg ataxia. He had normal power and sensation in his limbs.

Investigations

A CT of the brain on admission (3 hours and 20 minutes after onset) was normal, confirmed at review by a neuroradiologist. A stroke thrombolysis call was not made.

An MRI of the brain 24 hours after onset demonstrated right cerebellar infarction with diffusion restriction (Figures 40.1A–40.1C). A CT angiogram revealed a dissecting aneurysm of the right posterior inferior cerebellar artery, which was confirmed on an MR angiogram (Figure 40.1D) and catheter angiography (Figure 40.1E).

A transthoracic echocardiogram with bubble was normal. A 24-hour ECG monitor had normal sinus rhythm. A comprehensive search for other causes of acute ischaemic stroke was negative.

Management and Outcome

The patient improved and returned to work as a production engineer. He was treated with clopidogrel. At follow-up, blood pressure remained normal.

A further follow-up over three years with MR angiogram surveillance showed no change in the right posterior inferior cerebellar artery dissecting aneurysm. A multidisciplinary team suggested annual follow-up for five years.

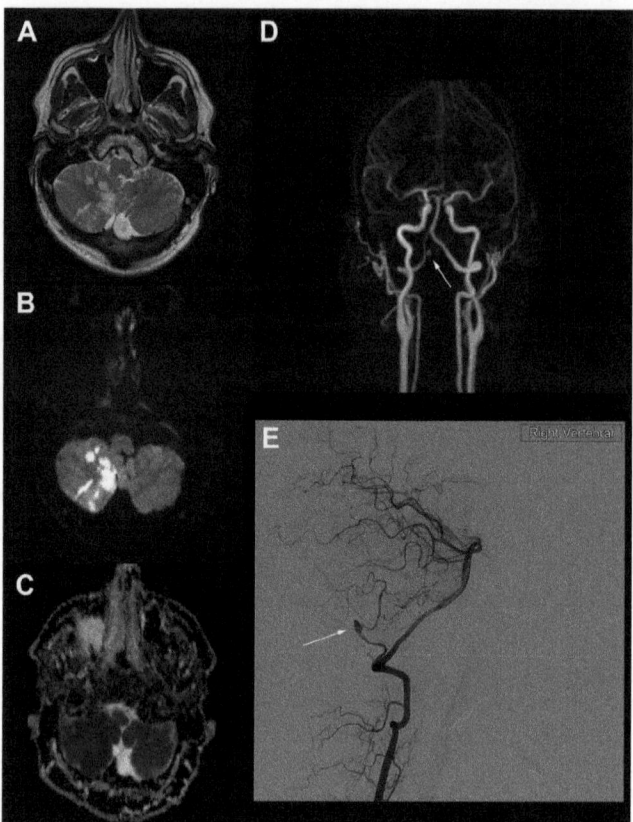

Figure 40.1 Axial (A) FLAIR T2, (B) diffusion-weighted and (C) ADC map MRI scans of the brain showing right cerebellar signal change and restricted diffusion consistent with acute infarction. (D) MR and (E) catheter angiograms showing a dissecting aneurysm in the right posterior inferior cerebellar artery (arrow).

Diagnosis: Right Cerebellar Infarction Secondary to Posterior Inferior Cerebellar Artery Dissecting Aneurysm

Comment

Defining Dizziness and Vertigo

Dizziness is defined as the sensation of disturbed or impaired spatial orientation without a false or distorted sense of motion. Such sensations include giddiness, light-headedness and non-specific dizziness, but are not vertigo.

Vertigo is the sensation of self-motion of the head/body when no self-motion is occurring or the sensation of distorted self-motion during an otherwise normal head movement.

Acute vertigo and dizziness are common symptoms, making up 3.5% of all emergency department attendances. The differential diagnosis and order of frequency at a tertiary centre emergency department are highlighted in Table 40.1.

Clinical Features of Acute Vestibular Syndrome

The history of an acute vestibular syndrome has limited utility in distinguishing peripheral lesions (vestibular neuronitis and Ménière's disease) from a central cause due to acute cerebral ischaemia. Only about 25% of patients with suspected peripheral vestibular disorders complain of vertigo. Lesions in the cerebellum present with both dizziness and vertigo, as occurred with our patient.

In addition, the symptom quality does not differentiate a peripheral from a central aetiology. The symptom duration is highly variable in central lesions. Peripheral lesions have a higher symptom intensity compared to a vestibular stroke but this is not clinically useful.

Table 40.1 Frequency of diagnosis in acute vertigo/dizziness

Frequency ranking	Cause of vertigo/dizziness
1	Benign paroxysmal positional vertigo – 25% of all presentations (posterior semi-circular canal most frequent sub-type)
2	Cardiovascular events (orthostatic hypotension, presyncope, cardiac arrhythmia)
3	Stroke or transient ischaemic attack
4	Acute unilateral vestibulopathy
5	Functional disorders
6	Vestibular migraine
7	Ménière's disease
8	Infections
9	Central nervous system inflammation
10	Intoxication
11	Metabolic disturbance (e.g. hyponatraemia)

Adapted from Zwergal and Dieterich [1] with permission from Wolters Kluwer.

While isolated vertigo/dizziness is not usually due to stroke, 16% of patients with a posterior inferior cerebellar artery-territory stroke complain of this symptom.

Clinical indicators to prompt consideration of vestibular stroke include acute onset with a trigger, no previous history of vertigo or dizziness, accompanying headache, focal neurological signs and symptoms, and a cardiovascular risk profile. Hearing loss can be ambiguous as it occurs in Menière's disease and in about half of patients with anterior inferior cerebellar artery infarction (as it supplies the labyrinthine artery) [1].

Targeted Examination in Acute Vestibular Syndrome

A bedside vestibular, ocular and postural examination may help distinguish a peripheral from a central cause of acute vertigo and dizziness. However, inability to walk or direction-changing (gaze-evoked) nystagmus should prompt consideration of stroke. The presence of a normal Head Impulse test, gaze-evoked Nystagmus or Test of Skew eye deviation (so-called HINTS testing) in a patient with acute vestibular syndrome suggests a pontomedullary and/or cerebellar stroke with both high sensitivity and specificity [2]. A bilaterally normal head impulse test in the presence of spontaneous nystagmus is the most sensitive indicator of central stroke aetiology, followed by gaze-evoked nystagmus in the opposite direction of the spontaneous nystagmus. Table 40.2 summarises the examination features of central and peripheral causes of an acute vestibular syndrome.

Table 40.2 Targeted physical examination to diagnose patients with acute vestibular syndrome

Specific examination	Peripheral (all must be present to diagnose vestibular neuritis)	Central (any one of these findings suggests posterior fossa stroke)
Nystagmus (straight ahead gaze and right and left gaze)	Dominantly horizontal, direction-fixed, beating away from affected side[a]	Dominantly vertical or torsional or dominantly horizontal, direction-changing on left/right gaze[b]
Test of skew (alternate cover test)	Normal vertical eye alignment and no corrective movement (i.e. no skew deviation)	Skew deviation (small vertical correction on uncovering the eye)[c]
Head impulse test	Unilaterally abnormal with head moving towards the affected side (presence of a corrective re-fixation saccade towards normal side)[d]	Bilaterally normal
Targeted neurological examination	No cranial nerve, brainstem, or cerebellar signs	Presence of limb ataxia, dysarthria, diplopia, ptosis, anisocoria, facial sensory loss (pain/temperature), unilateral decreased hearing
Gait and truncal ataxia	Able to walk unassisted or sit up in stretcher without holding on or leaning against bed or rails	Unable to walk unassisted or sit up in stretcher without holding on or leaning against bed or rails

[a] Inferior branch vestibular neuritis will present with downbeat-torsional nystagmus, but is a rare disorder.

[b] More than half of posterior fossa strokes will have direction-fixed horizontal nystagmus that, alone, cannot be distinguished from that typically seen with vestibular neuritis.

[c] More than half of posterior strokes will have no skew deviation, so, on this criterion alone, cannot be distinguished from vestibular neuritis.

[d] Strokes in the anterior inferior cerebellar artery territory may produce a unilaterally abnormal head impulse test that mimics vestibular neuritis, but hearing loss is usually present as a clue. If a patient has bilaterally abnormal head impulse test, this is also suspicious for a central lesion if nystagmus is present (as may be seen in Wernicke's syndrome).

Adapted from Edlow et al. [3] with permission from Elsevier.

Neuroimaging Diagnoses of PICA Dissection

Cerebral arterial dissection is a difficult diagnosis to make and is particularly difficult for posterior inferior cerebellar artery dissections. However, T1-volume isotropic turbo spin-echo acquisition (T1-VISTA) may enable visualisation of intra-mural haematoma to help in the diagnosis of dissection of the posterior inferior cerebellar artery and the vertebral artery.

Although there was no evidence of sub-arachnoid haemorrhage in our patient, it is important to be aware that posterior inferior cerebellar artery dissection may be associated with sub-arachnoid haemorrhage more often than vertebral artery dissection [4].

Evidence for Medical Management

The natural history of cervical artery dissection appears to be more benign than previously thought, with 12-month outcome showing less than 3% risk of recurrent stroke with either anti-platelet or anti-coagulant medication. Future trials will assess the harms and benefits of direct oral anti-coagulants.

Dissecting pseudo-aneurysms (blood collecting in the surrounding tissue) usually have a benign course. For our patient annual angiography surveillance had been recommended for five years. Empirical anti-platelet therapy has also been recommended.

Thrombolysis Treatment for Posterior Circulation Acute Ischaemic Strokes

Our patient did not receive intravenous thrombolysis as he was initially thought to have labyrinthitis. A retrospective calculation of his National Institutes of Health Stroke Scale (NIHSS) score was 2. Delays in diagnosing posterior circulation strokes may result from a wide range of presenting and sometimes non-specific symptoms. In addition, patients with posterior circulation strokes are more likely to be Face, Arms, Speech, Time (FAST)-negative and have lower NIHSS scores than anterior circulation strokes. Even among patients treated with intravenous thrombolysis, onset to door times and door to needle times are longer for patients with posterior circulation strokes compared to patients with acute anterior circulation ischaemic strokes.

References

1. Zwergal A, Dieterich M. Vertigo and dizziness in the emergency room. *Curr Opin Neurol.* 2020;33(1):117–25.

2. Krishnan K, Bassilious K, Eriksen E et al. Posterior circulation stroke diagnosis using HINTS in patients presenting with acute vestibular syndrome: a systematic review. *Eur stroke J.* 2019;4(3):233–9.

3. Edlow JA, Gurley KL, Newman-Toker DE. A new diagnostic approach to the adult patient with acute dizziness. *J Emerg Med.* 2018;54(4):469–83.

4. Matsumoto J, Ogata T, Abe H et al. Do characteristics of dissection differ between the posterior inferior cerebellar artery and the vertebral artery? *J Stroke Cerebrovasc Dis.* 2014;23(10):2857–61.

Learning Points

- Clinical assessment of patients with acute vestibular syndrome can distinguish central (stroke) from peripheral (vestibular neuritis) causes.
- HINTS testing has high sensitivity and specificity in diagnosing stroke in patients with acute vestibular syndrome.
- Diagnosis of posterior inferior cerebellar artery aneurysm is often difficult and may require repeated and detailed radiological investigation to identify a mural haematoma.

- In young patients, cervical arterial dissection is a common cause of ischaemic stroke, which usually has a low risk of stroke recurrence.

Patient's Perspective

1. **What was the impact of the condition?**

   a. Physical (e.g. job, driving, practical support)
   Co-ordination and balance problems.

   b. Psychological (e.g. mood, future, emotional well-being)
   Tired and low tolerance level.

   c. Social (e.g. meeting friends, home)
   Limited due to fatigue and tiredness.

2. **What can you no longer do?**
   I can easily get dizzy or sick if walking in circles.

3. **Was there any other change for you due to your medical condition?**
   I tire a lot more quickly. I have more headaches. My memory is not as good.

4. **What is/was the most difficult aspect of the condition?**
   The memory and fatigue issues.

5. **Was any aspect of the experience good or useful? What was that?**
   I now have a different way of looking at life.

6. **What do you hope for in the future for your condition?**
   1. More help to explain the condition and more encouragement to rehabilitate
   2. Better awareness of the cause of my symptoms so doctors and Emergency Department can respond faster.

41 Late Familial Falling

History

A 67-year-old right-handed man was referred from cardiology because of falls. He reported impaired balance for one year. He had become aware of increasing swaying of his body when he was walking. His family had noticed that his speech had become less clear.

In his past medical history, he had a bicuspid aortic valve and moderate aortic stenosis.

His only medication was betahistine 16 mg tid. He was a driver and a farmer. He drank very little alcohol. He did not smoke cigarettes.

Because of poor balance, his mother had been in a wheelchair from age 70 years until her death, aged 90 years. His maternal aunt was similarly affected. His maternal grandmother was also affected in the same way in the latter stages of her life. He had one brother and three daughters.

Examination

He had scanning dysarthria, horizontal gaze-evoked nystagmus and limb ataxia. Otherwise, examination was normal.

Investigations

An MRI of the brain showed moderately severe cerebellar atrophy extending laterally into the cerebellar hemispheres (Figure 41.1).

A diagnostic test was performed.

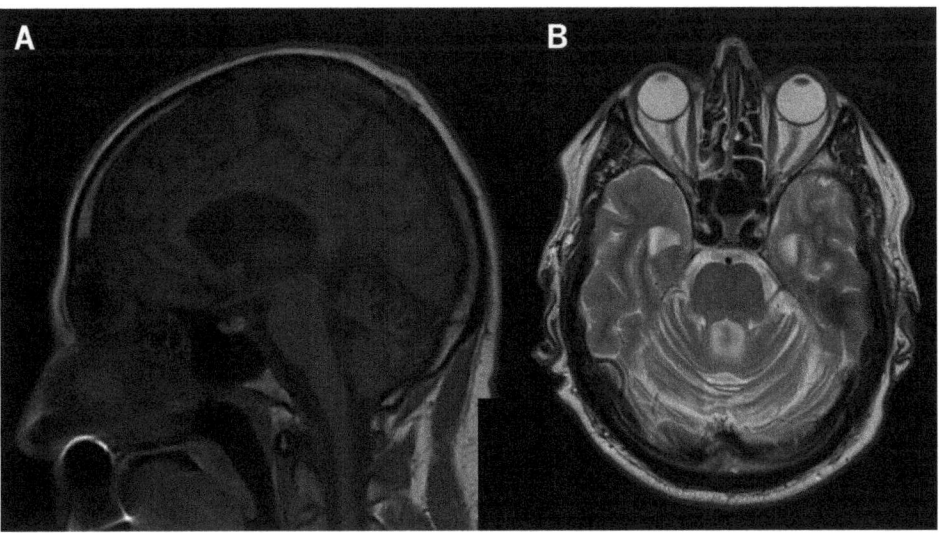

Figure 41.1 (A) Sagittal T1-weighted and (B) axial T2-weighted MRI scans of the brain showing bihemispheric moderate cerebellar atrophy.

Genetic Testing

Because of the family history, an initial genetic screen for spinocerebellar ataxias (SCAs) type 1, 2, 3 and 6 was requested. Spinocerebellar ataxia type 6 was diagnosed as the *CACNA1A* gene had 13 CAG repeats on allele 1 and 22 repeats on allele 2. (The normal range of CAG repeats in the CACNA1A gene is 4–18.)

Diagnosis: Spinocerebellar Ataxia Type 6

Management
He used a stick and, despite physiotherapy input, his Berg balance remained at 46/56. Exercises and stretches were advised. He was also referred to occupational therapy. He continued under cardiology follow-up due to his bicuspid aortic stenosis.

Comment
Dominant Ataxias
In 1993, Huda Zogbi and Harry Orr identified a heterozygous expansion in a CAG repeat encoding polyglutamine in the *ATXN1* gene in a family with a dominantly inherited ataxia. This condition is now called spinocerebellar ataxia type 1 (SCA 1). Polyglutamine expansions in other genes were subsequently found in other dominantly inherited ataxias – dentatorubral pallidoluysian atrophy, SCA 2, SCA 3, SCA 6, SCA 7 and SCA 17 [1]. Further dominant SCAs were genetically profiled as having repeat expansions in non-coding regions (e.g. SCA 8, SCA 10 and SCA 12).

Spinocerebellar ataxias are characterised by cerebellar degeneration, which may be accompanied by brainstem atrophy. Clinically, the core symptoms in SCA are gait ataxia, dysarthria and visual disturbances. However, additional features – cognitive impairment, limb and trunk ataxia, tremor, rigidity, bradykinesia, dystonia and hyper-reflexia may suggest a particular type of SCA.

It should be noted that the majority of SCAs are not caused by repeat expansions, although some of these have been described in one family only [2].

Spinocerebellar ataxias not caused by repeat expansions do not demonstrate anticipation (earlier disease onset and more severe phenotype in subsequent generations) and there is no cellular aggregation of toxic polyglutamines.

Epidemiology and Clinical Features of SCA 6
Spinocerebellar ataxia type 6 is an autosomal dominant ataxia with an estimated prevalence of 1 in 100,000, making up 15% of all cases of dominant inherited ataxia in the USA. It is usually a later onset progressive disorder, as with our patient. Age of onset varies from 19 to 73 years, with a mean of 43 to 52 years.

Spinocerebellar ataxia type 6 may initially appear as a pure ataxia. A previous classification labelled SCA 6 as autosomal dominant ataxia type III (i.e. pure cerebellar ataxia). However, in SCA 6, dysphagia and choking are common, hyper-reflexia and extensor plantar responses may develop in up to 50%, and dystonia and blepharospasm can occur in 25% of patients.

Offspring have a 50% risk of inheriting the CAG trinucleotide repeat. Prenatal testing and pre-implantation genetic testing are available for SCA 6.

Molecular Biology of *CACNA1A*
Spinocerebellar ataxia type 6 is one of three disorders due to mutations in the *CACNA1A* gene, which encodes an α1A subunit of the P/Q calcium channel Cav2.1 [1]. Spinocerebellar ataxia type 6 is due to small expansions of the CAG repeat (encoding polyglutamine) in exon 47. The other two disorders – familial hemiplegic migraine type 1 and episodic ataxia type 2 – are due to mutations in the *CACNA1A* gene, which cause a loss of channel function in

episodic ataxia type 2 and a gain of channel function in familial hemiplegic migraine type 1. The short expansions of polyglutamine from the CAG repeat in SCA 6 are in the cytoplasmic C-terminal tail and seem to have a role in channel regulation and in transcription regulation of other neuronal genes.

The affected range for full penetrance of SCA 6 is 20–33 CAG repeats. Nineteen CAG is termed an 'intermediate allele', predisposing to expansion into the abnormal range or a susceptibility factor with variable penetrance and expression [1].

Natural History of SCA 6

Spinocerebellar ataxia type 6 progresses faster in women than in men. Longer CAG repeats are associated with earlier disease, but length of CAG repeat or age of onset does not appear to affect progression in SCA 6. This may be due to small variations in repeat length or just slower disease progression in SCA 6 compared to SCA 1, SCA 2 and SCA 3 [3].

There is very limited evidence of effective treatment for SCA 6. Acetazolamide, a brain carbonic anhydrase inhibitor, may temporarily reduce impact of the condition. As polyglutamine SCAs share common pathogenic mechanisms, including mitochondrial dysfunction as well as proteasome and autophagy impairment, research may be directed at exploring genetic editing therapy. Such potential treatments have encouraged natural history studies, rating scale optimisation and biomarker development.

References

1.   Giunti P, Mantuano E, Frontali M, Veneziano L. Molecular mechanism of spinocerebellar ataxia type 6: glutamine repeat disorder, channelopathy and transcriptional dysregulation. The multifaceted aspects of a single mutation. *Front Cell Neurosci*. 2015;9:5.

2.   Müller U. Spinocerebellar ataxias (SCAs) caused by common mutations. *Neurogenetics*. 2021;22(4):235–50.

3.   Jacobi H, du Montcel ST, Bauer P et al. Long-term disease progression in spinocerebellar ataxia types 1, 2, 3, and 6: a longitudinal cohort study. *Lancet Neurol*. 2015;14(11):1101–8.

Learning Points

- A proportion of dominantly inherited ataxias known as the spinocerebellar ataxias are due to a trinucleotide CAG repeat (polyglutamine) expansion of several different genes.

- Spinocerebellar ataxia type 6 or SCA 6 is an adult-onset slowly progressive cerebellar ataxia accompanied by dysarthria and nystagmus.

- The trinucleotide expansion ataxias may demonstrate anticipation, that is, earlier disease onset and more severe phenotype in subsequent generations due to increased length of trinucleotide expansion. This has not been observed in SCA 6.

Patient's Perspective

1.   **What is/was the impact of the condition?**

    a. Physical (e.g. practical support)
    My balance, co-ordination, speech and writing are affected. I now struggle to dress myself, fall regularly and walk with a stick.

    b. Psychological (e.g. mood, emotional well-being)
    Psychologically I am not helped by people with little or no understanding of the condition. I find myself having to raise my voice to be heard and have to repeat myself. My mood swings.

    c. Social (e.g. meeting friends, home)
    I have a largely understanding family but few friends, just acquaintances. As my speech is deteriorating others can struggle to understand me. I avoid busy places as I appear intoxicated.

2. **What can you no longer do?**
   I have to be careful of surfaces for walking. I have to be close to toilet facilities due to bladder and bowel weakness.

3. **Was there any other change for you due to your medical condition?**
   A feeling of weakness and unsteadiness in my legs, particularly if I sit on a low seat. Tingling in my spine, restlessness in bed. When walking, I cannot focus to speak to anyone at the same time.

4. **What is/was the most difficult aspect of the condition?**
   Slowing everything down; each task takes more time.

5. **Was any aspect of the experience good or useful? What was that?**
   No, not applicable.

6. **What do you hope for in the future for your condition?**
   A cure.

42   Non-familial Falling

History

A 20-year-old male student complained of a balance problem for over a year. He had noticed poor balance in a shower on closing his eyes, falling on one occasion. He sometimes stumbled when walking. He had noticed that he sometimes stepped sideways to maintain his balance. He had fallen off a bicycle on a couple of occasions. He was sometimes unaware that he had crossed his legs. He felt that his writing had slowed. At times he thought that his speech was slurred, although this was not noticed by his family. He had had a couple of migraines over a few years. He drank very little alcohol, was a non-smoker and denied any illicit drug use. His three siblings and parents were alive and well.

Examination

Higher mental function was normal. He had a positive Romberg's sign with increasing swaying. He had finger–nose and heel–shin ataxia. He had no nystagmus. He denied any sensory loss but pin prick and proprioception were mildly impaired. Power was normal but reflexes were absent with flexor plantar responses.

Investigations

Initial investigations included an MRI of the brain, which was reported as normal.

Blood investigations included full blood count, ESR, CRP, electrolytes, liver function tests, thyroid profile, ferritin, B12, folate, coeliac serology and vitamin E, which were all normal or negative. Lactate, pyruvate and lipids were normal. Glutamic acid decarboxylase 65 and thyroperoxidase antibodies were negative. A lumbar puncture was unremarkable.

Visual evoked responses were normal. Median sensory evoked responses showed delayed cortical responses from both arms. It was not possible to record the cervical responses.

Nerve conduction studies demonstrated a severe, probably axonal peripheral neuropathy affecting sensory fibres with relative preservation of motor fibres. A sensory neuronopathy was suggested.

A triplet repeat ataxia gene screen for spinocerebellar ataxia types 1, 2, 3 and 6, Friedreich's ataxia and dentatorubral pallidoluysian atrophy was sent at the initial presentation.

Diagnosis: Friedreich's Ataxia
(Confirmed on Genetic Testing)

Management and Outcome

The student disability office was informed to help with practical issues at university. Physiotherapy, occupational and speech and language therapy with a neuro-rehabilitation team helped out in subsequent management. He was directed towards Ataxia UK (www.ataxia.org .uk).

A review of anti-oxidant role in Friedreich's ataxia prompted co-enzyme Q10 (400 mg) and vitamin E (2,000 IU) treatments.

Over the 15 years following his diagnosis, he had some falls, fracturing his right fibula on two occasions.

Comment

Epidemiology and Clinical Features of Friedreich's Ataxia

Friedreich's ataxia has a prevalence of 1 in 40,000 and is the most commonly inherited ataxia among individuals of European ancestry. The average age of onset is 10–15 years. Friedreich's ataxia causes progressive ataxia of limbs and gait, dysarthria, cardiomyopathy and an increased rate of diabetes mellitus. The main sites of neuropathology in Friedreich's ataxia are:

1. dorsal root ganglia
2. dentate nuclei of the cerebellum
3. posterior columns
4. spinocerebellar tracts
5. corticospinal tracts
6. peripheral nerves.

The heart and pancreas are other sites of pathology in Friedreich's ataxia with cardiomyopathy being the most common cause of premature death [1].

Genetics

Friedreich's ataxia is an autosomal recessive disorder. The genetic cause of the disease was identified in 1996 as a homozygous GAA triplet repeat (56–1300) expansion in intron 1 of *Frataxin* (*FXN*) [2]. It was soon recognised that 96% of Friedreich's ataxia patients are homozygous for the GAA triplet repeat, while 4% of Friedreich's ataxia patients are compound heterozygous for a GAA expansion in one allele and have a *FXN* point mutation in the other allele.

A phenotype–genotype correlation was found in Friedreich's ataxia: the number of GAA repeats in the smaller allele has an inverse correlation with age of onset and some other clinical features (presence of cardiomyopathy, diabetes mellitus, scoliosis and time from onset to wheelchair mobility) [3].

Pathology

Frataxin is largely found in mitochondria and is highly expressed in dorsal root ganglia, the spinal cord, cerebellar dentate nuclei, the cerebral cortex, pancreas, heart and skeletal muscle, reflecting the main sites of pathology. Frataxin, a 210 amino acid polypeptide, is cleaved to a 130 amino acid protein from which different isoforms are produced. Frataxin is part of a complex, which assembles iron-sulphur (Fe-S) clusters in the mitochondrial matrix. The Fe-S clusters are co-factors for proteins in the Krebs cycle and in mitochondrial respiratory complexes I, II and III. Deficiency in frataxin results in reduced mitochondrial adenosine triphosphate (ATP) production.

Excess iron has been found in the dentate nuclei of the cerebellum of patients with Friedreich's ataxia.

Treatment Research

Potential therapies lie in restoring frataxin levels in key tissues. Iron chelators that cross the blood–brain barrier (deferiprone) have not proven to be effective. Indeed, the evidence-base for effective treatment to alter the natural history of Friedreich's ataxia is scant, but novel research continues, including activation of the impaired nuclear factor erythroid 2-related factor 2 (Nrf2) signalling, which improves mitochondrial function.

Causes of Sensory Neuronopathy

Primary degeneration of the dorsal root ganglia and their projections causes a sensory neuronopathy. The sensory ganglia contain the cell bodies of the sensory nerves. These can be damaged in general medical and paraneoplastic disorders. Reduction in sensory nerve action potentials is present with normal conduction velocity. Recognised causes of sensory neuronopathy/ganglionopathy are shown in Table 42.1.

Sensory neuronopathies are a group of disabling peripheral nerve disorders. The first reported cases by Derek Denny-Brown in 1948 involved two patients with bronchial carcinoma in whom the dorsal root ganglia were affected with sparing of the ventral motor roots. Inflammatory, genetic, infective, paraneoplastic, vitamin deficiency (E and B12) and excess (B6) as well as mitochondrial disease can all affect the dorsal root ganglia neurones.

Table 42.1 Causes of sensory neuronopathy

Category	Cause
Immune/inflammatory	Sjögren's syndrome Systemic lupus erythematosus Rheumatoid arthritis Gluten sensitivity Autoimmune hepatitis CANOMAD syndrome – chronic ataxic neuropathy ophthalmoplegia IgM paraprotein cold agglutinins disialosyl antibodies Anti-fibroblast growth factor receptor 3 antibodies
Infective	HIV Human T-cell lymphotropic virus type 1 Epstein–Barr virus Measles Varicella zoster virus (localised) Zika
Paraneoplastic (anti-Hu syndrome)	Small-cell lung cancer Lymphoma Bronchial carcinoma Breast cancer Neuroendocrine tumours

Table 42.1 (Cont.)

Category	Cause
Medication	Cisplatin/oxaliptan/doxorubicin Checkpoint inhibitors
Vitamin deficiency or excess	Vitamin B6 (pyridoxine) toxicity Nicotinic deficiency Vitamin E, Vitamin B12 deficiency
Hereditary	Friedreich's ataxia Fabry disease Hereditary sensory and autonomic neuropathy CANVAS syndrome – cerebellar ataxia, neuropathy and vestibular areflexia Spinocerebellar ataxias 1, 2, 3, 4 and 7 Fragile X-associated tremor and ataxia syndrome
Mitochondrial disorders	DNA Polymerase γ or *POLG* mutations

Compiled from a number of sources including Gwathmey [4], Amato and Ropper [5] and Fargeot and Echaniz-Laguna [6].

References

1. Pousset F, Legrand L, Monin M-L et al. A 22-year follow-up study of long-term cardiac outcome and predictors of survival in Friedreich ataxia. *JAMA Neurol.* 2015 Nov.;72(11):1334–41.

2. Campuzano V, Montermini L, Moltò MD et al. Friedreich's ataxia: autosomal recessive disease caused by an intronic GAA triplet repeat expansion. *Science.* 1996 Mar.;271(5254):1423–7.

3. Dürr A, Cossee M, Agid Y et al. Clinical and genetic abnormalities in patients with Friedreich's ataxia. *N Engl J Med.* 1996 Oct.;335(16):1169–75.

4. Gwathmey KG. Sensory neuronopathies. *Muscle Nerve.* 2016;53:8–19.

5. Amato AA, Ropper AH. Sensory ganglionopathy. *N Engl J Med.* 2020;383;1657–62.

6. Fargeot G, Echaniz-Laguna A. Sensory neuronopathies: new genes, new antibodies and new concepts. *J Neurol Neurosurg & Psychiatry.* 2021;92:398–406.

Learning Points

- Friedreich's ataxia is the most commonly inherited ataxia among individuals of European ancestry.

- The genetic cause of Friedreich's ataxia is a homozygous GAA triplet repeat expansion or compound heterozygous GAA repeat and a pathogenic mutation in the *Frataxin* gene – inherited as an autosomal recessive trait.

- Frataxin deficiency leads to a reduction in iron-sulphur cluster biogenesis, which is important in mitochondrial ATP generation.

- Cerebellar atrophy is not a common finding in Friedreich's ataxia.

Patient's Perspective

1. **What was the impact of the condition on you?**

   a. **Physical (e.g. practical support)**
   Initially I still felt pretty well and strong physically, but particularly in the last three years, I have felt weaker, physically limited in what I was able to do and too disabled to do things I wanted to do. The gradual decline has meant that stopping doing some things in case my balance failed and caused me injury, has solidified into physical inability. This is particularly true of sports. For a while after

diagnosis in 2007 I walked unaided, then used a large umbrella, then a walking stick from 2015 and started using a frame indoors from March this year (2020). Outdoors a walking stick and on someone's elbow.

b. **Psychological (e.g. mood, emotional well-being)**
After the initial shock, uncertainty set in and never really left. Not only had my health prospects changed, my career was gone. I have since found it hard to plan or imagine what life will be like in the future, and my confidence has taken a knock. Life is not what I had looked forward to when I started college with high hopes, but I suppose most people could say that.

c. **Social (e.g. meeting friends, home)**
Giving up sports and outdoor pursuits meant losing touch with some people pretty quickly, and having to reassure new acquaintances about unusual symptoms meant that I found the company of existing friends – from before diagnosis – much more comfortable and probably supportive too, given that some were training medically and had more idea than most what ataxia was. Meeting friends has been difficult since college since I haven't really belonged to any social institution. I found a very positive voluntary project to get involved in for a few years and enjoyed the social aspects, but since it closed and my health has declined I don't go out much in the evenings ever since moving back home except with family, who have been very supportive.

2. **What can or could you not do because of the condition?**
My balance, co-ordination and stamina are diminishing. I can swim and usually walk, but normal mobility is gone so most sports are beyond me. I can't do some household chores and gardening, DIY and hiking/long walks in even moderate terrain without assistance, or solitary walks. Most personal tasks I managed before dislocating my shoulder. Working would be difficult and very tiring now.

3. **Was there any other change for you due to your medical condition?**
I can't drive so independent travel – daily or for leisure – is very difficult. I'm lucky that my siblings have organised a number of trips abroad in the last years, giving me something to look forward to. I have noticed my sleep is much worse, though this is at least partly due to indiscipline on my part. I've always been a night owl, and used to enjoy the cool and quiet of long late-evening walks while I still could.

4. **What is/was the most difficult aspect of the condition for you?**
The uncertainty of the rate of progression – planning has been difficult, both daily energy (and sleep) and longer term; what can I take on, manage, aim for and achieve. This ties into independence too. I guess this was just the coincidence of when I was diagnosed – right as I was getting used to living independently and enjoying my own space and freedom, the medium and longer term prospects of it changed drastically.

5. **Was any aspect of the experience of the condition good or useful? What was that?**
Patience with myself – perhaps too much!
I can take a different outlook on things, and freed of normal expectations I have had more time to enjoy things at my own pace, catching up on reading, films and cultural and intellectual pursuits that I skipped in college – probably because these are sedentary. Can sometimes appreciate still being able to do something, and the ephemeral and impermanent nature of life. The appreciation of recovery of function after recent injuries. Accepting the unpredictable beyond my control may have helped this year.

6. **What do you hope for in the future for people with this condition?**
I am hopeful that the importance of understanding mitochondria to our metabolism and health will lead to a therapy of some sort to slow progression or lessen the worst symptoms.

History

A 52-year-old left-handed woman and driver presented with a one-year history of intermittent but progressive left leg tremor. Prior to assessment, the right leg had also developed an intermittent but less prominent tremor. She had no tremor when walking but was aware of the leg tremor on standing still. She had also noticed a left arm tremor, particularly on pouring liquids. A painful left shoulder had prevented her from lying on her left side in bed at night. She had noticed that dressing had become slower and more challenging.

Sleep could be disturbed but there was no suggestion of lashing out or vivid dreams. She had no falls. She did not have constipation. She had no speech or swallowing problems. She denied loss of smell.

She had previously been a gym instructor. A maternal grandmother had had a tremor in her ninth decade.

Past medical history included coeliac disease and the frozen left shoulder. Medication was co-codamol, naproxen, amitriptyline and cyanocobalamin tablets. She had no known drug allergies. She drank a glass of wine at night.

Examination

The patient was alert and orientated, and able to provide her medical history. Pulse was 90 beats per minute and blood pressure was 144/91 mmHg. There was hypomimia. She had a decreased range of movement of her left shoulder. At rest, she had a leg tremor. There was no postural or intention arm tremor. Walking was associated with a decreased arm swing. There was bradykinesia (decrementing amplitude and speed) at pincer movements and foot-tapping, worse on the left than the right. There was no rigidity or cogwheeling. Limb power was normal. Co-ordination, reflexes and sensation were all intact.

Diagnosis: Idiopathic Parkinson's Disease

Investigations

A dopamine transporter (DaT) scan had shown decreased putamen uptake in both hemispheres consistent with a Parkinsonian syndrome (Figure 43.1).

Management

Co-beneldopa (a mixture of 4 parts by mass of levodopa to one part benserazide hydrochloride) was prescribed and increased to 100/25 mg tid with good benefit; there was less bradykinesia. Rasagiline 1 mg per day was subsequently added.

She returned to work on a part-time basis and continued to drive after informing the Driver and Vehicle Licensing Agency of the diagnosis of Parkinson's disease.

Comment

Parkinson's Disease Epidemiology and Pathology

Parkinson's disease can present with asymmetric bradykinesia, resting tremor, rigidity and postural instability. The diagnosis rests on the presence of bradykinesia combined with rest

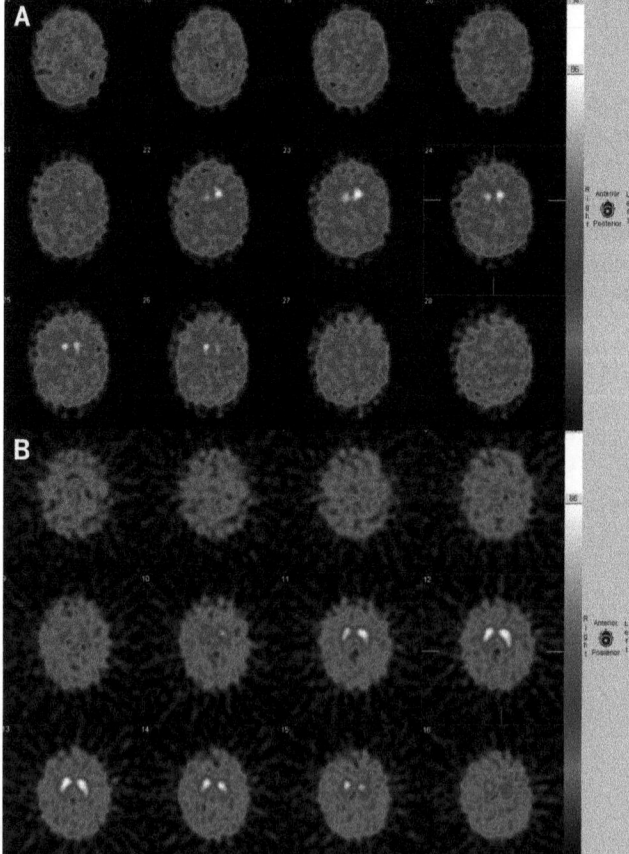

Figure 43.1 An I[123]-ioflupane single-photon emission computerised tomography or DaT scan showing (A) decreased isotope in the putamen bilaterally of patient with Parkinson's disease and (B) a normal control in which the isotope shows up as two symmetrical crescent-shaped areas of equal intensity.

tremor, rigidity, or both. This progressive neurodegenerative disease affects approximately 1% of the population over 65 years, making it the second most common neurodegenerative disorder after Alzheimer's disease. There is evidence that the incidence, prevalence and years lived with disability of Parkinson's disease are increasing, although the reasons for this are not fully understood [1].

Progressive neuronal loss in the nigrostriatal pathway is the fundamental pathology in idiopathic Parkinson's disease with degeneration of the substantia nigra pars compacta and the presence of insoluble alpha-synuclein-containing cytoplasmic inclusions known as Lewy bodies. The clinical diagnosis of Parkinson's disease has always required demonstration of a motor syndrome. However, the 2015 Movement Disorder Society criteria also prompt consideration of non-motor symptoms, including hyposmia, autonomic dysfunction, sleep and psychiatric problems [2]. Patients can present exclusively with non-motor symptoms, which can delay diagnosis compared to patients presenting with motor manifestations. Heterogenous presentations and progression as well as variation in patient priorities all prompt a call for precision medicine [1].

Pre-clinical (neurodegeneration has started but no clinical signs or symptoms are present), prodromal (when signs and/or symptoms are present but are insufficient to diagnose clinical Parkinson's disease) and clinical Parkinson's disease are all recognised.

Diagnostic Criteria for Parkinson's Disease

Diagnostic accuracy of Parkinson's disease by experts is consistently around 76–90%, the higher estimate being achieved by the time of death. There are two levels of diagnostic certainty: clinically established Parkinson's disease and clinically probable Parkinson's disease. The clinical steps in the diagnosis of Parkinson's disease [2] are outlined. These are provided in detail to reflect the emphasis on the clinical diagnosis.

Step 1

Step 1 involves confirming the presence of parkinsonism (i.e. bradykinesia plus rest tremor and/or lead-pipe rigidity). Bradykinesia is slowness of movement and decrement in amplitude or speed (or progressive hesitations or halts) as movements continue. Movements assessed usually include finger-tapping, hand movements, pronation-supination, toe-tapping and foot-tapping.

Rigidity is described as lead-pipe resistance. This is a velocity-independent resistance to passive movement around a joint that is not due to a failure to relax. Cogwheeling may reflect rigidity with co-existent tremor. Cogwheeling in the absence of lead-pipe rigidity does not fulfil minimum requirements for rigidity.

Rest tremor at 4–6 Hz occurs in a fully resting limb and is suppressed during movement initiation. Kinetic and postural tremors alone do not qualify as parkinsonism criteria. Although a re-emergent hand tremor is described after prolonged posture in parkinsonism, to meet criteria, the tremor must also occur during rest.

Step 2

Step 2 involves confirming absence of absolute exclusion criteria. They include unequivocal cerebellar abnormalities (as can occur in multiple system atrophy), downward gaze supranuclear gaze palsy or selective slowing of downward vertical saccades (as seen in progressive supranuclear palsy), a diagnosis of probable behavioural variant frontotemporal dementia or primary progressive aphasia within the first five years of disease, parkinsonism features restricted to the lower limbs for more than three years (suggestion of vascular parkinsonism), drug-induced parkinsonism due to dopamine receptor blocker or dopamine-depleting agent, absence of observable response to high-dose levodopa (≥600 mg a day) despite at least moderate severity of disease, unequivocal cortical sensory loss, clear limb ideomotor apraxia or progressive aphasia (features seen in corticobasal degeneration syndrome). Although not required for diagnosis, normal functional neuroimaging of the presynaptic dopaminergic system is another exclusion criterion. Finally, an alternative condition known to produce parkinsonism and plausibly connected to the patient's symptoms is also an exclusion criterion [2].

Step 3

In step 3, the criteria stipulate that no red flags and two or more supportive criteria must be present. The red flags include rapid progression of gait impairment requiring wheelchair within five years of onset, absence of progression of motor symptoms or signs over five years or more unless stability is related to treatment, early bulbar dysfunction – dysphonia, dysarthria or severe dysphagia within the first five years of disease, diurnal or nocturnal inspiratory stridor or frequent inspiratory sighs and severe autonomic failure within the first five years of disease. Severe autonomic failure includes orthostatic hypotension (30 mmHg systolic or 15 mmHg diastolic drop in blood pressure on standing at three minutes in the absence of dehydration, medication or other disease explaining autonomic dysfunction) or severe urinary incontinence or retention in the first five years of disease (prostate disease must be excluded in men).

Other red flags are recurrent falls due to impaired balance within three years of disease onset, the presence of disproportionate anterocollis or contractures of hand or feet within the first 10 years of disease and absence of common non-motor features of disease despite disease of five years duration – sleep dysfunction (sleep-maintenance insomnia, excessive daytime somnolence, rapid eye movement (REM) sleep behaviour disorder), autonomic dysfunction (constipation, daytime urinary urgency or symptomatic orthostasis), hyposmia, psychiatric illness (depression, anxiety or hallucinations), unexplained pyramidal tract signs and bilateral symmetrical parkinsonism throughout the disease course.

The supportive criteria include a clear and dramatic response to dopaminergic therapy, the presence of levodopa-induced dyskinesia, rest tremor of a limb documented on clinical examination, at least one positive result from a diagnostic test that has over 80% specificity for Parkinson's disease from other parkinsonian conditions (e.g. age- and sex-adjusted olfactory loss) or metaiodobenzylguanidine scintigraphy clearly documenting cardiac sympathetic denervation.

Summary of Movement Disorder Society Diagnostic Criteria for Parkinson's Disease

Clinically established Parkinson's disease requires steps 1 and 2 plus no red flags and two or more supportive criteria.

Clinically probable Parkinson's disease requires steps 1 and 2 plus EITHER one red flag and one or more supportive criteria OR two red flags and two or more supportive criteria.

Differential Diagnosis of Parkinsonism

Accuracy of a diagnosis of Parkinson's disease varies with disease duration, patient age, clinician experience and improvement in our understanding of Parkinson's disease. Even for step 1, repeated movements (i.e. search for bradykinesia) can be difficult to elicit due to other conditions such as arthritis, pyramidal weakness, depression, dyspraxia, cerebellar disease, dystonia, obsessional slowness and other cognitive deficits.

The differential diagnosis includes other causes of parkinsonism (Table 43.1). Diagnostic inaccuracy can be attributed to other neurodegenerative pathologies such as multiple system atrophy and progressive supranuclear palsy or the absence of a progressive parkinsonian disorder such as essential tremor. The most common mimics are tremor disorders, drug-induced parkinsonism, vascular parkinsonism and the Parkinson-plus or atypical parkinsonian disorders [3].

The causes of Parkinson's disease include both genetic and environmental factors (which may be historic) and their interactions. It is estimated that 3–5% of patients with Parkinson's disease have monogenic Parkinson's disease. Presentation under the age of 40 years may be the best clue to a genetic cause. Mutations in *SNCA* (earlier age of onset, faster progression and rapid cognitive decline), *LRRK2*, *PRKN*, *PINK1* and *GBA* are known causes of genetic Parkinson's disease. *PRKN* mutations account for most cases of juvenile (age of onset of less than 20 years) Parkinson's disease. Genetic risk variants also account for a proportion of Parkinson's disease [1].

Some toxins have been recognised as causes of parkinsonism, such as MPTP (1-methyl-4-phenyl-1,2,3,6-tetrahydropyridine), produced during manufacture of a synthetic opioid and pesticides.

Progression in Parkinson's disease is inevitable but variable. Clinically, frequent aggressive dreams in newly diagnosed Parkinson's disease patients have been shown in at least one study to hasten motor and cognitive decline, as has REM sleep behaviour disorder.

Dopamine Transporter Scan

A DaT scan (ioflupane[123] single-photon emission computerised tomography) is not required to diagnose idiopathic Parkinson's disease. However, for some patients, diagnosis and management can be helped with a DaT scan, particularly for atypical presentations and in distinguishing early parkinsonism from essential tremor. Its clinical utility, at least in the published literature, suggests that management may be changed in half of the patients tested and diagnosis altered in a third of patients.

Table 43.1 Some causes of parkinsonism

Category	Example (pathology)
Atypical parkinsonian disorders	Dementia with Lewy bodies (α-synuclein Lewy bodies) Progressive supranuclear palsy (tauopathy) Multiple system atrophy (α-synucleinopathy) Corticobasal syndrome (tauopathy)
Secondary causes of parkinsonism	Normal pressure hydrocephalus Drugs (anti-psychotic drugs, cinnarizine, valproate) Vascular parkinsonism
Genetic forms of parkinsonism	Familial PD (*LRRK2, PRKN, PINK1* and *DJ-1*) Huntington's disease Wilson's disease Spinocerebellar ataxias 2, 3 and 17 Fragile X-associated tremor/ataxia syndrome Frontotemporal dementia *POLG* mutations
Tremors	Essential tremor Dystonic tremor

Treatments for Parkinson's Disease

While current pharmacological therapy emphasises symptomatic treatment with drugs that enhance the effect of dopamine, a search for disease-modifying treatments for idiopathic Parkinson's disease has, to date, been elusive. It is now generally accepted that there is no therapeutic rationale for postponing symptomatic treatment.

Levodopa (a precursor of dopamine) is the first-line and often the best treatment. Multidisciplinary teamwork (neurologist, specialist nurse and physiotherapist) can optimise management. Determining the cause of the motor-anxiety loop seen in Parkinson's disease may direct more effective non-motor therapies.

The non-pharmacological aspects of managing Parkinson's disease are very important for a chronic progressive disease. High-intensity aerobic exercise has an emerging supportive evidence base. Education about exercise, driving implications, risk of impulse control disorders and psychosis are very important.

References

1.   Bloem BR, Okun MS, Klein C. Parkinson's disease. *Lancet*. 2021;397(10291):2284–303.
2.   Postuma RB, Berg D, Stern M et al. MDS clinical diagnostic criteria for Parkinson's disease. *Mov Disord*. 2015;30(12):1591–601.
3.   Ali K, Morris HR. Parkinson's disease: chameleons and mimics. *Pract Neurol*. 2015;15(1):14–25.

Patient's Perspective

1.   **What is the impact of the condition on you?**
    a. Physical (e.g. practical support, work, activities of daily living)
    The impact was physical, causing uncontrollable shaking in both my legs.
    b. Psychological (e.g. mood, emotional well-being)
    Emotionally it was difficult to deal with, but since I have been on the medication, it is more bearable.
    c. Social (e.g. meeting friends, home)
    I found this very difficult and I was very self-conscious. Being in lockdown (due to COVID-19 pandemic) didn't help. It also knocked my confidence at work.

2.   **What can you not do because of the condition?**
    I can't stand too long, which is a problem with work as I would have carried out a lot of workshops in my work. I also have problems turning my head, which is very painful.

3.   **Has there been any other change for you due to the condition?**
    As you can see from my handwriting it has got worse. My left knee keeps locking.

4.   **What is/was the most difficult aspect of the condition for you?**
    Nighttime is the most difficult as I cannot stop the shaking in bed. I take amitriptyline at night, which helps but I end up getting up out of bed around 3am.

5.   **Was any aspect of the experience good or useful? What was that?**
    No.

6.   **What do you hope for in the future for people with your condition?**
    I hope that a cure is found.

History

A 40-year-old woman developed progressive unsteadiness and slurring of speech, triggering admission to hospital. She had a long history of systemic lupus erythematosus (discoid rash, photosensitivity, anti-dsDNA and leucopenia) for which she had received a lot of immuno-suppressive medication.

Other past medical history included focal onset epilepsy (déjà vu feeling, confused or 'weird smells') with secondary generalisation from the age of 13 years. An MRI of the brain had been reported as normal and an EEG showed a moderate excess of slow waves over both temporal regions. At one stage, she had been five years free of seizures on carbamazepine 400 mg per day. When seizures recurred, carbamazepine was increased, then lamotrigine and levetiracetam were added. Generalised events had stopped three years prior to her presentation with unsteadiness and slurred speech, although she continued to have déjà vu feelings.

Medication

Lupus medication included prednisolone, often 50 mg od, hydroxychloroquine 200 mg bd, mepacrine 200 mg od and tacrolimus 6 mg bd, started two months before onset of unsteadiness.

Other medication included levetiracetam 1500 mg bd, carbamazepine 400 mg bd, lamotrigine 250 mg mane and 200 mg nocte, diazepam 2 mg od, ranitidine 150 mg od, oxybutynin 5 mg bd, alendronic acid 70 mg per week, calcium/vitamin D, sertraline 100 mg od and co-trimoxazole 960 mg three times per week.

Previous immunosuppressant medication for lupus had included rituximab, belimumab (inhibitor of B cell-activating factor), golimumab, cyclophosphamide and mycophenolate, all of which had been either ineffective or not tolerated.

Examination

Skin was intact. Visual acuity was 6/9 bilaterally. She had bilateral horizontal gaze-evoked nystagmus. She had marked ataxia and dysarthria. There were no other neurological abnormalities.

Investigations
Blood Investigations

HIV 1 and 2 specific antibody, antigen (p24) and syphilis immunoassay were negative. Full blood count revealed a normocytic anaemia and lymphocyte count of 0.44/nL with a pan-lymphopenia (CD3, CD4, CD8 and CD 19 all below normal). A nuclear autoantibody screen had shown positive anti-Ro 60 and anti-La antibodies. Lupus anti-coagulant, vasculitic screen (C-ANCA, P-ANCA and MPO-ANCA and PR3-ANCA), anti-cardiolipin IgG and IgM anti-bodies and beta2-glycoprotein-1 IgG and IgM antibodies were negative. No paraprotein was detected on plasma protein electrophoresis. Immunoglobulin M was reduced at <0.1 g/L (normal range 0.5–1.9 g/L).

Neuroimaging

MRI brain imaging demonstrated right middle cerebellar peduncle and smaller left middle cerebellar peduncle lesions as well as rostral pontine high signal (Figures 44.1A and 44.1B). Within six weeks, a further MRI scan of the brain revealed disease progression (Figures 44.1C and 44.1D).

Cerebrospinal Fluid

The lumbar puncture findings are recorded in Table 44.1.

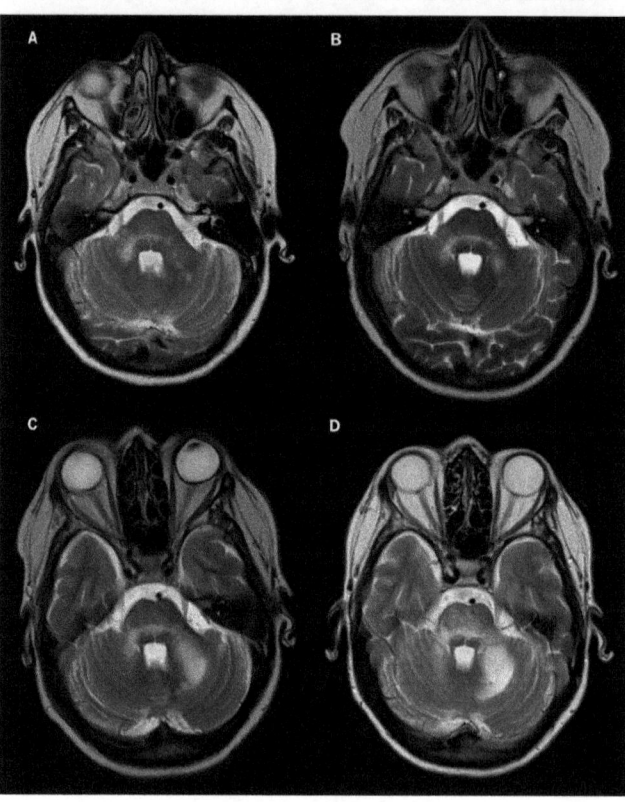

Figure 44.1 (A and B) An axial T2-weighted MRI scan of the brain showing abnormal signal in the dorsal pons extending along the middle cerebellar peduncles into the medial cerebellar hemispheres. Six weeks later, (C and D) an axial T2-weighted MRI scan of brain shows that these lesions had progressed, particularly into the left medial cerebellum.

Table 44.1 Lumbar puncture findings

	First lumbar puncture	Second lumbar puncture – three weeks later
Opening pressure	Not measured	8 cmCSF
White cell count	1/μL	0
Red cell count	26/μL	326
CSF glucose	2.8 mmol/L	2.6 mmol/L

Table 44.1 (Cont.)

	First lumbar puncture	Second lumbar puncture – three weeks later
Serum glucose	4.3 mmol/L	
CSF protein	0.71 g/L	0.59 g/L
Oligoclonal bands	Positive	
CSF infective panel	Herpes simplex virus 1 and 2, varicella zoster virus, parechovirus, enterovirus and Epstein–Barr virus – PCR – all negative	
Cryptococcal antigen	Negative	

CSF, cerebrospinal fluid

JC (John Cunningham) virus DNA (229 genome copies/ml) and JC virus polyoma virus antibody titre 1:40 were detected from the first lumbar puncture. JC virus polyoma virus antibody titre 1:40 was also found in the second lumbar puncture.

Diagnosis: Progressive Multifocal Leukoencephalopathy

Management

Further deterioration in speech and balance ensued over the next few months reflecting the neuroimaging progression on serial MRI brain scans. Swallowing difficulties arose due to severe oropharyngeal dysphagia with choking and food pooling in her mouth. A percutaneous endoscopic gastrostomy feeding tube was inserted for nutrition.

With a diagnosis of progressive multifocal leukoencephalopathy, all immunosuppressants were stopped and prednisolone was switched to maintenance hydrocortisone (15 mg mane and 5 mg nocte).

When the patient stablised, hydroxychloroquine 100mg bd and mepacrine 100 mg nocte were continued as the only immunosuppressants. Mirtazapine was added in view of some anecdotal evidence at the time of possible efficacy in progressive multifocal leukoencephalopathy.

Although stable, she still required a hoist for transfers. She had severe dysarthria, ongoing visual disturbance (oscillopsia). Her MRI scan of the brain showed no further progression. Rehabilitation was commenced.

Six years after her initial ataxia presentation, she still had oscillopsia, but mobilised with a walker. Swallowing had improved and the percutaneous gastrostomy tube was removed. She had had no generalised seizures but still experienced some déjà vu events. She continues under neurological and orthoptic follow-up. Her lupus has remained quiescent.

Comment

The JC Virus and Clinical Manifestations

Progressive multifocal leukoencephalopathy, first described in 1958, is a rare disease of the brain caused by the polyomavirus JC (named after John Cunningham). It is a lytic infection of brain glial cells in severely immunosuppressed individuals. The JC virus is a double-stranded DNA virus from the Polyomaviridae family, and it is found only in humans. It was first isolated from a patient with Hodgkin's lymphoma in 1971. In the presence of cellular immunodeficiency, the JC virus can undergo genetic rearrangements in the non-coding regions and transform into a neurotropic virus, which crosses the blood–brain barrier and infects oligodendrocytes and astrocytes via the 5-HT_{2a} serotonin receptor to cause progressive multifocal leukoencephalopathy. The JC virus is found in glial cells, lymphocytes, kidney epithelial cells and plasma cells. The JC virus causes asymptomatic and persistent infection in immunocompetent, healthy people and is intermittently excreted in the urine.

The manifestations of progressive multifocal leukoencephalopathy due to demyelination include motor weakness, sensory deficit, hemianopia, cognitive deficit, dysphasia and co-ordination/gait difficulties. Our patient's posterior fossa abnormalities accounted for ataxia as her predominant presenting feature.

Other clinical manifestations of the JC virus include granule cell neuronopathy, encephalopathy and meningitis.

Diagnostic Criteria for Progressive Multifocal Leukoencephalopathy

The diagnosis of progressive multifocal leukoencephalopathy requires clinical, radiological and virological evidence, as shown in Table 44.2 [1]. Virological evidence comprises viral DNA or proteins from a brain biopsy (in situ hybridisation or immunohistochemistry of JC virus proteins) or detection of JC virus DNA via PCR from cerebrospinal fluid (CSF).

Risk Factors for Progressive Multifocal Leukoencephalopathy

Progressive multifocal leukoencephalopathy is associated with CD4+ or CD8+ T-cell lymphopenia or a reduction of immune surveillance within the central nervous system. AIDS, haematological malignancies (lymphoma, leukaemia), post-transplant immunosuppression and rheumatological diseases are risk factors for progressive multifocal leukoencephalopathy. In addition, drugs, which suppress the immune system including the biological agents or monoclonal antibodies such as natalizumab for multiple sclerosis and Crohn's disease, and rituximab for lupus and efalizumab for psoriasis, are recognised iatrogenic causes of progressive multifocal leukoencephalopathy. Although AIDS is the most common global cause of progressive multifocal leukoencephalopathy, immunomodulatory or immunosuppressant drugs cause an increasing proportion of cases. For neurologists, the emergence of progressive multifocal leukoencephalopathy in multiple sclerosis patients on disease-modifying therapy has highlighted the need to stratify the risk of progressive multifocal leukoencephalopathy for patients prescribed natalizumab [2].

Lupus per se, even without any drug treatment/immunosuppressant, has a recognised association with progressive multifocal leukoencephalopathy [3]. Our patient also had prolonged immunosuppression for lupus.

Prognosis of Progressive Multifocal Leukoencephalopathy

In the era before highly active anti-retroviral treatment became available for HIV infection, progressive multifocal leukoencephalopathy was often fatal, but that trend has reversed and

Table 44.2 Diagnostic criteria for progressive multifocal leukoencephalopathy

Category	Clinical features	Imaging features	Cerebrospinal fluid PCR for JC virus
Definite	✔	✔	✔
Probable	✔	Negative	✔
	Negative	✔	✔
Possible	✔	✔	Not done or negative
	Negative	Negative	✔
Not PML	Negative	Negative	Negative
	✔	Negative	Negative
	Negative	✔	Negative

PML, progressive multifocal leukoencephalopathy

Adapted from Berger et al. [1] with permission from Wolters Kluwer.

HIV patients with progressive multifocal leukoencephalopathy now survive longer than non-HIV patients with progressive multifocal leukoencephalopathy.

Potential Treatments for Progressive Multifocal Leukoencephalopathy

Progressive multifocal leukoencephalopathy is often fatal if the JC virus is not restrained. Mirtazapine (blocker of $5HT_{2A}$ receptors used for the JC virus to gain access to glial cells), mefloquine (an anti-malarial drug reported to inhibit the JC virus in vitro) and cidofovir (a nucleotide analogue with anti-JC virus activity in a mouse model) have all been considered possible therapies for progressive multifocal leukoencephalopathy either individually or in combination. However, a study of mefloquine failed to show any evidence of efficacy.

More recently, because immune reconstitution facilitates control of progressive multifocal leukoencephalopathy, as shown with anti-retroviral therapy in AIDS cases, there is hope of future therapies harnessing this principle. Since 2019 (after our patient's diagnosis), a range of targeted approaches has been reported as potential therapies.

1   Adoptive transfer of human leucocyte antigen-matched JC virus-specific T-cells. BK-virus specific T-cells from healthy, related donors can be stimulated ex vivo with BK antigens. (BK is the initials of the patient in whom the virus was first detected in 1971.) Infusion of these BK-specific T-cells into patients with progressive multifocal leukoencephalopathy promotes cross-reactive neutralisation of the JC virus because the BK and JC viruses are similar polyomaviruses. Very few centres can provide virus-specific T-cell allogenic transfer.

2   Exploitation of T-cell exhaustion with immune checkpoint inhibition. Engagement of programmed cell death protein 1 (PD-1) on the surface of T-cells down-regulates immune responses. In the presence of chronic infection, PD-1 expression may impair viral clearance. Increased expression of PD-1 and programmed death ligand 1 (PDL-1) on CD4+ and CD8+ T-cells have been found in blood, CSF and autopsy lesions in patients with progressive multifocal leukoencephalopathy. PD-1 blockade with pembrolizumab has been proposed as a treatment by upregulating immune activity if there are sufficient JC virus-specific CD4+ T-cells.

3   A combination of BK virus-specific T-cells and PD-1 blockade has been proposed.

4   Interleukin 7 is an important cytokine in T-cell biology that can decrease expression of PD-1 on T-cells and increase antigen-specific responses. Human recombinant interleukin 7 has shown benefit for immune-deficit patients with progressive multifocal leukoencephalopathy. Interleukin 15 may be helpful as it stimulates natural killer cells and CD8+ T-cells.

5   Passive (intravenous immunoglobulin) and active immunisation strategies may have a role in stabilising progressive multifocal leukoencephalopathy.

Treatment of progressive multifocal leukoencephalopathy is a major clinical challenge as improved immunity risks an immune reconstitution inflammatory syndrome, in which paradoxical worsening of neurological symptoms is associated with enhancing mass lesions and oedema on MR imaging. Immune checkpoint inhibition appears to have a low frequency of both immune reconstitution inflammatory syndrome and immune-mediated adverse effects (e.g. colitis and pneumonitis) probably due to the severe immunodeficiency in progressive multifocal leukoencephalopathy. On the other hand, attempts to use recombinant human interleukin 7 in patients with progressive multifocal leukoencephalopathy were associated with severe immune reconstitution inflammatory syndrome.

Natalizumab and Progressive Multifocal Leukoencephalopathy

Between 2006 and 2021, natalizumab has been implicated in 853 cases of progressive multifocal leukoencephalopathy (3.86 per 1,000 patients). A risk stratification of serological testing for JC virus has lowered the risk of natalizumab-associated progressive multifocal leukoencephalopathy.

In summary, immunotherapies have led to an increase in the incidence of progressive multifocal leukoencephalopathy. Although there are increasingly newer options for the treatment of the disease which aim for a balance in effective and safe immune function restoration, management remains challenging.

References

1. Berger JR, Aksamit AJ, Clifford DB et al. PML diagnostic criteria: consensus statement from the AAN neuroinfectious disease section. *Neurology*. 2013;80(15):1430–8.

2. Major EO, Yousry TA, Clifford DB. Pathogenesis of progressive multifocal leukoencephalopathy and risks associated with treatments for multiple sclerosis: a decade of lessons learned. *Lancet Neurol*. 2018;17(5):467–80.

3. Henegar CE, Eudy AM, Kharat V et al. Progressive multifocal leukoencephalopathy in patients with systemic lupus erythematosus: a systematic literature review. *Lupus*. 2016;25(6):617–26.

Learning Points

- Progressive multifocal leukoencephalopathy is due to activation of the JC virus.

- Genetic rearrangements in immunocompromised patients lead to neurotropic JC virus infecting oligodendrocytes and astrocytes to cause progressive multifocal leukoencephalopathy.

- Emerging targeted treatments have a goal of re-invigorating T-cell immune activity to reduce viral load either via a Trojan horse appearance with BK virus-specific T-cell infusion or blockade of the programmed cell death pathway to increase T-cell activity.

- Treatment of progressive multifocal leukoencephalopathy may result in immune reconstitution inflammatory syndrome – paradoxical worsening of neurological deficits associated with MRI brain-enhancing mass lesions and oedema.

Patient's Perspective

1. **What was the impact of the condition on you?**

   a. Physical (e.g. job, driving, practical support)
   Not able to walk unassisted, being confined to a wheelchair most of the time. Unable to carry out simple tasks. Having visual and balance/co-ordination difficulties.

   b. Psychological (e.g. mood, emotional well-being)
   Can be up and down. Mostly down feelings of guilt, e.g. what changes my partner and son have had to make to their own lives to help with mine.

   c. Social (e.g. meeting friends, home)
   I lack the social skills I once had with friends and family apart from my partner and son. I do not socialise any more, feel too embarrassed of my disabilities and my speech.

2. **What could you not do because of the condition?**
   Climb stairs, walk unaided for any distance, difficulty with reading – cannot read or focus on most things. The inability to carry out everyday tasks such as making a cup of tea or cooking some food. I can't do a lot for myself and I need a lot of assistance.

3. **Was there any other change for you due to your medical condition?**
   Changes to my surroundings at home – adaptations for ground floor facilities, the introduction of care agency to help with some needs (to relieve some pressure on my partner and son).

4. **What is/was the most the difficult aspect of the condition for you?**

   My sight – I have double and blurred vision all the time. The balance and co-ordination issues also cause a lot of difficulty in everyday life – probably will never be able to walk properly because of these issues.

5. **Was any aspect of the experience good or useful? What was that?**

   No aspect or experience of my condition was good although my partner would say that it has humbled him and taught him to appreciate more and take less for granted.

6. **What do you hope for in the future for people with this condition?**

   I would hope for better understanding and monitoring so that action could be taken quicker to reduce the long-term effects of PML.

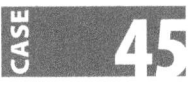

History

A 40-year-old man was referred for neurological assessment. He had had a five-year history of progressive slurred speech, difficulty initiating swallowing of both liquids and solids, choking episodes and poor balance.

In his past medical history, he had asthma, gastro-oesophageal reflux and vitamin B12 deficiency. His only medication was omeprazole and B12.

He had two siblings who were well. His father had deafness and diabetes mellitus.

Examination

He was tall and thin. He had marked slurring dysarthria with slow tongue movements. Smooth pursuit eye movements and vestibulo-ocular reflex were impaired. There was bilateral horizontal, gaze-evoked nystagmus. Saccades were of normal speed and latency but were hypermetric. He had heel-shin ataxia and a broad-based ataxic gait. Scleral telangiectasia were noted (Figure 45.1A). He had brisk reflexes but plantar responses were flexor.

On Folstein Mini-Mental State Examination, he scored 24/30. His Rivermead behavioural memory test score was 9/12, suggesting moderate difficulty with some memory function.

Investigations

Duodenal biopsy revealed no evidence of coeliac disease. Pulmonary function tests were normal. At lumbar puncture, there was an opening pressure of 7 cm of cerebrospinal fluid (CSF). The CSF had 430 red cells/μL, 0 white cells/μL, protein 0.32 g/L. The CSF glucose was 4.0 mmol/L (with plasma glucose 5.8 mmol/L) and cytology was normal. There was no evidence of restricted oligoclonal bands.

There was no evidence of autonomic failure; there was normal beat-to-beat heart rate variation including with Valsalva manoeuvre and no postural drop in blood pressure. Nerve conduction studies and EMG were normal.

A paraneoplastic antibody screen (Yo, Hu and Ri) was negative. Organic acids, very long chain fatty acids and α-fetoprotein were normal. Syphilis serology was negative. Serum protein electrophoresis and immunoglobulins were normal. Lactate and pyruvate were normal. Lysosomal enzyme screen was negative.

Genetic testing for spinocerebellar ataxia (SCA) types 1, 2, 3, 6 and 7, dentatorubral pallidoluysian atrophy and Friedreich's ataxia were negative. The mitochondrial *A3243 G* and *T8993 G/C* mutations were negative. Muscle biopsy showed only focal atrophy. There was no evidence of a mitochondrial disorder. An MRI scan of the brain revealed diffuse cerebellar atrophy (Figures 45.1B and 45.1C).

Videofluoroscopy showed decreased control for fluids in the oral stage 3. Residue in the valleculae on soft solids was cleared effectively with the chin tuck technique.

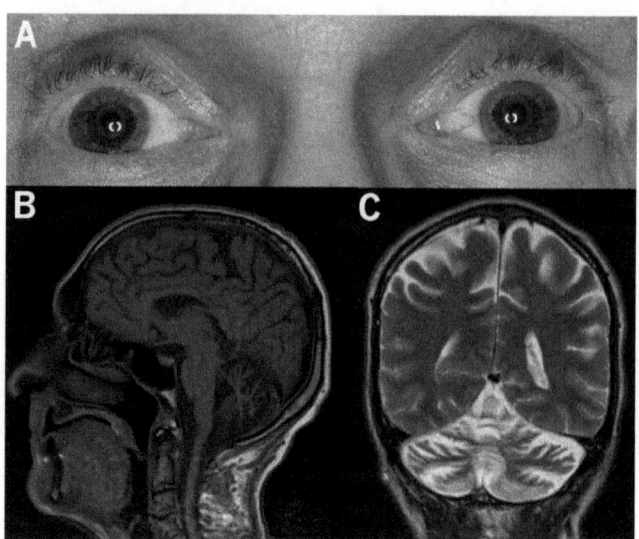

Figure 45.1 (A) Scleral telangiectasia. (B) Sagittal T1 and (C) coronal T2-weighted MRI scan of the brain showing diffuse cerebellar atrophy

Fifteen years later, an Addenbrooke's Cognitive Examination score was 51/100. His ataxia progressed. The Scale for the Assessment and Rating of Ataxia went from 16/40 to 26/40 over five years.

Molecular analysis of a 98 gene ataxia panel revealed a homozygous c.132dupA p.(Asp45fs) mutation in anoctamin 10. (*ANO 10*)

Diagnosis: Anoctamin 10 Ataxia or SCAR 10

Comment

Ataxias

Lack of co-ordination or ataxia occurs in many neurological disorders from multiple sclerosis and stroke to infection. Progressive ataxia, as in this patient, can result in a label of 'idiopathic ataxia' or a delayed diagnosis. Advances in molecular genetics have helped identify many underlying genetic diagnoses of ataxia [1].

Algorithm for Investigating Ataxia

Because the ultimate diagnosis of an ataxia may be markedly delayed or even not established, steps for investigating ataxia in patients have been published [1]. A systematic investigation plan should follow a strategy to obtain the following information.

1 Age of onset and associated signs may be important clues.
2 Mode of inheritance (N.B. autosomal recessive ataxias may have no family history). Adolescent onset and a family history has markedly increased the diagnostic yield from next-generation sequencing [2] – see step 7.
3 MRI brain features (N.B. cerebellar atrophy is not usually present in Friedreich's ataxia, but is prominent feature in anoctamin 10 or SCAR 10 ataxia).
4 Biomarker screening. Examples include low vitamin E (hereditary ataxia with vitamin E deficiency and abetalipoproteinaemia), increased α-fetoprotein in ataxia telangiectasia and ataxia with oculomotor apraxia type 2, increased cholestanol in cerebrotendinous xanthomatosis. Low albumin occurs in ataxia with oculomotor apraxia type 1 and SCA with axonal sensorimotor neuropathy.
5 Genetic analysis. The repeat expansions make up 40–50% of dominant ataxias. Importantly, the repeat expansions are not usually detected in panel or genome screening. The age of onset often correlates with the number of CAG repeats and the SCA 6 is a late onset condition. The usual repeat expansion analysis includes SCA 1, 2, 3, 6, 7, 12 and 17 and dentatorubral-pallidoluysian atrophy.
   Ataxia panel testing has emerged as a useful tool to examine the multiple genetic causes of ataxia. A 98 gene panel yielded anoctamin 10 as the cause of ataxia in our patient. Importantly, a genetic panel may not contain the most recently identified genetic causes of ataxia.
6 Deeper phenotyping of the associated signs. The cerebellum appears to have a role in cognition. The cerebellar cognitive affective syndrome was defined in 1998. Neuropathy and parkinsonism can provide additional clues.
7 Whole exome sequencing has increased the diagnostic rate of ataxias. The genetic ataxias have a high phenotypic overlap and the responsible genetic mutations include hundreds of genes. Despite the advances in technology, there is a ceiling of successful molecular diagnosis from whole exome sequencing (approximately 50%).
8 Whole genome sequencing is being rolled out by NHS England and is likely to increase diagnostic yield. However, the use of whole genome screening can throw up variants of uncertain significance; such inconclusive results have to be interpreted cautiously.

The algorithm for investigating ataxia has suggested levels of investigation, as outlined in Table 45.1 [1]. These have been itemised for our patient who was initially investigated in 2004 before a request for the gene panel in 2015 yielded the genetic cause of his ataxia.

Table 45.1 Investigation algorithm of ataxia

Investigations	Results from patient
Primary care	
Serum urea, creatinine and electrolytes	Normal
Full blood count	Normal
ESR/CRP	Normal
Liver enzymes	Normal
Thyroid profile	Normal
Folate and B12	Normal
Plasma glucose	Normal
Chest X-ray	Normal
Secondary care (first line)	
α-fetoprotein	2.7 KU/L
Blood film	Normal
Caeruloplasmin and copper	Normal
Coeliac disease screen	Normal
Serum creatine kinase	Normal
Genetic screening for Friedreich's ataxia, fragile X tremor-ataxia syndrome, SCA 1, 2, 3, 6, 7 (12 and 17)	Friedreich's atataxia, SCA 1, 2, 3, 6 and 7 negative
Lactate	Normal
Lipid-adjusted vitamin E and lipoproteins	Normal
Lumbar puncture (cell counts, protein, glucose, cytology, oligoclonal bands, lactate, ferritin)	<1 white cell/μL, 430 red cells/μL, protein 0.32 g/L, glucose (CSF) 4.0 mmol/L, oligoclonal bands (OCB) negative
MRI of the brain and cervical spine	Cerebellar atrophy
Hu/Yo and other paraneoplastic antibodies, glutamic acid decarboxylase (GAD) antibody, voltage-gated calcium channel antibody	Negative
CT scan of chest, abdomen and pelvis	Normal
14-3-3 and other CSF proteins (prion diseases)	Not done
Secondary care (second line)	
Cholestanol	Not done
Plasma oxysterols	Not done
Bile acids	Not done
Coenzyme Q10 (ubiquinone),	Muscle ubiquinone 320 pmol/mg (normal range 140–580)

Electroencephalography	Not done
Very-long-chain fatty acids	Normal
Muscle biopsy	Focal atrophy
Ophthalmology/optical coherence tomography	Not done
Peripheral nerve conduction studies	Normal. Electromyography (EMG) normal.
Phytanic acid	Not done
Remaining genetic tests (next generation sequencing),	98 gene panel for ataxia 2016 autosomal recessive ANO10-related condition (c.132dupA p.(Asp45fs)) SPG7 heterozygous c.1529C>T p.(Ala510Val)
Total body PET scan	Not done
White cell enzymes	Lysosomal enzyme screen negative

Adapted from de Silva et al. [3]. Reproduced under the Creative Commons License (http://creativecommons .org/publicdomain/zero/1.0/).

Anoctamin 10

In 2010, Sascha Vermeer and colleagues identified anoctamin 10 (a putative calcium-dependent chloride channel) mutations in patients with autosomal recessive cerebellar ataxia (ARCA) [4]. The gene was identified in remotely consanguinous parents in a Dutch family by single nucleotide polymorphism-based linkage analysis followed by targeted Sanger sequencing [4]. Since then, many publications have identified other mutations throughout the world (Europe, Japan and China) and confirmed the phenotype (ataxia, dysarthria, spasticity and sometimes executive and attentional issues). By 2020, more than 50 patients had been reported. The disorder has been classified as ARCA 3 (i.e. without an accompanying neuropathy) and subsequently called SCAR 10.

A previous phenotypic classification of ARCAs was based on the presence and type of co-existent neuropathy; ARCA 1 had a pure sensory neuropathy, ARCA 2 had a sensorimotor axonal neuropathy and ARCA 3 had no associated neuropathy (e.g. SCAR 10). Another attempt to phenotypically classify ARCAs based on additional phenotypes is shown in Figure 45.2. Anoctamin 10 (ANO10) has 13 exons and 660 amino acids. The original mutation was identi-fied in exon 10, a substitution of leucine by arginine at codon 510 (p.Leu510Arg).

ANO10 has the highest expression in the brain, particularly in the frontal and occipital cortices as well as the cerebellum. Expression is also higher in the adult compared to the foetal brain, consistent with the late age of onset. The *ANO10* product is known as TMEM16 K (transmembrane 16 K) and may be a calcium-activated chloride channel. Deranged calcium signalling in Purkinje cells is a recognised cause of cerebellar ataxia.

Phenotype of *ANO10* Ataxia

Homozygosity for the truncating p.Leu384fs mutation, which has been identified in Roma gypsies, may denote earlier onset and more cognitive decline. In most cases, however, *ANO10* ataxia is a slowly progressive spastic ataxia. Age of onset varies from 6 to 53 years and most patients remain ambulant 25 years after onset. Extensor plantar responses and cognitive decline are variable.

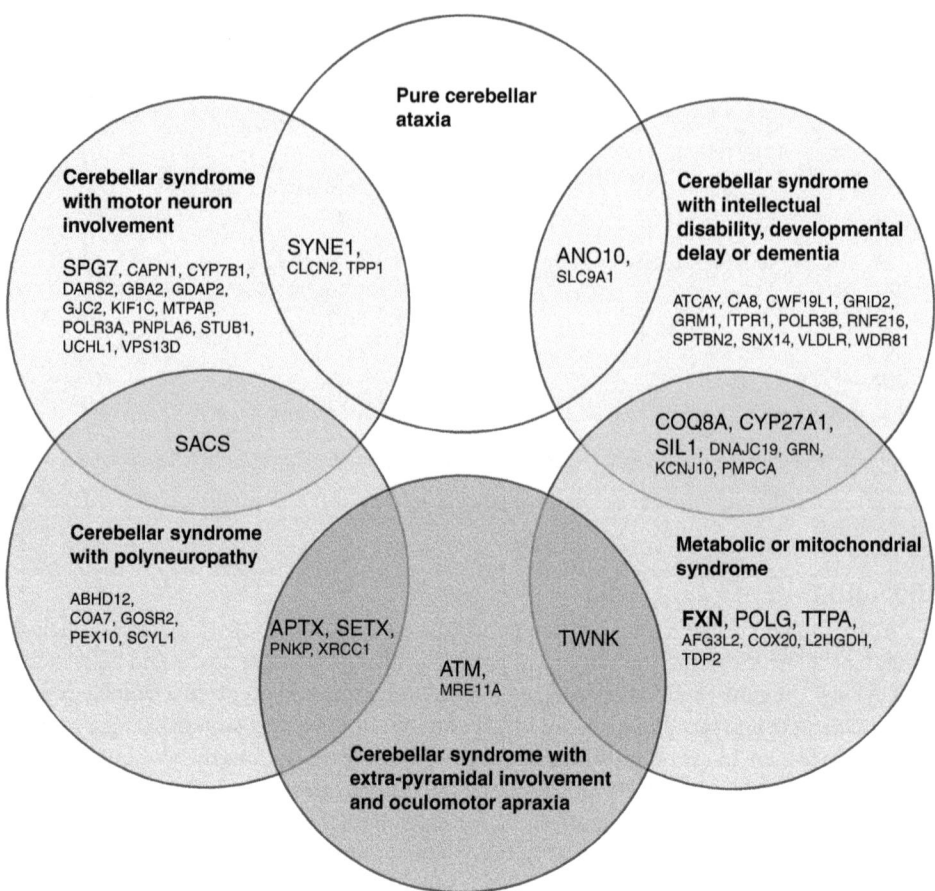

Figure 45.2 Clinical classification of autosomal recessive ataxias. The gene associated with each primary recessive ataxia is classified according to the most frequent clinical syndrome described for this disorder. Note that some disorders have more complex or variable phenotypes and are placed in the overlapping areas between two categories. Genes presented in larger font represent the most prevalent ataxias. Adapted from Beaudin et al. [5]. Reproduced under the Creative Commons License (http://creativecommons.org/licenses/by/4.0/).

Lower motor neurone involvement (denervation) and downbeat nystagmus are common but not invariable features. Conjunctival vessel tortuosity has also been observed in *ANO10* ataxia.

The c.132dupA mutation has been implicated in a range of cognitive impairment in *ANO10* ataxia. This mutation has a heterozygous carrier rate of 1 in 184 in different ethnic groups.

Low levels of co-enzyme Q10 have been reported in some ataxias, including *ANO10* ataxia. However, very few reports have included descriptions of the use of co-enzyme Q10 treatment. Although the results have been equivocal, the concept of a molecular diagnosis facilitating a specific treatment remains a goal in researching and managing genetic ataxias.

References

1.   de Silva RN, Vallortigara J, Greenfield J et al. Diagnosis and management of progressive ataxia in adults. *Pract Neurol.* 2019;19(3):196–207.

2. Németh AH, Kwasniewska AC, Lise S et al. Next generation sequencing for molecular diagnosis of neurological disorders using ataxias as a model. *Brain*. 2013;136(10):3106–18.

3. de Silva R, Greenfield J, Cook A et al. Guidelines on the diagnosis and management of the progressive ataxias. *Orphanet J Rare Dis*. 2019;14:51.

4. Vermeer S, Hoischen A, Meijer RPP et al. Targeted next-generation sequencing of a 12.5 Mb homozygous region reveals ANO10 mutations in patients with autosomal-recessive cerebellar ataxia. *Am J Hum Genet*. 2010;87(6):813–9.

5. Beaudin M, Matilla-Dueñas A, Soong B-W et al. The classification of autosomal recessive cerebellar ataxias: a consensus statement from the society for research on the cerebellum and ataxias task force. *Cerebellum* 2019;18(6):1098–125.

Learning Points

*   Autosomal recessive ataxia may have no family history.
*   Autosomal recessive cerebellar ataxia types 1–3 classify ataxias according to the presence and type of neuropathy.
*   Mutations in anoctamin 10 cause autosomal recessive cerebellar ataxia type 3 (without neuropathy).
*   Algorithmic investigation of ataxia has emerged but clinical clues can help navigate the investigation ladder.

Patient's Perspective

1. **What is/was the impact of the condition?**
    a. Physical (e.g. job, driving, practical support)
    I slowed down. I had been a baker. I now have to use crutches or a rollator. I moved into my mother's house.
    b. Psychological (e.g. mood, future, emotional well-being)
    I got down a lot, especially because of my speech.
    c. Social (e.g. meeting friends, home)
    I feel locked in the house. I previously walked the dog.

2. **What can you no longer do?**
    I cannot go for walks. I have difficulty getting up from a chair. I feel as if I have no support in my legs.

3. **Has there been any other change for you due to your condition?**
    I can no longer drive.

4. **What is the most difficult aspect of the condition?**
    I have difficulty judging distances. I find it hard having to let people do things for me.

5. **Was any aspect of the experience good or useful? What was that?**
    Nothing.

6. **What do you hope for in the future for your condition?**
    I just take it day by day …

46 A Neurological Miscarriage

History

A 24-year-old right-handed woman who smoked six cigarettes per day had a sudden onset of pins and needles in her left arm and leg with associated weakness. She had difficulty carrying objects.

Past medical history was unremarkable.

Medication had included the combined oral contraceptive pill at the time of symptom onset.

Examination

She was cognitively and systemically normal. Limbs had normal tone and power but there was decreased left arm and left leg pin prick sensation. Left limb reflexes were brisker than right limb reflexes. Plantar responses were flexor.

After a second similar event 11 months later, there was a mild left pyramidal distribution of weakness in her left leg and a left extensor plantar response.

Investigations

A full blood count demonstrated a mild thrombocytopenia (119×10^9/L). An MRI of the brain (Figure 46.1) was reported as showing white matter lesions including a lesion in the splenium of the corpus callosum. The brainstem and cerebellum were normal. A transthoracic echocardiogram was normal. At lumbar puncture, cerebrospinal fluid (CSF) had less than 1 white cell/μL, 170 erythrocytes/μL. Cerebrospinal fluid glucose was 3.1 mmol/L, plasma glucose 6.0 mmol/L and CSF protein was 0.23 g/L. Oligoclonal bands were not detected. Visual evoked responses and somatosensory evoked potentials were normal. An EEG showed occasional runs of suspicious sharpened slow waves suggestive but not diagnostic of an epileptic process.

A diagnostic test was performed.

A nuclear autoantibody screen was negative. Lupus anticoagulant was weakly positive. Anticardiolipin antibodies (aCLs) revealed an elevated IgG of 108 GPLU/mL (normal range <10 GPLU/mL) and normal IgM of 4.9 GPLU/mL (normal range <7 GPLU/mL). Repeat aCLs more than three months later still had an elevated IgG of >120 GPLU/mL but normal IgM of 5.1 MPLU/mL. Factor V Leiden was negative and prothrombin 20210A mutation was negative.

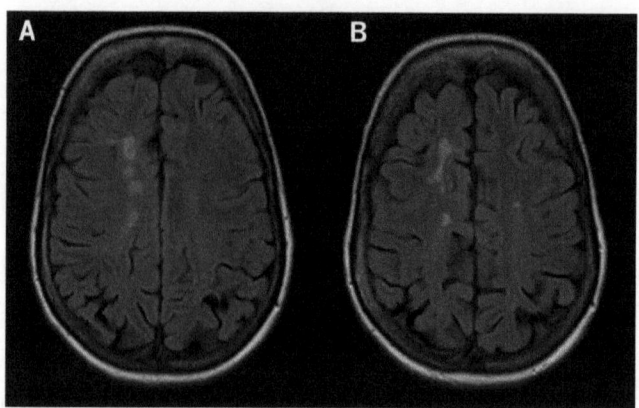

Figure 46.1 (A and B) An axial T2 FLAIR MRI scan of the brain showing high signal in the subcortical white matter predominantly in the right hemisphere

Diagnosis: Primary Antiphospholipid Syndrome

Management

Following a diagnosis of antiphospholipid syndrome, she was advised to take aspirin 75 mg per day. She then became pregnant and enoxaparin was added. When 20 weeks pregnant, she had a tonic-clonic seizure. She had a stillbirth at 25 weeks. A post-mortem report recorded placental infarction attributed to antiphospholipid syndrome but no foetal abnormality.

Further tonic-clonic seizures occurred. After the stillbirth, warfarin was started. A further pregnancy ended in miscarriage at nine weeks. Another pregnancy occurred and warfarin was switched to low-molecular-weight heparin 1 mg/kg with 75 mg of aspirin per day. She gave birth to twins. Following delivery, she switched back to warfarin.

Epilepsy was managed with lamotrigine chosen because of evidence of its efficacy in focal onset seizures and low teratogenicity risk. She had no further seizures over the next ten years.

Comment

Definition or Diagnostic Criteria

The antiphospholipid syndrome is defined by obstetrical (miscarriages after the tenth week of gestation or recurrent early miscarriages, intrauterine growth restriction or severe preeclampsia) and thrombotic events (venous – usually leg deep venous thrombosis and cerebral venous sinus thrombosis or arterial – usually acute ischaemic stroke, and microvascular) in the presence of persisting antiphospholipid antibodies (on two or more occasions at least 12 weeks apart) [1].

The antiphospholipid antibody tests include aCLs (IgG or IgM) detected by enzyme-linked immunosorbent assay, lupus anticoagulant that paradoxically detects antibodies that prolong in vitro clotting time, and anti-β_2-glycoprotein 1 (IgG or IgM) detected by enzyme-linked immunosorbent assay.

The lupus anticoagulant test correlates better with clinical events (thrombosis or adverse pregnancy outcome) than the aCL or β_2-glycoprotein 1 antibodies. A high-risk profile is defined as a positive lupus anticoagulant test with or without a moderate-to-high titre of aCL or β_2-glycoprotein 1 IgG or IgM. An entity known as catastrophic antiphospholipid syndrome involves thrombosis in and failure of multiple organs; this condition has a high mortality.

The revised Sapporo classification criteria [1] do not include other recognised clinical manifestations of the antiphospholipid syndrome, which are cognitive dysfunction and subcortical white matter changes, thrombocytopenia, haemolytic anaemia, renal vascular lesions, cardiac valve vegetations or thickening or nodules, livedo reticularis or racemosa and recurrent and painful skin ulceration [2].

Pathogenesis

Antiphospholipid antibodies bind to β_2-glycoprotein 1, a plasma protein, which avidly binds to phospholipid surfaces. This promotes the expression of prothrombotic cellular adhesion molecules (E-selectin and tissue factor) and supresses the tissue factor pathway inhibitor, reduces activated protein C activity (an endogenous anticoagulant) and activates complement [2].

A two-hit hypothesis for thrombosis has been proposed with initial endothelial disruption followed by thrombus formation [3]. An oxidised form of β_2-glycoprotein 1 (disulphide bridges in domains I and V) is more immunogenic than the free thiol variant of β_2-glycoprotein 1. It has been proposed that β_2-glycoprotein 1 immune complexes then form on the cell surface to exert their pathogenicity [3].

Epidemiology

There is a limited literature on the epidemiology of primary antiphospholipid syndrome. False positive or transient antiphospholipid antibody tests have impeded epidemiological study. The antiphospholipid antibody syndrome is, however, not an uncommon cause of acute ischaemic stroke in young patients. For example, young women under 50 years with acute ischaemic stroke have a 17% chance of harbouring a positive lupus anticoagulant compared to 0.7% of controls. Conventional risk factors such as the oral contraceptive pill and smoking increase the thrombotic risk.

Management

Management of (traditional) risk factors – smoking, hypertension, diabetes mellitus and hypercholesterolaemia – is important. The background risk of antiphospholipid-antibody-positive patients in the absence of other risk factors has been estimated to be 1% per year. Secondary prevention of arterial (if moderate-to-high risk) or venous thrombosis has evidence that warfarin with an international normalised ratio (INR) target of 2–3 is beneficial. There is no high-quality evidence to manage recurrent thrombosis, despite use of warfarin. Direct oral anticogulants continue to be tested and compared to warfarin.

The current strategy for obstetric management involves low-dose aspirin plus prophylactic dose of unfractionated or low-molecular-weight heparin for the prevention of pregnancy-related complications. For our patient, this was not successful, and so a decision was made to use warfarin until she became pregnant and then switch to high-dose enoxaparin.

The long-term risk of thrombosis in women with obstetrical antiphospholipid syndrome is lower than the risk in women who present with thrombosis-defined antiphospholipid syndrome. In the absence of other risk factors, some authors do not recommend long-term anticoagulation in women with obstetrical antiphospholipid syndrome [2].

Epileptic seizure control was another requirement for our patient. Lamotrigine in focal epilepsy has been shown to be superior to other anti-epileptic drugs, possibly because it is better tolerated. For women, the associated low teratogenicity documented in pregnancy registries makes it a preferred anti-epileptic drug in women during pregnancy.

Isolated Antiphospholipid Antibodies

It is not clear whether primary prevention thromboprophylaxis should be used in asymptomatic patients. A thrombosis rate of 1.7 thromboses per 100 patient years has been reported among a heterogenous population including patients with systemic lupus erythematosus. Triple-positive asymptomatic patients with antiphospholipid antibodies may be at higher risk than single-positive patients. Low-dose aspirin has been suggested for asymptomatic patients with a high-risk profile, which includes the presence of lupus anticoagulant (most related to thrombosis), double or triple antiphospholipid antibody positivity, but the evidence is not strong and aspirin-induced bleeding may have a higher risk than antithrombotic benefits.

References

1. Miyakis S, Lockshin MD, Atsumi T et al. International consensus statement on an update of the classification for definite antiphospholipid syndrome (APS). *J Thromb Haemost*. 2006;4:295–306.

2. Garcia D, Erkan D. Diagnosis and management of the antiphospholipid syndrome. *N Engl J Med*. 2018;378(21):2010–21.

3. Giannakopoulos B, Krilis SA. The pathogenesis of the antiphospholipid syndrome. *N Engl J Med*. 2013;368(11):1033–44.

Learning Points

- Antiphospholipid syndrome is in the differential diagnosis of ischaemic stroke, particularly in a young individual.
- Mid-trimester miscarriage is a recognised feature of antiphopshoplipid syndrome.
- Warfarin has been the drug of choice to prevent recurrent thrombotic events in antiphospholipid syndrome while direct oral anticoagulants continue to be evaluated.
- Obstetric management of patients with antiphospholipid syndrome may require appropriate anti-epileptic and anticoagulant medication.

Patient's Perspective

1. **What was the impact of the condition?**

    a. Physical (e.g. practical support)
    After the first episode going from a fully capable person to needing help with something as simple as washing dishes or even walking was very daunting. I wasn't able to shower/wash on my own. I relied on my family and friends to help with day-to-day tasks.

    b. Psychological (e.g. mood, emotional well-being)
    Left me feeling very vulnerable, frustrated, scared and sometimes down. I was annoyed, embarrassed and stressed.

    c. Social (e.g. meeting friends, home)
    Being quite an outgoing person, this had a great impact on my social life. I was afraid that my condition would have limited our outings.

2. **What can or could you not do because of the condition?**
    At the beginning I lost the strength in my left side; this left me unable to do basic daily activities. Even my work as an office administrator suffered. Wanting to start a family seemed unlikely.

3. **Was there any other change for you due to your medical condition?**
    Continuous hospital and doctor appointments took me away from work on numerous occasions, and I was temporarily banned from driving, so I couldn't drive to the appointments. My memory isn't what it used to be, which is very unsettling.

4. **What is/was the most difficult aspect of the condition for you?**
    The loss of two babies.
    Thankfully with trying different medications and a lot of needles, we succeeded and had twins! But it wasn't easy. Whole change of lifestyle.

5. **Was any aspect of the experience of the condition good or useful? What was that?**
    It was a relief to know that there was a name for the condition and that doctors know what to do to help. I am very grateful for this.

6. **What do you hope for in the future for people with this condition?**
    As so far there is no chance of cure, it would be beneficial to have more people aware of the condition and of the great impact it can have on those who have it.

47 Am I Repeating Myself?

History

A 71-year-old right-handed, semi-retired, self-employed man went to a gym one morning at 08:10 hrs. He started his usual light exercise routine. He recalled using a foot press and then nothing more until his wife arrived in the gym.

His wife explained that she received a telephone call from her husband at 09:15 hrs. His speech did not make sense to her. He said things such as 'What colour is our car?' and 'I can't find my keys'. He had used a key fob to get into the gym but he repeatedly said 'I can't find my keys'. He then seemed to find the keys in his pocket. He asked his wife 'Where are you?' When his wife arrived at the gym, she said that he once more explained that he could not find his keys. He kept returning to a bowl, where other keys had been left. She then advised him to check his own pocket, where he found the keys. She decided that they should go to hospital and, en route to hospital, he asked further questions 'Did you phone me?', 'Did I really phone you?' and he questioned her about the phone call on four or five occasions. His wife asked him the day of the week and the month. He could not answer these questions but he knew the year. He also had no recall that there had been another man in the gym with him.

The episode of amnesia lasted approximately 85 minutes. A CCTV review confirmed the search for keys. He had been pacing around putting his hands on his face and then on the back of his neck.

Examination

No cognitive deficits were identified when he arrived in hospital. His pulse was 68 beats per minute and blood pressure was 131/69 mmHg. Neurological examination was normal.

Investigations

An MRI scan of the brain and EEG were unremarkable.

Diagnosis: Transient Global Amnesia

Management
An explanation of the benign outcome and reassurance were provided. The patient was informed that there was no driving restriction.

Comment

Diagnostic Criteria and Epidemiology
Patients with transient global amnesia are frequently referred to general neurology and neurovascular clinics. It is a rewarding diagnosis both for the patient and the neurologist. The patient can be reassured of a benign entity with no sinister stroke sequelae [1] (except a low recurrence rate of transient global amnesia) as well as no driving ban for drivers, while the neurologist determines the diagnosis based entirely on features from the history including eye-witness evidence to fulfil diagnostic criteria [2]. The neurologist may also wonder at the transient inability to acquire, store or retrieve new or relatively new information. Attention, reasoning, language and visuospatial abilities remain intact in the presence of a devastating neuropsychological dysfunction of memory.

The features of transient global amnesia have at their core a clear episode of anterograde amnesia lasting less than 24 hours [2]. In their original paper in 1990, John Hodges and Charles Warlow suggested that witnessed attacks must confirm no impairment of consciousness or loss of personal identity. Amnesia should be the only focal neurological symptom with no evidence of a recent epileptic seizure or head injury [2].

Although first reported in the 1950s, transient global amnesia was probably recognised in the 1880s. There have been a number of case series documented in the literature [2]. Our own case series from Altnagelvin hospital highlights many features documented in other patients attending a district general hospital. The incidence of transient global amnesia has been estimated to be 3.4–10.4 per 100,000 per year. It occurs most commonly in the seventh decade, and is almost equally common in both sexes. The recurrence rate of transient global amnesia is reported to be less than 10% in studies with up to 10 years follow-up.

Differential Diagnosis
Transient epileptic amnesia is the main differential diagnosis. Recurrent and atypical symptoms of confusion and language disorder are clues to a diagnosis of transient epileptic amnesia in addition to absence of hippocampi diffusion-weighted imaging lesions on appropriately timed MRI brain scanning. In the absence of MRI brain support, the accuracy of a clinical diagnosis of transient global amnesia may reflect the level of training or experience and the number of diagnostic questions asked by the clinician.

Putative Pathophysiology
The exact aetiology of transient global amnesia is not certain. Venous congestion, ischaemia and migrainous phenomena have all been implicated but not confirmed. Spreading depolarisation may underpin the mechanism.

Transient global amnesia demonstrates that short-term or working memory is separate from long-term memory store. The anterograde amnesia may be independent of retrograde

Table 47.1 Case series of patients with transient global amnesia from Altnagelvin hospital

Clinical feature	Findings
Number	49
Male:female ratio	27:22
Mean age (SD)	63.1 (10.3) years
Mean duration amnesia (SD)	184 (125) minutes
Recognised trigger (N = 56 transient global amnesia events)	38 (68%)
Physical/emotional trigger	26/12
Mean follow-up years	8.8
Number of patients with one recurrence (two recurrences)	6 (1)

amnesia, as anterograde amnesia is always severe but the retrograde amnesia is variable (days to decades) and importantly, is recoverable. Long-established memories are more robust than recent memory entries; this is known as Ribot's law of retrograde amnesia.

Intriguingly, procedural memories for perceptual and motor skills can be acquired during episodes of transient global amnesia, highlighting the selective deficit of the condition. Diffusion-weighted MRI of the brain has shown usually small unilateral CA1 hyperintensities with correlated restricted diffusion in the hippocampus in up to 85% of affected patients. Diffusion-restricted lesions (which can be left, right or bilateral) are most likely to be detected 12–24 hours after symptom onset. Thin-sliced MR imaging can reduce partial-volume effects. The lesions appear to be entirely reversible.

Precipitating events have been recognised in case series of transient global amnesia. Emotional stress, physical effort and water contact/temperature change have been reported immediately before an attack. Anxiety-provoking issues (conflict at work or home, health-related problems) and exhaustion have been described as remote events. Physical and emotional triggers may be identified in over 60% of patients with transient global amnesia.

Altnagelvin Hospital Case Series of Transient Global Amnesia

A case series of 49 consecutive patients with transient global amnesia attending one neurologist in our general hospital over 14 years highlights features, including the frequency of potential triggers of the condition (Table 47.1). As already reported in the literature, physical exertion including sex may be a trigger. Short-lasting transient global amnesia (<60 minutes) which has recently been reported [3] was also observed in our cohort. Three episodes among the Altnagelvin cohort had amnesia recorded for just 60 minutes. A recurrence rate of 12.2% was recorded over a mean follow-up of 8.8 years.

References

1. Mangla A, Navi BB, Layton K, Kamel H. Transient global amnesia and the risk of ischemic stroke. *Stroke*. 2014;45(2):389–93.

2. Hodges JR, Warlow CP. Syndromes of transient amnesia: towards a classification. A study of 153 cases. *J Neurol Neurosurg Psychiatry*. 1990;53(10):834–43.

3. Romoli M, Tuna MA, Li L et al. Time trends, frequency, characteristics and prognosis of short-duration transient global amnesia. *Eur J Neurol*. 2020;27(5):887–93.

Learning Points
- Transient global amnesia is a benign condition in which a mild reversible retrograde amnesia accompanies a permanent period of anterograde amnesia lasting usually one to several hours.
- Executive functioning is retained in transient global amnesia.
- Physical and emotional triggers can be identified in most episodes of transient global amnesia.
- Thin-sliced diffusion MRI brain scans are most sensitive in picking up punctate medial temporal lobe or hippocampal diffusion hyperintensities 12–24 hours after the onset of symptoms.

Patient's Perspective
1. **What was the impact of the condition?**
   a. Physical (e.g. job, driving, practical support)
   It stopped me from finishing a workout in a gym. I was trying to understand why I was there. I don't remember what I did for approximately one hour. I made a phone call to my wife during that time (period), but I don't remember it. I had to put in a code to open the phone.
   b. Psychological (e.g. mood, future, emotional well-being)
   Anxious, confused, loss of confidence, frightened but curious. I was relieved when my wife came.
   c. Social (e.g. meeting friends, home)
   I haven't gone back to the gym; I lost my confidence. I need support to do this. Socially, it (transient global amnesia) has not affected me otherwise.

2. **What could you not do because of the condition?**
   I couldn't go to the swimming pool, gym or walk alone. I couldn't drive for several days due to anxiety that it would happen again.

3. **Was there any other change for you due to your medical condition?**
   None.

4. **What was the most difficult aspect of the condition for you?**
   The uncertainty of not knowing what was happening. Loss of control was frightening, the Accident & Emergency doctor being baffled and continuously saying 'It's a strange one'.

5. **Was any aspect of the experience good or useful? What was that?**
   It put life into perspective for me, compassion for others with dementia etc. Support from my wife, family and friends. The explanation of the condition was reassuring and a relief.

6. **What do you hope for in the future for people with this condition?**
   I hope for a greater medical and public awareness of this condition (signs and symptoms and awareness of antecedents).

A Raspberry Causing Trouble

History

A 31-year-old female primary school teacher had a post-partum tonic-clonic seizure. This was in the context of HELLP syndrome (haemolysis, elevated liver enzymes and a low platelet count).

She first developed epileptic seizures at the age of 14 years. For the next five years, she had focal seizures (right arm shaking and loss of language). Milder episodes involved a feeling of impending doom before tingling in her right hand radiated up her right arm to her right shoulder with associated dysphasia. Over a number of years, she had been tried on carbamazepine, levetiracetam and lamotrigine. Off medication she could go for up to five years with no events. When assessed on this occasion, her only medication was clobazam 10 mg/day. She did not drink alcohol or smoke cigarettes. Following this presentation she had a subsequent pregnancy, having three children in total.

Examination

She had a normal general and neurological examination. In particular, she had no skin lesions such as port wine stain or café au lait spots.

Investigations

An MRI scan of the brain showed a left parietal abnormality (Figure 48.1).

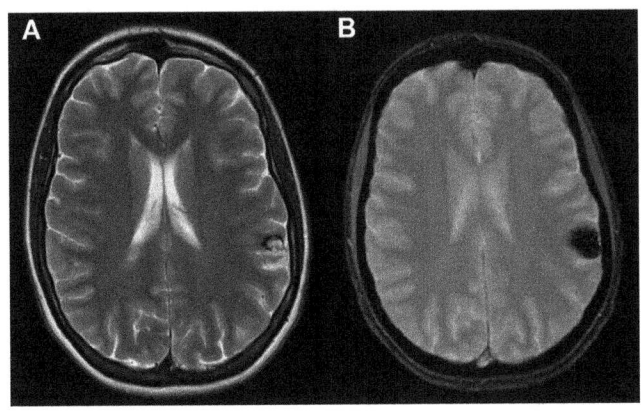

Figure 48.1 (A) A T2-weighted and (B) susceptibility weighted axial MRI scan of the brain showing low signal in left parietal cortex consistent with a cavernoma

Diagnosis: Focal (or Localisation-Related) Seizures – Aware, Motor, Sensory and Dysphasia with Secondary Generalisation Secondary to Left Parietal Cavernous Haemangioma

Management
She was assessed twice by neurosurgery. After considering the evidence, including the upfront risk of surgery versus the known risk of haemorrhage, she declined surgical intervention.

Comment
Most of the focal or localisation-related epilepsies have a known or presumed structural cause. Focal onset epilepsies of childhood such as benign epilepsy of childhood with centrotemporal spikes and Panayiotopoulos syndrome are of unknown cause but may have a genetic component.

Definition and Epidemiology of Cerebral Cavernous Malformations
Cerebral cavernous malformations (CCMs) or cavernomas are collections of structurally abnormal, fragile and leaky slow-flow capillaries first reported by Hubert von Luschka in 1854. Macroscopically they are bluish mulberry-like lesions also likened to a raspberry. They predominate in the central nervous system – brain and spinal cord. Cerebral cavernous malformations usually occur as a single lesion, which may or may not be associated with a developmental venous anomaly. They are present in 0.4–0.6% of the general population and 80% are supratentorial.

Cerebral cavernous malformations are mostly sporadic or non-hereditary and often asymptomatic. Previous brain irradiation is a risk factor for CCM formation. Familial CCMs are less frequent but inherited as autosomal dominant from three recognised genes – *CCM1 (KRIT1)*, *CCM2 (MGC4607)* and *CCM3 (PDCD10)* [1].

Cerebral cavernous malformations can cause epileptic seizures, stroke due to symptomatic haemorrhage or new focal neurological deficit without evidence of haemorrhage on MRI. Cerebral cavernous malformations have an MRI prevalence of 1 in 625 neurologically asymptomatic people.

Epileptic Seizures and CCMs
As patients with incidental CCMs have a 4% risk of seizure over five years, there is no role for prophylactic anti-seizure medication [1]. The five-year risk of epilepsy in adult CCM patients presenting with a seizure is 94%, but 47% can achieve two-year seizure remission. Treatment is therefore usually advised after a first-presenting epileptic seizure. Among these patients, medical therapy has a 50–60% chance of conferring seizure freedom [2]. Surgical resection can achieve post-operative seizure freedom in about 75%, but surgery can be associated with new neurological deficits [1]. Patients with ongoing seizures may not have had the epileptogenic zone correctly defined and resected.

Haemorrhage Risk of CCMs

The natural history of CCM is dynamic – that is, there may be temporal clustering of haemorrhage [1]. Brainstem location increases the risk of haemorrhage among patients presenting without intracerebral haemorrhage or focal neurological deficit (3.8% in non-brainstem CCM patients versus 8% in patients with brainstem CCM over five years). Previous presentation with intracerebral haemorrhage or focal neurological deficit increases the risk further (18.4% in non-brainstem CCM and 30.8% in brainstem CCM patients over five years). Long-term antithrombotic therapy does not increase haemorrhage risk.

In addition to brainstem location, increased bleeding has been recognised with CCMs due to *CCM3* mutations. An MRI classification known as the Zabramski classification was described in 1994; type I (hyperintense CCM on both T1- and T2-weighted MRI sequences reflecting subacute haemorrhage and haemosiderin core) and type II (popcorn appearance with mixed signal intensity on both T1- and T2-weighted MRI sequences due to multiple haemorrhages at different stages) lesions have increased bleeding risk [1]. Type III lesions represent chronic haemorrhage and type IV lesions are multiple punctate microhaemorrhages. The classification is, however, not often used clinically.

Pregnancy and CCM

There is no known increase in the risk of intracerebral haemorrhage from CCM in pregnancy or by mode of delivery.

Management of CCMs

Surgical treatment guidelines from the US Angioma Alliance Scientific Advisory Board Clinical Experts panel have been published [2]. The guidelines do not recommend resection of asymptomatic CCMs except when a CCM is easily accessible and located in a non-eloquent area in an appropriately selected patient (to reduce haemorrhage risk, psychological burden and long-term follow-up or when anticoagulation is required).

Early surgical resection of CCM in patients with symptomatic epilepsy should be considered. (Our patient has had two neurosurgical assessments to consider resection for this indication.) An acceptable morbidity and mortality of resection of a symptomatic but easily accessible CCM is the two-year morbidity and mortality from living with a CCM. Symptomatic or prior haemorrhage from a deep CCM has a higher surgical morbidity and mortality, equivalent to living with the CCM for 5–10 years. The guidelines suggest that for the more aggressive course of brainstem CCM, it may be reasonable to offer surgical resection after a second symptomatic bleed.

Neurosurgical excision or stereotactic radiosurgery has a reported incidence of death, non-fatal symptomatic intracerebral haemorrhage or non-fatal new or worse non-haemorrhagic functional neurological deficit of about 6 per 100 person-years. There is a need for a randomised controlled trial comparing different treatment modalities to include stereotactic radiosurgery. The US Angioma Alliance Scientific Advisory Board Clinical Experts panel does not recommend radiosurgery for asymptomatic CCMs. Radiosurgery can be considered for solitary CCM in an eloquent area with a previous haemorrhage when there is a high and unacceptable surgical risk.

Pregnancy and Anti-epileptic Drugs

The childbirth rate in women with epilepsy is 20–40% lower than that of the general population.

There are no randomised controlled trials of anti-epileptic drugs and pregnancy outcomes. National and international pregnancy registries provide the best available evidence of drug safety in pregnancy. High recruitment to such registries may mitigate against selection bias. The UK and Ireland pregnancy register (started in 1996) as well as the European and International Registry of Anti-epileptic Drugs and Pregnancy (EURAP – launched in Europe in 1999) have provided teratogenicity risks for a number of anti-epileptic drugs. Teratogenicity is a concern particularly with prenatal exposure to valproate; 10% of exposed fetuses have a major congenital malformation. Polytherapy combinations with valproate further increase teratogenicity risk. Congenital malformations due to valproate may be due to inhibition of histone deacetylases. Valproate not only has a dose-dependent teratogenicity risk, but also has been associated with impaired cognitive development and autism (30–40%).

In 2018, the Medicines and Health Regulatory Authority in the UK mandated more restricted prescribing of valproate in women of childbearing age, requiring formal declaration of risk communication and permanent pregnancy prevention plans.

Levetiracetam, lamotrigine and oxcarbazepine have a teratogenicity risk similar to the risk observed in unexposed mothers (2–3%; Table 48.1). However, lamotrigine, carbamazepine, valproate and phenobarbital have a dose-dependent association with major congenital malformations, an important consideration for early pregnancy dosing. Lamotrigine at 325 mg/day or less was associated with the lowest frequency of major congenital malformation [3].

At the time of our patient's third pregnancy, there were only four monotherapy clobazam cases recorded in the UK and Ireland Epilepsy in Pregnancy Register and none of these was associated with malformation. Since then however, several cases have been reported raising concern that clobazam may be teratogenic. National registries and pregnancies registries will be investigating this issue.

Although folic acid supplementation did not reduce the odds of major congenital malformations in pregnancies exposed to anti-epileptic drugs, studies have demonstrated that

Table 48.1 Prevalence of major congenital malformations in offspring exposed prenatally to one of eight different anti-epileptic monotherapies

	Dose range (mg/day)	Number of pregnancies exposed	Number of major congenital malformation events	Prevalence of major congenital malformation events (95% CI)
Lamotrigine	25–1,300	2,514	74	2.9% (2.3–3.7)
Carbamazepine	50–2,400	1,957	107	5.5% (4.5–6.6)
Valproate	100–3,000	1,381	142	10.3% (8.8–12)
Levetiracetam	250–4,000	599	17	2.8% (1.7–4.5)
Oxcarbazepine	75–4,500	333	10	3.0% (1.4–5.4)
Phenobarbital	15–300	294	19	6.5% (4.2–9.9)
Topiramate	25–500	152	6	3.9% (1.5–8.4)
Phenytoin	30–730	125	8	6.4% (2.8–12.2)

Adapted from Tomson et al. [3] with permission from Elsevier.

periconceptual folic acid is associated with better cognitive outcomes and fewer autistic traits in children of mothers taking anti-epileptic medication. It is for this reason that neurologists advise folic acid 5 mg/day pre-conceptually and throughout pregnancy in women taking anti-epileptic medication.

References

1. Munakomi S, Torregrossa F, Grasso G. Natural course, clinical profile, and treatment strategies for cerebral cavernous malformations. *World Neurosurg.* 2022;159:373–80.

2. Akers A, Al-Shahi Salman R, Awad IA et al. Synopsis of guidelines for the clinical management of cerebral cavernous malformations: consensus recommendations based on systematic literature review by the Angioma Alliance Scientific Advisory Board Clinical Experts panel. *Clin Neurosurg.* 2017;80(5):665–80.

3. Tomson T, Battino D, Bonizzoni E et al. Comparative risk of major congenital malformations with eight different antiepileptic drugs: a prospective cohort study of the EURAP registry. *Lancet Neurol.* 2018;17(6):530–8.

Learning Points

- Cerebral cavernous malformations can be asymptomatic or cause epileptic seizures, intracerebral haemorrhage or focal neurological deficits without imaging evidence of haemorrhage.

- Sporadic CCMs are usually a single lesion. Familial CCMs are often multiple and due to mutations in three genes (*CCM1*, *CCM2* and *CCM3*).

- Surgical management of symptomatic CCMs in non-eloquent and easily accessible areas is recommended for epilepsy due to CCM epileptogenicity.

- Causative *CCM3* mutations and MRI appearances reflecting multiple subacute haemorrhages and/or brainstem location are all associated with increased haemorrhagic risk.

- Valproate is not advised for women of childbearing age due to an almost 10% teratogenicity risk and 30–40% risk of impaired cognitive development in the foetuses exposed to valproate during gestation.

Patient's Perspective

1. **What was the impact of the condition on you?**

   a. Physical
   Apart from when I was taking a seizure, the physical impact of the condition on my wider lifestyle was minimal. During the seizures, however, I would lose my ability to formulate sentences and would often have fallen and/or pinched at my body. This would have lasted for a minute or two (usually), then I was back to normal very quickly.

   b. Psychological (e.g. mood, emotional well-being)
   Experiencing my first seizure at 14, and having the seizures continue through my teenage years definitely had a profound psychological impact on me. My family and friends were wonderful, but in their attempts to "protect" me, they tended to play down my condition, or in some cases, deny it completely. This caused significant confusion for me as I tried to make sense of it all. I remember many occasions where I would meet new people, take a seizure in their company, then struggle to explain or articulate to them what had just happened. This caused significant embarrassment and stress which I bottled up as I didn't want to burden my family with it. It wasn't until I was 30 years old and had my second baby that I actually started to take ownership of the condition and accept that I didn't need to feel shame. At that time I took a grand mal seizure and was referred to a neurologist. This was a turning point for me as my condition was finally explained to me as an adult (not as a teenager chaperoned by parents!). Therefore I was able to understand it all so much better and accept it – hence manage it better also! In hindsight, I wish I had the power of this information and insight when I was younger.

   c. **Social (e.g. meeting friends, home)**
I kept a group of friends who were extremely protective of me and looked after me when I took seizures. They made excuses for my seizures to others, however, and whilst this was, what we felt was right at the time, I really feel now that more openness and transparency about my condition would have been so much better for us all.

2. **What can or could you not do because of the condition?**
I couldn't go anywhere on my own as a young adult. I cannot drive.

3. **Was there any other change for you due to your medical condition?**
Interestingly, my seizures always seemed to follow my menstrual cycle. During my three pregnancies I never experienced one seizure!

4. **What is/was the most difficult aspect of the condition for you?**
I have come to terms with not being able to drive. So for me, the most difficult aspect is the regret of not being better informed and empowered as a young girl.

5. **Was any aspect of the experience good or useful? What was that?**
It has probably given me some grit!

6. **What do you hope for in the future for your condition?**
Information, education, awareness and no shame.

History

Over six days, an 81-year-old man had eight episodes of slurred speech with numbness in his right hand. On the second occasion, his family also noticed that he had right facial weakness. Each episode lasted approximately 10 minutes.

Less than a year later, he had two episodes of left hand and forearm weakness with a sensory change lasting 8–10 minutes on two consecutive days. Clinically he fully recovered and remained independent in his daily activities. He stopped driving.

Past medical history included an intracerebral haemorrhage following thrombolytic therapy for an acute myocardial infarction 23 years earlier. He also had an old right hemisphere cortical infarction. He had a permanent pacemaker in situ for trifascicular block with collapse. Three years before his first presentation (with slurred speech and a numb right hand), he developed atrial fibrillation. Clopidogrel was switched to rivaroxaban. He had chronic kidney disease with an estimated glomerular filtration rate of 40 mL/min/1.72m^2.

Other medication included simvastatin 40 mg od, ramipril 5 mg od and bisoprolol 3.75 mg od.

Examination

He had an irregular pulse of 66 beats per minute. General and neurological examinations were normal.

Investigations

His cardiac pacemaker was deemed not to be MRI-compatible. A CT brain scan showed an old right frontal infarct and right temporal low density from previous thrombolysis-related haemorrhage. No other abnormality was initially reported. However, a review of the imaging suggested a convexity subarachnoid haemorrhage in the left hemisphere from the first presentation (Figure 49.1A).

From the second presentation, a further convexity subarachnoid haemorrhage was identified in the right hemisphere (Figure 49.1B).

An ECG confirmed atrial fibrillation. Doppler ultrasound of the carotid system (prior to the imaging review) showed no flow disturbance.

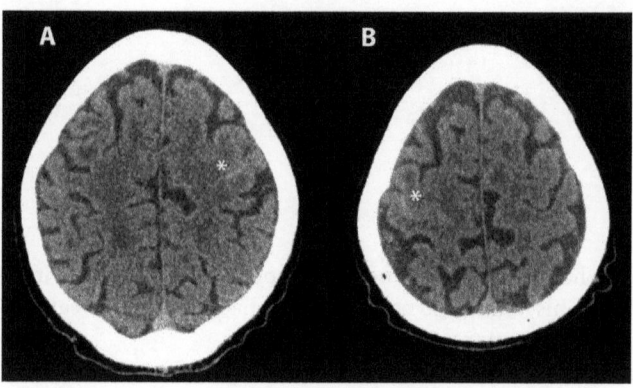

Figure 49.1 CT brain scans showing convexity subarachnoid haemorrhage in the (A) left hemisphere and (B) right hemisphere. An asterisk highlights the blood

Diagnosis: Transient Focal Neurological Episodes Due to Sulcal Subarachnoid Haemorrhage Secondary to Cerebral Amyloid Angiopathy ('Amyloid Spells')

Management

CHA$_2$DS$_2$VASc score was 6, meaning that this patient had a 9.7% risk of ischaemic stroke/transient ischaemic attack (TIA)/systemic embolism per year (Table 49.1). With one parenchymal haemorrhage and two convexity haemorrhages, his risk of further brain haemorrhage was as high as 10.5%. He was offered randomisation to a clinical trial, but he chose to remain on rivaroxaban. He has subsequently been referred for consideration of left atrial appendage closure.

Comment
What Is Cerebral Amyloid Angiopathy?

Deposition of amyloid-β protein (predominantly Aβ-40) in small- to medium-sized arteries, arterioles and capillaries in the cortex and overlying leptomeninges defines cerebral amyloid angiopathy (CAA). Cerebral amyloid angiopathy prevalence increases with age and the main clinical feature is lobar haemorrhage (sporadic, anticoagulant- and thrombolysis-related). Lobar intracerebral haemorrhages increased in the UK in over 75-year-olds between the 1980s and early 2000s, suggesting an increasing role of CAA in intracerebral haemorrhage. Other clinical phenotypes of CAA include transient focal neurological episodes (as happened in our patient), dementia and rapid cognitive decline.

In addition, a rare encephalopathy along with rapid cognitive decline, behaviour change, headache and seizures has been associated with CAA-related inflammation. Cohorts of such patients suggest that immunosuppressive treatment improves outcomes. The clinical features

Table 49.1 The CHA$_2$DS$_2$VASc score for our patient

Risk factor	Score	Patient
Congestive heart failure/LV dysfunction	1	1
Hypertension >140/90 mmHg	1	0
Age ≥75 years	2	2
Diabetes mellitus	1	0
Stroke/TIA/TE	2	2
Vascular disease (prior myocardial infarction, peripheral arterial disease or aortic plaque)	1	1
Age (65–74 years)	1	0
Sex category (i.e. female gender)	1	0
Total		6

LV: left ventricular; TE: thromboembolism

Adapted from Lip et al. [1] with permission from Elsevier.

are similar to adverse effects identified in patients who received active Aβ vaccination in a trial for Alzheimer's disease, leading to the suspension of such treatment. Passive immunisation with aducanumab (a drug approved by the FDA in the USA for mild-moderate Alzheimer's disease) has also been associated with similar radiological appearances known as amyloid-related imaging abnormalities (ARIAs), which include cerebral oedema (ARIA-E) and cerebral microhaemorhage (ARIA-H).

Following the identification of apolipoprotein E (*APOE*) ε4 allele as a dose-dependent risk factor for sporadic Alzheimer's disease, the same allele was implicated as a dose-dependent risk factor for vascular Aβ40 deposition in CAA. However, a neuropathologist in Glasgow, UK, Professor James Nicoll, demonstrated that the less frequent *APOE* ε2 allele, which has a protective role in Alzheimer's disease, paradoxically plays a role in CAA-related haemorrhage via a range of vasculopathic complications. Subsequent work has shown an over-representation of *APOE* ε4 in lobar cerebral microbleeds and *APOE* ε2 in superficial siderosis due to CAA.

There are rare genetic forms of CAA due to mutations in amyloid precursor protein (e.g. Dutch-type hereditary CAA) and also in other proteins such as transthyretin and cystatin C.

What Are Amyloid Spells?

Transient focal neurological episodes or 'amyloid spells' due to CAA have been documented since the 1980s. These episodes are focal, usually motor or sensory, of short duration (usually less than 30 minutes) and are often recurrent and stereotyped, and can mimic TIAs, migraine aura or seizures. Positive (transient paraesthesias) and negative phenomena (focal weakness and dysphasia) have been recorded [2], but most appear to be spreading or migrating sensory disturbances that correlate with the anatomical location of convexity subarachnoid haemorrhage. Amyloid spells have been closely associated with convexity subarachnoid haemorrhage or cortical superficial siderosis [3]. Electroencephalography recording has supported the idea that the semiology reflects a spreading depression.

Distinguishing amyloid spells from TIAs is challenging without imaging, although migratory symptoms, sensory disturbances and recurrent stereotyped events occur more frequently in patients with convexity subarachnoid haemorrhage than in patients with TIA.

Causes of Sulcal or Convexity Subarachnoid Haemorrhage

In addition to CAA, other recognised causes of non-traumatic acute sulcal or convexity subarachnoid haemorrhage include reversible cerebral vasoconstriction syndrome, central nervous system (CNS) vasculitis, hyperperfusion and endocarditis.

The modified Boston CAA criteria recognise sulcal haemorrhage or cortical superficial siderosis as features of CAA (Table 49.2). A more recent clinical and MRI-based diagnosis of CAA and its clinical spectrum is more sensitive and includes non-haemorrhagic features (Boston criteria version 2; Table 49.3). The aetiology of remote intracerebral haemorrhages following thrombolytic therapy is increasingly recognised as due to CAA. In addition to the previous thrombolysis-related haemorrhage, our patient had two haemorrhages fulfilling the criteria for probable CAA.

Balancing Risk of Haemorrhage versus Embolism

The CHA_2DS_2VASc score (Table 49.1) predicts risk of ischaemic stroke in non-anticoagulated patients with atrial fibrillation. Scores can be calculated to predict risk of embolism and stroke. Although there are observations that suggest that transient focal neurological events due to

CAA are risk factors for intracerebral haemorrhage, the size of this risk is not well established. It is also unclear if the risk changes with time. In contrast, the CHA_2DS_2VASc (score 0–9) has been validated as a useful predictive tool. For our patient, the risks of haemorrhage versus embolism (including ischaemic stroke) appeared similar. He was therefore referred for consideration of left atrial appendage closure.

Left Atrial Appendage Closure

Left atrial appendage closure may permit substitution of anticoagulation therapy for the lower bleeding risk of antiplatelet therapy. There is emerging evidence that transcatheter left atrial appendage closure may have a role in such patients who carry a high bleeding risk [4]. Studies have shown similar thromboembolic event rates but significantly reduced bleeding events compared to anticoagulation therapy.

Table 49.2 Modified Boston criteria for attributing intracranial haemorrhage to CAA

Category of classification	Definition
Definite CAA	Post-mortem examination showing • lobar, cortical or corticosubcortical haemorrhage/microbleed • severe CAA with vasculopathy • absence of other diagnostic lesion.
Probable CAA with supporting pathology	Clinical data and pathological tissue from evacuated haematoma or cortical biopsy showing • lobar, cortical or corticosubcortical haemorrhage/microbleed • some degree of CAA in specimen • absence of other diagnostic lesion.
Probable CAA	Clinical data and MRI or CT demonstrating • multiple haemorrhages/microbleeds restricted to lobar, cortical or corticosubcortical regions (cerebellar haemorrhage allowed) OR • single lobar, cortical or corticosubcortical haemorrhage/microbleed and focal or disseminated superficial siderosis AND • age of ≥55 years AND • absence of other cause of haemorrhage or superficial siderosis.
Possible CAA	Clinical data and MRI or CT demonstrating • single lobar, cortical or corticosubcortical haemorrhage/microbleed OR • focal or disseminated superficial siderosis AND • age of ≥55 years AND • absence of other cause of haemorrhage or superficial siderosis.

Adapted from Linn et al. [5] with permission from Wolters Kluwer.

Table 49.3 Boston criteria version 2.0 for sporadic CAA

1. Definite CAA
Full brain post-mortem examination demonstrating:
- spontaneous intracerebral haemaorrhage, transient focal neurological episodes, convexity subarachnoid haemorrhage, or cognitive impairment or dementia
- severe CAA with vasculopathy
- absence of other diagnostic lesion.

2. Probable CAA with supporting pathology
Clinical data and pathological tissue (evacuated haematoma or cortical biopsy) demonstrating:
- presentation with spontaneous intracerebral haemorrhage, transient focal neurological episodes, convexity subarachnoid haemorrhage, or cognitive impairment or dementia
- some degree of CAA in specimen
- absence of other diagnostic lesion.

3. Probable CAA
For patients aged ≥50 years, clinical data and MRI demonstrating:
- presentation with spontaneous intracerebral haemorrhage, transient focal neurological episodes, or cognitive impairment or dementia
- at least two of the following strictly lobar haemorrhagic lesions on $T2^*$-weighted MRI, in any combination: intracerebral haemorrhage, cerebral microbleeds, or foci of cortical superficial siderosis or convexity subarachnoid haemorrhage

OR
- one lobar haemorrhagic lesion plus one white matter feature (severe perivascular spaces in the centrum semiovale or white matter hyperintensities in a multispot pattern)[a]
- absence of any deep haemorrhagic lesions (i.e. intracerebral haemorrhage or cerebral microbleeds) on $T2^*$-weighted MRI
- absence of other cause of haemorrhagic lesions[b]
- haemorrhagic lesion in cerebellum not counted as either lobar or deep haemorrhagic lesion.

4. Possible CAA
For patients aged ≥50 years, clinical data and MRI demonstrating:
- presentation with spontaneous intracerebral haemorrhage, transient focal neurological episodes, or cognitive impairment or dementia
- absence of other cause of haemorrhage[b]
- one strictly lobar haemorrhagic lesion on $T2^*$-weighted MRI: intracerebral haemorrhage, cerebral microbleeds, or foci of cortical superficial siderosis or convexity subarachnoid haemorrhage

OR
- one white matter feature (severe visible perivascular spaces in the centrum semiovale or white matter hyperintensities in a multisport pattern)[a]
- absence of any deep haemorrhagic lesions (i.e. intracerebral haemorrhage or cerebral microbleeds) on $T2^*$-weighted MRI
- absence of other cause of haemorrhagic lesions[b]
- haemorrhagic lesion in cerebellum not counted as either lobar or deep haemorrhagic lesion.

[a] Notable changes from the modified Boston criteria

[b] Other causes of haemorrhagic lesion: antecedent head trauma, haemorrhagic transformation of an ischaemic stroke, arteriovenous malformation, haemorrhagic tumour and CNS vasculitis. Other causes of cortical superficial siderosis and acute convexity subarachnoid haemorrhage should also be excluded.

Reprinted from Charidimou et al. [6] with permission from Elsevier.

References

1. Lip GYH, Nieuwlaat R, Pisters R, Lane DA, Crijns HJGM. Refining clinical risk stratification for predicting stroke and thromboembolism in atrial fibrillation using a novel risk factor-based approach: the euro heart survey on atrial fibrillation. *Chest.* 2010;137(2):263–72.

2. Charidimou A, Peeters A, Fox Z et al. Spectrum of transient focal neurological episodes in cerebral amyloid angiopathy: multicentre magnetic resonance imaging cohort study and meta-analysis. *Stroke.* 2012;43(9):2324–30.

3. Smith EE, Charidimou A, Ayata C, Werring DJ, Greenberg SM. Cerebral amyloid angiopathy-related transient focal neurologic episodes. *Neurology.* 2021;97(5):231–8.

4. Nakajima Y. Effectiveness and safety of transcatheter left atrial appendage closure. *J Cardiol.* 2022;79(2):186–93.

5. Linn J, Halpin A, Demaerel P et al. Prevalence of superficial siderosis in patients with cerebral amyloid angiopathy. *Neurology.* 2010;74(17):1346–50.

6. Charidimou A, Boulouis G, Froschet MP et al. The Boston criteria version 2.0 for cerebral amyloid angiopathy: a multicentre, retrospective, MRI-neuropathology diagnostic accuracy study. *Lancet Neurol.* 2022; 21:714–24.

Learning Points

- Cerebral amyloid angiopathy increases with age and has a broad spectrum of phenotypes including intracerebral haemorrhage (microbleeds and macrobleeds), transient focal neurological events dementia and an autoimmune encephalopathy known as CAA-related inflammation.

- Gyral or convexity subarachnoid haemorrhage and superficial siderosis are associated with transient focal neurological events, which may precede lobar haemorrhage.

- Apolipoprotein E or *APOE* ε4 alleles are associated with vascular Aβ deposition (CAA) and the *APOE* ε2 allele with vasculopathic complications leading to haemorrhage.

- Left atrial appendage closure in patients with atrial fibrillation and haemorrhagic features of CAA may reduce recurrent haemorrhagic risk.

Patient's Perspective

1. **What was the physical impact of the condition on you?**
   I stopped driving. Then I thought, 'I can do without driving', so I sold my car.

2. **Did the condition affect your mood or emotional well-being?**
   Not after I decided to sell my car.

3. **Had the condition any impact on you socially (e.g. meeting friends, home)?**
   No restrictions. My son takes me out when I want.

4. **What can you no longer do?**
   I like gardening. I enjoy pruning my roses. I can still do my gardening activities except I no longer dig the garden, but that is more to do with my arthritic knees.

5. **What do you hope for in the future?**
   I hope to be able to go on living and doing what I can still do.

50 Following the Eyes

History

A 46-year-old man who had experienced a one-day history of a moderate global headache was found by his son after a fall and noted to have a left-sided weakness. He had slurred speech. He was admitted to hospital at 05:20 hrs. In hospital, he had an initial Glasgow Coma Scale of 3, which subsequently improved. A CT scan of the brain was reported as normal. A neurology opinion was sought at 15:30 hrs.

Past medical history included having shrapnel in his torso from a bullet injury.

Examination

He had small unreactive pupils, was markedly dysarthric and had hiccups during the examination. He had vertical nystagmus and a left internuclear ophthalmoplegia (right eye abducting nystagmus and his left eye failed to adduct on attempting to look to the right). There was no ptosis. He had facial symmetry and normal hearing. Tongue movements were slow. His arm and leg strength were normal but both plantars were extensor.

Investigations

MRI was contraindicated due to shrapnel. Review of the CT scan of the brain on admission suggested a hyperdense basilar artery (Figure 50.1A). A CT angiogram of the neck vessels to the circle of Willis showed basilar artery occlusion, which was confirmed at catheter angiography (Figure 50.1B) and shown to be secondary to a left vertebral artery dissection.

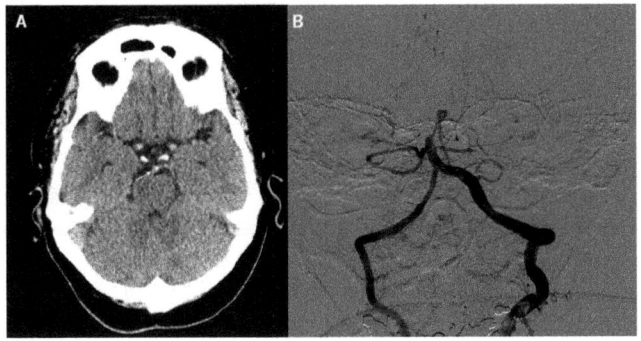

Figure 50.1 (A) A non-contrast CT brain scan on admission demonstrates a hyperdense distal basilar artery (arrow). (B) A catheter angiogram confirms basilar artery occlusion

Diagnosis: Basilar Artery Thrombosis (Secondary to Left Vertebral Artery Dissection)

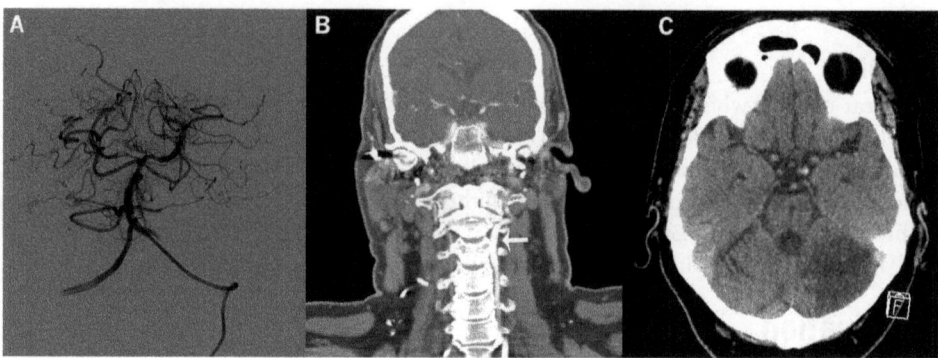

Figure 50.2 (A) A catheter angiogram shows basilar artery recanalisation. (B) A CT angiogram of neck vessels demonstrates patent left vertebral artery with stents in situ (arrow). (C) A non-contrast CT scan of the brain showing left paramedian pontine and left cerebellar hemisphere infarctions

Management

Aspirin and subcutaneous enoxaparin were given at the acute general hospital. The patient was then transferred to a neuroscience centre where he had clot retrieval to achieve recanalisation of the basilar artery (Figure 50.2A). Stents were inserted into the dissected left vertebral artery, the source of the basilar clot (Figure 50.2B). He had a fluctuating level of consciousness, vomited and required intubation and ventilation for a short period of time. He was treated with dual antiplatelet therapy for six months (aspirin and clopidogrel).

A follow-up CT brain scan showed infarction of the left cerebellum and left median pons (Figure 50.2C). A CT angiogram had shown a patent vertebrobasilar system.

Nine months later, he was independent with only mild residual ataxia (heel-toe walking and mild dysarthria).

Comment

Posterior Circulation Strokes

Posterior circulation ischaemic stroke syndrome may be due to stenosis, thrombosis or embolic occlusion of posterior circulation arteries (i.e. the vertebral arteries, basilar artery and posterior cerebral arteries; Figure 50.3).

Basilar artery thrombosis accounts for 1% of all ischaemic strokes and 5% of large vessel occlusive strokes. The wide spectrum of features in presentations of basilar artery thrombosis can be challenging for the neurologist, but a low threshold for proceeding to a CT angiogram can help achieve an early diagnosis. Basilar artery thrombosis has a poor prognosis; 68% of patients are disabled (modified Rankin score 4 or 5) or dead at one month. Stuttering neurological deficits, an apparently normal CT brain (if hyperdense basilar artery not actively considered or seen) and at times a deceptively low stroke severity score (National Institute of Health Stroke Score; NIHSS) were all present in this patient. The NIHSS gives more weight to symptoms of anterior circulation stroke.

Clinical Features of Basilar Artery Thrombosis

In the circle of Willis, the basilar artery provides short paramedian or perforating arterial branches to the paramedian aspects of the base of the pons and pontine tegmentum (Figure 50.3). Occlusion of a single paramedian artery can cause a lacunar syndrome (pure motor, pure sensory, ataxic hemiparesis, sensorimotor stroke and dysarthria-clumsy hand syndrome make up five of over 20 described lacunar syndromes). Disturbances in eye movement can occur as witnessed in our patient. The 'locked-in syndrome' occurs with bilateral infarction or haemorrhage at the base of the pons [1].

When an embolus impacts in the rostral or distal basilar artery, a wide variety of symptoms and signs can emerge as a 'top of the basilar syndrome'. Louis Caplan documented pupillary abnormalities, eye movement abnormalities, altered level of alertness and amnesia due to thalamic infarction [3]. Agitation and visual hallucinations can also occur. The hallucinations are vivid, colourful and sometimes distorted images of animals or people. They are known as *peduncular hallucinosis* and were first described by Jean Lhermitte in 1922. He reported a 72-year-old woman with a midbrain and pontine infarction. The hallucinations may be a release phenomenon due to damage of the reticular activating system.

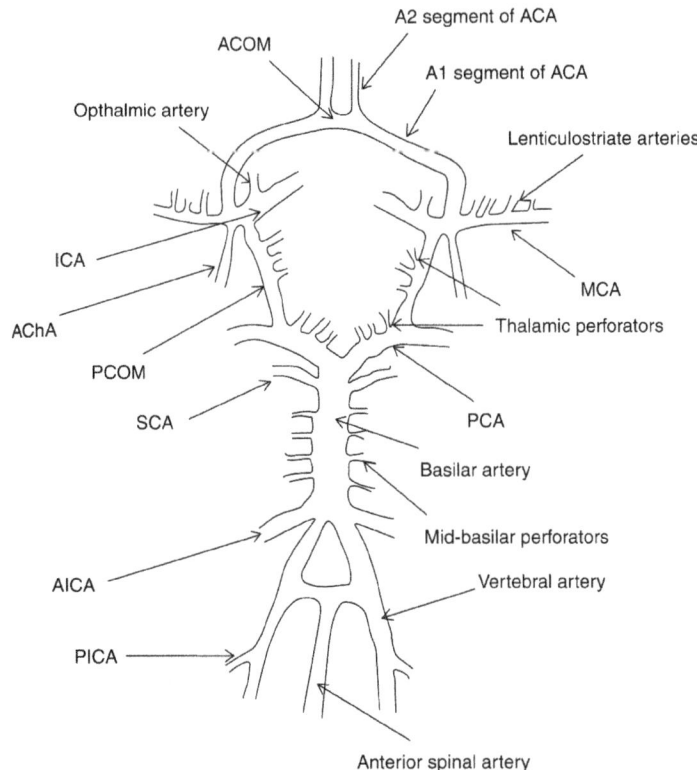

Figure 50.3 Schematic drawing of the circle of Willis. (ACA, anterior cerebral artery; AChA, anterior choroidal artery; ACOM, anterior communicating artery; AICA, anterior inferior cerebellar artery; ICA, internal carotid artery; MCA, middle cerebral artery; PCA, posterior cerebral artery; PCOM, posterior communicating artery; PICA, posterior inferior cerebellar artery; SCA, superior cerebellar artery) Reprinted from Tarulli [2] with permission from Cambridge University Press.

Lower and middle basilar artery involvement occurs when pontine paramedian perforators and short circumferential branches are occluded. In this way, corticospinal tract lesions cause unilateral or bilateral limb weakness, while corticobulbar tract lesions cause dysarthria, dysphonia and dysphagia. In addition, involvement of the paramedian pontine reticular formation can result in horizontal gaze palsy, internuclear ophthalmoplegia, nystagmus and pinpoint pupils. Ischaemia of the medial lemniscus causes sensory deficits.

The anterior inferior cerebellar artery (AICA) supplies the lateral pons, the anterior inferior cerebellum, the labyrinth and cochlea. An AICA infarct may result in hemifacial sensory loss, facial weakness, Horner's syndrome, limb ataxia and an acute vestibular syndrome with deafness. Such an infarct can result in an abnormal video-head impulse test – an exception to the usual interpretation of an abnormal head impulse test, suggesting a peripheral lesion.

The superior cerebellar artery supplies the lateral midbrain and superior cerebellum (superior vermis and dentate nucleus). Superior cerebellar infarction may result in a fourth cranial nerve palsy, ipsilateral hemifacial sensory loss, contralateral body hemisensory loss, Horner's syndrome, truncal and gait ataxia, dysarthria, nausea and vomiting.

Evidence-Based Management

Intravenous Thrombolysis

Early time-sensitive recanalisation has been shown to be key to improved prognosis from acute ischaemic stroke. Intravenous thrombolysis for acute ischaemic stroke had its first positive randomised controlled trial in 1995. Posterior circulation ischaemic strokes were under-represented in trials of intravenous thrombolysis. Patients with posterior circulation ischaemic stroke make up between 12 and 19% of all intravenous thrombolysis-treated ischaemic stroke patients. For basilar artery occlusion, a good outcome (defined as a modified Rankin score of 0–2) has been achieved in 21–53% of patients.

Endovascular Therapy

The first robust evidence of the benefit of endovascular therapy or mechanical thrombectomy for large vessel anterior circulation strokes emerged in 2015; prior to 2015, the evidence for endovascular therapy was not present due to long delays from onset to treatment, older-generation devices and inadequate patient selection. For posterior circulation strokes, there are registry data showing that these patients may have a longer therapeutic time window of up to 24 hours for intervention [4]. Trial evidence for endovascular therapy for basilar occlusion first emerged in 2022.

It is recognised that recanalisation benefits patients with a target perfusion mismatch profile independent of time for both endovascular therapy and intravenous thrombolysis – so-called tissue-dependent as opposed to time-dependent treatment.

Collateral circulation is recognised as an important factor for salvaging at-risk or ischaemic brain as collaterals have been associated with better outcome from basilar artery occlusion.

More evidence of benefit from endovascular intervention for basilar artery thrombosis may emerge in appropriately selected patients with good initial collateral vessels. As with anterior circulation endovascular therapy, advanced imaging may therefore improve patient selection to avoid futile recanalisation.

References

1. Schulz UG, Fischer U. Posterior circulation cerebrovascular syndromes: diagnosis and management. *J Neurol Neurosurg Psychiatry*. 2017;88(1):45–53.

2. Tarulli A. *Neurology: A Clinician's Approach*. Cambridge: Cambridge University Press; 2011.

3. Caplan LR. *Caplan's Stroke*. Third edition. Boston: Butterworth-Heinemann; 2000.

4. Zi W, Qiu Z, Wu D et al. Assessment of endovascular treatment for acute basilar artery occlusion via a nationwide prospective registry. *JAMA Neurol*. 2020;77(5):561–73.

Learning Points

- Compared to other types of acute ischaemic stroke, basilar artery thrombosis has a poor prognosis.

- Basilar artery thrombosis can present with a wide spectrum of features including coma, locked-in, hemiparesis, oculomotor abnormalities, facial palsy, bulbar symptoms, homonymous hemianopia and cortical blindness.

- Delays in diagnosing basilar artery thrombosis may be due to failure to recognise the clinical syndrome, a stuttering onset and an underestimation of stroke severity as measured by NIHSS.

- Recognition of basilar artery thrombosis should prompt consideration of urgent intravenous thrombolysis and endovascular therapy.

- In acute ischaemic stroke, endovascular therapy evidence for basilar artery thrombosis has lagged behind the evidence for anterior circulation large vessel occlusion.

Patient's Perspective

1. **What was the impact of the condition?**
   a. Physical (e.g. job, driving, practical support)
   I am still weak on my left side. Balance is very poor, worse at times when walking.
   b. Psychological (e.g. mood, emotional well-being)
   I got very quick-tempered and would be a lot more emotional.
   c. Social (e.g. meeting friends, home)
   I go out less as people think I am drunk due to bobbling and balance problem.

2. **What can or could you not do because of your condition?**
   I can no longer canoe or parachute.

3. **Was there any other change for you due to your medical condition?**
   I don't smoke anymore (as I don't remember I did).

4. **What was the most difficult aspect of the condition?**
   My balance problem remains the most challenging aspect of this condition.

5. **Was any aspect of the experience good or useful? What was that?**
   I lost part of my memory in that I didn't remember that I smoked!

6. **What do you hope for in the future for people with this condition?**
   I hope people can be happy and enjoy their second chance to change for the better.

History

A 43-year-old male farmer was found face-down near a slurry pit. A relative found him unresponsive with agonal breathing. Basic life support was started. There was a restoration of spontaneous circulation and spontaneous breathing, but he still had a Glasgow Coma Scale of 3. His pupils were fixed and dilated. A Helicopter Emergency Medical Service intubated and ventilated him at the scene. It was estimated that his loss of consciousness had been no more than 10 minutes. He was transferred to an Emergency Department.

He had an unremarkable past medical history. He did not smoke cigarettes and did not drink alcohol.

He was extubated and a neurology consultation was requested on day 5.

Examination

He was cardiovascularly stable. He had spontaneous eye opening but did not track (eye response score 3 out of 4). There was limited communication; he raised his thumb for approval/confirmation (motor response score 4 out of 4). Pupil and corneal reflexes were now intact (brainstem reflexes score 4 out of 4). He had a regular breathing pattern (respiration score 4 out of 4). Total Full Outline of UnResponsiveness or FOUR score was 15 out of 16. He could move all four limbs. He had normal sensation and reflexes.

Investigations

A CT of the brain was reported as unremarkable. Ten days later, an MRI of the brain demonstrated symmetrical T2 and FLAIR increased signal in the fronto-parieto-temporal cortex, subcortical white matter and basal ganglia (putamina and caudate nuclei). The symmetrical areas of signal abnormality included the perirolandic cortex. The perirolandic cortex, peripheral putamina and external capsules demonstrated diffusion restriction (Figure 51.1). Two EEGs six days apart revealed diffuse fast (beta 13–30 Hz) and slow activity but no focal abnormalities.

Management

He deteriorated on day 6 and required re-intubation. He was treated for an aspiration pneumonia and had a tracheostomy.

After two months, he was fit for transfer to a local rehabilitation ward and then a regional rehabilitation centre. Dysarthria gradually improved. He progressed from using a steady aid to crutches/rollator. His Berg balance score (named after Katherine Berg), a measure of static and dynamic balance, improved to 47 out of 56. He was independent in upper limb function and personal care.

More than a year later, he was keen to drive but required a road driving assessment. He had ongoing input from a multidisciplinary community brain injury team. His initial driving assessment was unsuccessful, but more than two years after his collapse, he passed a driving assessment.

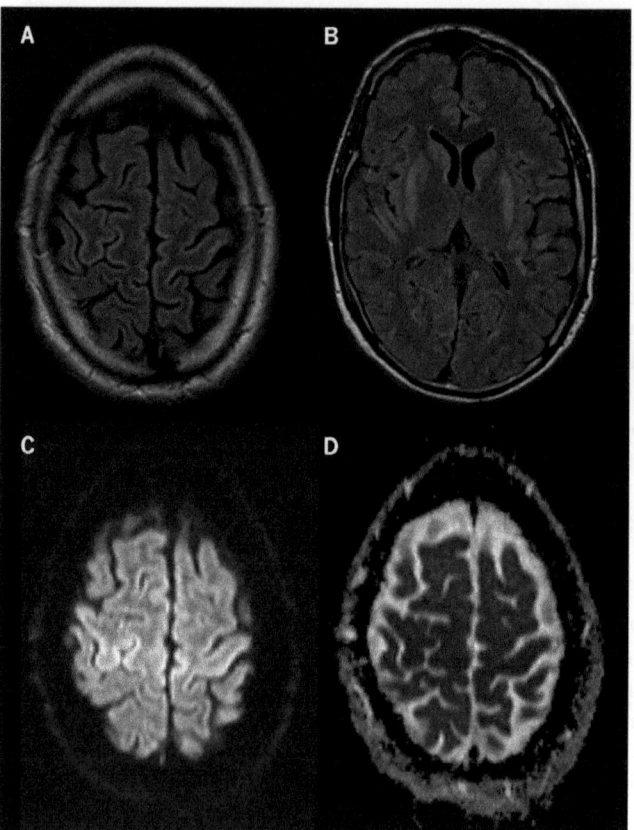

Figure 51.1 An axial T2 FLAIR MRI scan of the brain showing subtle increase in signal in (A) perirolandic cortex and (B) basal ganglia bilaterally. The perirolandic areas demonstrate (C) increased signal on a diffusion scan and (D) low signal on the corresponding apparent diffusion coefficient map

Diagnosis: Hypoxic Ischaemic Encephalopathy Secondary to Slurry Gas Asphyxiation

Comment

Acute Global Hypoxia or Ischaemia

Major causes of a rapid reduction of the oxygen content of blood or sudden reduction in blood flow to the brain result in acute global hypoxia and ischaemia. Obstruction of the airways (drowning, choking or suffocation), massive obstruction of the cerebral arteries (strangulation) and sudden decrease in cardiac output (asystole, severe arrhythmias, vasodepressor syncope, pulmonary embolism and massive systemic haemorrhage) may all cause acute global hypoxic ischaemia. It takes just six to eight seconds to lose consciousness if the cerebral circulation is stopped completely. Consciousness is lost in a few more seconds if blood flow continues but oxygen is not supplied.

Total ischaemic anoxia lasting more than four minutes results in the death of neurones; the neurones in the cerebral cortex (hippocampus) and cerebellum (Purkinje cells) are most vulnerable.

Out of hospital, cardiac arrests are common in the UK (55 per 100,000 per year). A return of spontaneous circulation is achieved in 30%, and when resuscitation is attempted, just 9% survive to hospital discharge. Cardiac origin arrests have better outcomes: 54% return of spontaneous circulation and 29% survival to discharge [1].

FOUR Score

Because of shortcomings of the Glasgow Coma Scale (devised for head injury), Eeclo F. M. Wijdicks and colleagues devised a validated coma score, which includes measurement of brainstem reflexes. The Full Outline of UnResponsiveness or FOUR score is an accurate predictor of survival outcome in cardiac arrest; at days three to five after cardiac arrest, a FOUR score of >8 is associated with more than 90% survival [2]. Our patient had a FOUR score of 15 on day 5 (Table 51.1). The FOUR score can be applied to patients with and without endotracheal intubation.

Table 51.1 Patient scores from FOUR

Clinical feature	Score	Patient –day 5
Eye response		
Eyelids open or opened, tracking or blinking to command	4	
Eyelids open but not tracking	3	3
Eyelids closed but open to loud voice	2	
Eyelids closed but open to pain	1	
Eyelids remain closed with pain	0	

Motor response

Thumbs-up, fist or peace-sign	4	4
Localising to pain	3	
Flexion response to pain	2	
Extension response to pain	1	
No response to pain or generalised myoclonus status	0	

Brainstem reflexes

Pupil and corneal reflexes present	4	4
One pupil wide and fixed	3	
Pupil or corneal reflexes absent	2	
Pupil and corneal reflexes absent	1	
Absent pupil, corneal and cough reflex	0	

Respiration

Not intubated, regular breathing pattern	4	4
Not intubated, Cheyne–Stokes breathing pattern	3	
Not intubated, irregular breathing	2	
Breathes above ventilator rate	1	
Breathes at ventilator rate or apnoea	0	

Adapted from Wijdicks et al. [3] with permission from Wiley.

Epidemiology of Slurry Accidents

Farm accidents are common. The agriculture sector has the highest death rate and serious injury of any industry in the UK. Slurry pit accidents can be one of the most dangerous areas of a farm. In Northern Ireland, four slurry pit-related deaths were reported between 1968 and 1985 [4] while 15 slurry pit-related fatalities were reported between 1997 and 2017. While some of these resulted from falling into slurry pits and drowning, many have been due solely to inhalation of slurry gases or environmental asphyxiation. It is recognised, however, that a combination of such events can occur; inhalation of slurry gases can cause a fall into a slurry tank. The reported number of slurry accidents is inevitably an underestimate as many non-fatal and non-injurious cases of slurry gas poisoning may not be reported.

Mechanism of Action

Decomposition of slurry releases methane, carbon dioxide, ammonia and hydrogen sulphide (H_2S). At low concentrations, H_2S has a rotten egg smell, but this is not detected at high concentration (over 100 parts per million) due to olfactory fatigue. At concentrations of over 500–1,000 parts per million, H_2S can be immediately fatal. H_2S appears to inhibit complex IV of the mitochondrial respiratory chain and induce apoptosis. Agitated slurry is associated with release of all four gases. Environmental asphyxiation can ensue as slurry gases are heavier than air and so displace oxygen. Once oxygen level drops to 4%, a person loses consciousness within two breaths and death is rapid. The MRI scan in our patient suggested environmental asphyxiation caused a hypoxic ischaemic encephalopathy insult.

Guidance on the safe handling of slurry is provided by the Health and Safety Executive in Great Britain (www.hse.gov.uk/pubns/ais9.pdf) and Northern Ireland (www.hseni.gov.uk/articles/slurry-working-safely-slurry).

References

1. The Resuscitation Council. Epidemiology of cardiac arrest guidelines authors out of hospital cardiac arrest (OHCA) in the UK in-hospital cardiac arrest (IHCA) in the UK. Available from: www.resus.org.uk/library/2021-resuscitation-guidelines/epidemiology-cardiac-arrest-guidelines.

2. Fugate JE, Rabinstein AA, Claassen DO, White RD, Wijdicks EFM. The FOUR score predicts outcome in patients after cardiac arrest. *Neurocrit Care*. 2010 Oct.;13(2):205–10.

3. Wijdicks EFM Bamlet WR, Maramattom BV, Manno EM, McClelland RL. Validation of a new coma scale: the FOUR scale. *Ann Neurol*. 2005;58(4):585–93.

4. Spiers M, Finnegan OC. Near death due to inhalation of slurry tank gases. *Ulster Med J*. 1986;55(2):181–3.

Learning Points

- Slurry pits are an important source of farm accidents.
- Gases from agitated slurry pits (H_2S, carbon dioxide, ammonia and methane) can cause environmental asphyxiation.
- Hypoxic ischaemic brain injury from cardiac arrest can be reduced with efficient resuscitation.
- The FOUR score is an accurate predictor of survival outcome in cardiac arrest.

Patient's Perspective

1. **What was the impact of the condition on you?**

   a. Physical (e.g. practical support, home, work)
   Slow process. I gradually gained independence. Initially I could do nothing alone.

   b. Psychological (e.g. mood, emotional well-being)
   Loss of my independence impacted my emotional well-being. I had to find a new 'normal' for me.

   c. Social (e.g. meeting friends, home)
   I cannot bear noise in large crowds. I need a one-to-one talk with friends. I am conscious of my speech being different as I sound different.

2. **What could you not do because of the condition?**
   I could not do anything – stand, dress, feed or toilet myself.

3. **Was there any other change for you due to your medical condition?**
   There was a big change in my lifestyle. I cannot go to work and I cannot walk unaided.

4. **What is/was the most difficult aspect of the condition for you?**
   My balance is challenging; I cannot walk unaided. 'Everything' for me is now slow (e.g. reaction times and movement).

5. **Was any aspect of the experience good or useful? What was that?**
   I have met a lot of people on my journey. Life has changed dramatically, but I am thankful for my life. I spend more time now with my family.

6. **What do you hope for in the future for your condition?**
   For people to set goals and meet them, positivity and improvements in medical knowledge.

52 From Skin to Brain

History

A 51-year-old right-handed man had a witnessed generalised tonic-clonic seizure. He had bowel incontinence and had bitten the left side of his tongue. Five months earlier, he had wakened up on the floor of his apartment and on that occasion, he had also had bowel incontinence. He had come round with his face on the floor. He had not sought medical attention for that episode.

Three years before, a skin lesion had been removed from his abdominal wall. A melanoma was diagnosed, resulting in a wider excision. Breslow thickness (depth of the melanoma from the surface of the skin to the deepest point of the tumour) was 1.0 mm, stage pT1a (Figure 52.1).

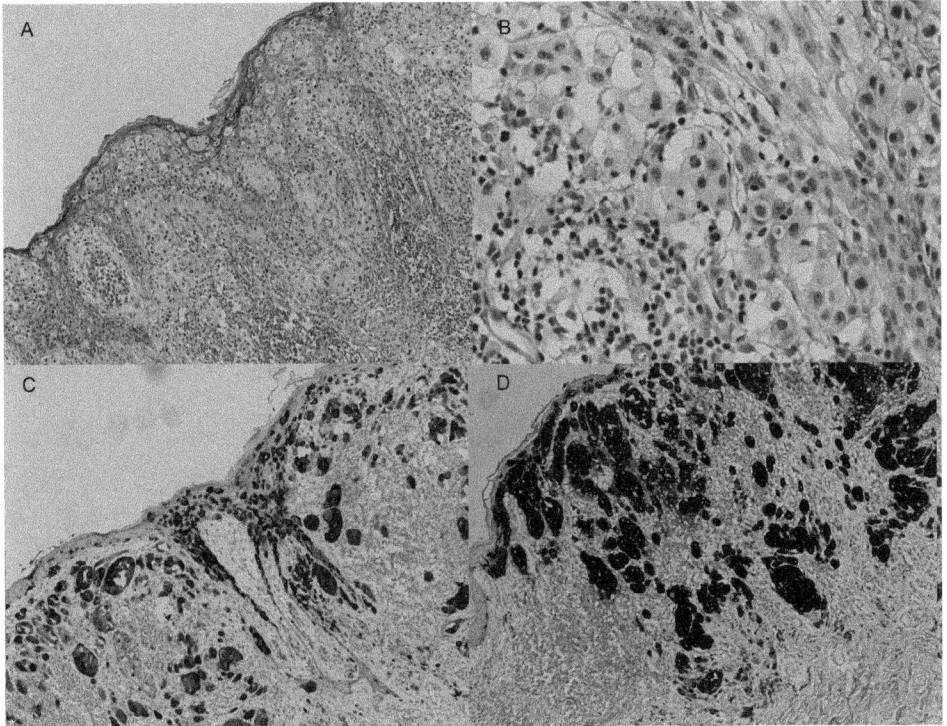

Figure 52.1 (A) Histology of the primary pigmented skin lesion excision shows numerous atypical melanocytes in confluent nests and as single cells. These occupy the dermis and dermoepidermal junction with a pagetoid (buckshot-like) scatter into the overlying atrophic epidermis. There is a lack of melanocytic maturation with depth and an associated lymphocytic inflammatory infiltrate. (B) A closer ×20 objective magnification shows epithelioid melanocytes with relatively abundant cytoplasm containing melanin pigment. The nuclei are enlarged and pleomorphic with many bearing a notable cherry-red nucleoli. (C) Melan A immunohistochemistry shows diffuse positivity within the melanocytes. (D) HMB45 immunohistochemistry demonstrates an abnormal diffuse expression throughout the lesion, which reflects the lack of normal melanocyte maturation and this is in keeping with malignant melanoma

He was on no medication. He drank ten pints of beer four times per month.

Examination

He had an amblyopic left eye with 6/60 vision. Visual acuity on the right was 6/6 unaided. The remainder of the neurological examination was normal. He had no palpable nodes in axillae or groins.

Investigations

A CT scan of the brain showed numerous intra-axial lesions within the cerebral (Figures 52.2A and 52.2B) and cerebellar hemispheres as well as the brainstem. An MRI scan of the brain confirmed the CT brain findings with paramagnetic melanotic effect (bright on T1 and dark on T2) with enhancing lesions (Figures 52.2C and 52.2D).

An MRI scan of the spine identified three left axillary lesions. A CT scan of the chest abdomen and pelvis demonstrated significant left axillary and mediastinal lymph adenopathy with bilateral inguinal lymph nodes. An ultrasound-guided left axillary soft tissue biopsy was performed.

The lymph node biopsy confirmed metastatic melanoma (Figure 52.3) and was BRAF codon 600 mutation positive.

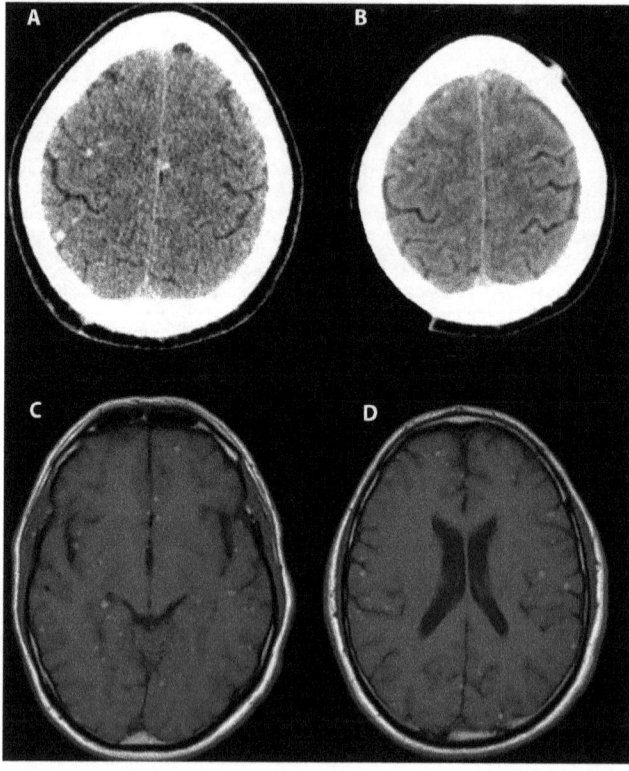

Figure 52.2 (A and B) A non-contrast CT scan of the brain showing multiple high-signal lesions in both hemispheres. (C and D) An axial non-contrast T1 MRI scan of the brain confirms multiple high-signal cerebral lesions

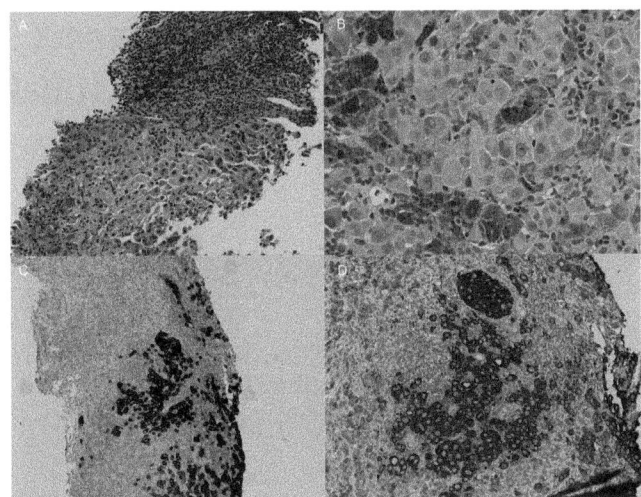

Figure 52.3 (A) Histology of the lymph node core shows infiltration by sheets, nests and single epithelioid cells with abundant eosinophilic cytoplasm and associated melanin pigment. (B) A closer ×20 magnification of the infiltrating cells shows them bearing large pleomorphic nuclei and notable cherry-red nucleoli. The diffuse and strong positivity for (C) melan A and (D) HMB45 immunohistochemistry are consistent with metastatic malignant melanoma

Diagnosis: Epilepsy Secondary to Cerebral Melanoma Metastases on Background of Left Axillary, Mediastinal and Bilateral Inguinal Melanoma Metastases

Management

Levetiracetam was started. Safety advice and UK Driver and Vehicle Licensing Agency (DVLA) regulations were explained.

After appropriate counselling, he was treated with pembrolizumab with dexamethasone cover as a palliative treatment. He received 43 cycles over 30 months.

He remained stable over the next three years off treatment. He returned to work as an electrician.

Comment

Brain Metastases

Melanoma frequency is increasing. It is a recognised cause of brain metastases. Breast, lung, colon and kidney cancers are other causes of brain metastases. Brain melanoma metastases tend to occur at the grey–white matter junction and vascular border zones in the cerebral hemispheres, particularly the frontal lobes.

However, advanced melanoma disease is less lethal because of advances in immunotherapy and targeted therapies since 2011 [1]. Treatment for metastatic melanoma has changed dramatically since then.

Melanoma Treatment

Standard surgical approaches are now markedly less invasive than previously advocated [1]. Safety margins depend on melanoma thickness and sentinel node biopsy can help in staging, as reported in 2017 by the American Joint Committee on cancer staging.

Of all solid tumours, melanoma has one of the highest mutational burdens. Drugs targeting the mitogen-activated protein kinase (MAPK) pathway (BRAF and MEK inhibitors) have improved the outcome for patients with metastatic melanoma. BRAF inhibition with dabrafenib plus the MEK inhibitor trametinib have improved survival in patients with unresectable or metastatic melanoma with *BRAF* V600E or V600K mutations. *BRAF* mutations occur in approximately 50% of patients with melanoma brain metastases, of which 90% are *BRAF* Val600Glu or V600E and 5% are Val600Lys or V600K. *BRAF* mutations cause constitutive activation of MAPK, which leads to proliferation, invasion and metastatic potential. Melanoma brain metastases can have additional variants not expressed in the primary lesion with interlesional and intralesional genomic heterogeneity [2].

The immune surveillance hypothesis of the 1950s led to clinical advances in inmmunooncology. In 2018, James P. Allison and Tasuku Honjo won the Nobel prize in physiology and medicine for their work on cancer immunotherapy. James P. Allison in California observed along with others that the T-cell protein known as cytotoxic T-lymphocyte antigen 4 (CTLA-4) functions as a brake on T-cells. In 1994, he used CTLA-4 antibodies to inhibit the brake in cancer in mice, and ultimately in 2010 an important clinical study showed promising results in advanced melanoma. Tasuku Honjo in Kyoto university had discovered that programmed cell death protein 1 (PD-1) was a surface protein on T-cells. Animal experiments had suggested that PD-1 blockade had a potential role in cancer treatment.

Receptor-ligand molecules, which dampen immune responses are known as immune checkpoints. Inhibitors of immune checkpoints of CTLA-4 can harness the immune system. The monoclonal antibody ipilimumab blocks CTLA-4 and was approved for treatment of advanced melanoma in 2011. Ipilimumab extended survival, although immune-based toxic effects (rash, thyroiditis, hepatitis and colitis) have been a limitation of CTLA-4 blockade.

Another checkpoint inhibitor emerged in the form of the pathway of PD-1, an inhibitory receptor expressed on activated tumour-specific CD4+ helper and CD8+ killer T-lymphocytes. The anti-PD-1 drug, nivolumab, demonstrated regression in a substantial proportion of advanced cancers including melanoma. Nivolumab or the combination of nivolumab and ipilimumab provided longer overall survival in advanced melanoma than ipilimumab alone. However, the combination of nivolumab and ipilimumab has a 14% risk of neurological immune-related adverse events (e.g. myositis, myasthenia gravis, acute and chronic inflammatory demyelinating polyradiculoneuropathy, aseptic meningitis and transverse myelitis).

The most common side effects of immune checkpoint inhibitors are dermatological and gastroenterological. Reported neurological adverse effects are three times more likely to affect the neuromuscular system (myositis, Guillain–Barré syndrome/peripheral neuropathies and myasthenia gravis) than the central nervous system (encephalitis and less frequently cerebellitis and myelitis) [3].

Pembrolizumab, another PD-1-blocking drug, used in our patient, has demonstrable antitumour activity and tolerability in advanced melanoma. Neurological immune-related adverse effects from monoclonal PD-1 antibodies occur in about 3% of treated patients.

It is recognised that somatic mutations alter the vulnerability of cancer cells to T-cell immunotherapy. Loss-of-function mutations in effector genes for CD8+ T-cells have been associated with resistance to cancer immunotherapy.

Advances in oncology have resulted in improved patient survival. Previously, patients with melanoma brain metastases had an overall one-year survival of approximately 20%; with the advances in systemic therapy patients with melanoma brain metastases now have over 80% one-year survival [2].

Uveal Melanoma

Uveal melanoma is distinct from cutaneous melanoma with different molecular drivers and tumour microenvironment. As a result, uveal melanoma is known to be less responsive to immune checkpoint inhibition. Fifty per cent of patients with uveal melanoma develop metastases, frequently in the liver with a median one-year survival of about 50%. However, even for uveal melanoma, molecules called immune-mobilising monoclonal T-cell receptors against cancer (ImmTAC) hold promise. An engineered high-affinity T-cell receptor targets a peptide-HLA complex on the target-cell surface. The same protein is fused to an anti-CD3 single chain variable fragment-activating domain. CD3 then recruits and activates polyclonal T-cells, releasing cytokines against the target cells. Tebentafusp is one such bi-specific protein or ImmTAC, which improves uveal melanoma survival. Oliver Sacks, the famous author and neurologist, died from metastatic uveal melanoma in 2015.

Fitness to Drive with Epilepsy and Metastatic Brain Melanoma

The UK guidance for medical doctors to assess fitness to drive is provided and updated by the DVLA (www.dvla.gov.uk/fitnesstodrive). There is guidance on different scenarios such as unprovoked seizures, permitted seizures and withdrawal of anti-epileptic medication. The first chapter deals with neurological disorders. Epilepsy features prominently as 'epilepsy is the most common cause for collapse at the wheel'. The guidance also includes a section on metastatic brain disease treated by immunotherapy or other targeted therapies. Relicensing for such patients with supratentorial brain disease can be considered one year after completion of primary treatment (or one year after starting targeted therapy if no other primary treatment for the intracranial disease has been given) if there is clinical and imaging evidence of disease stability or improvement, with no deterioration either intracranially or elsewhere in the body. If these criteria cannot be met, the DVLA state that driving must cease for two years.

References

1. Curti BD, Faries MB. Recent advances in the treatment of melanoma. *N Engl J Med.* 2021;384:2229–40.
2. Salvati L, Mandalà M, Massi D. Melanoma brain metastases: review of histopathological features and immune-molecular aspects. *Melanoma Manag.* 2020;7(2):MMT44.
3. Marini A, Bernardini A, Gigli GL et al. Neurologic adverse events of immune checkpoint inhibitors: a systematic review. *Neurology.* 2021;96(16):754–66.

Learning Points

- Melanoma can metastasise to the brain. Other cancers, which metastasise to the brain include lung, breast, colon and kidney.
- Better treatments for metastatic melanoma have emerged since 2011, particularly with immune checkpoint inhibitors.
- Cancer immunotherapy can improve overall long-term survival in a proportion of patients with melanoma metastases.
- Patients who want to drive but have epilepsy and brain metastases must be aware of the driving regulations for both conditions, and in the UK inform the DVLA.

Patient's Perspective

1. **What was the impact of the condition – seizures due to melanoma?**
   a. **Physical**
   Initially I struggled getting used to side effects of medication, i.e. levetiracetam. I experienced dizziness and headaches. I felt it affected my thought processes at times, which frustrated me.
   b. **Psychological (e.g. mood, future, emotional well-being)**
   I realised fairly early on that this was going to be a life-changing experience. I was anxious and worried; however I accepted the situation as best I could as ultimately, there was nothing I could do to change it.
   c. **Social (e.g. meeting friends, home)**
   I have a very close family and supportive friends who have been on this journey with me. This has helped me immensely.
2. **What could you not do because of the condition?**
   I could not drive, do safety critical work or work at heights.
3. **Was there any other change for you due the condition?**
   Frustration and irritation at times.
4. **What is/was the most difficult aspect of the condition for you?**
   Getting the diagnosis and the realisation of the consequences.

5. **Was any aspect of the experience good or useful? What was that?**

   I do not believe any aspect of the experience of this condition was good but it made me make some lifestyle changes, which I feel may be useful. These include diet and more daily exercise.

6. **What do you hope for in the future for this condition?**

   This is a difficult question for me to answer as my seizures were secondary to a diagnosis of melanoma. What I hope for the future for people diagnosed with melanoma would be more focused follow-ups, e.g. skin examinations plus imaging to detect the risk or early metastases.

   Neurologically my seizures are well controlled on levetiracetam and while I do not like taking medication on a daily basis, I realise I must continue. I hope for the future that there may be additional treatment options available that could possibly give insight re: the likelihood of a seizure occurring, through technology, thereby avoiding taking medication.

Presentation 1

History

A 34-year-old student nurse with a history of autoimmune polyendocrine syndrome type 1 with diabetes mellitus experienced stereotyped 'bizzing' sensations (not a noise) in her head with subsequent loss of consciousness. Within six months, four such events occurred. An eye-witnessed account suggested that she reached out to clutch or grab an object, her speech became confused and then she went rigid and blue. She frothed at the mouth with noisy respirations. There was twitching of her hands. The episodes typically lasted 90 seconds. She had bitten her tongue on two occasions but had not been incontinent. She was confused and disorientated for 90 minutes after the episodes. She had sustained at least one head injury as a consequence of the collapses. In two of the events, a blood glucose was recorded as normal. Corrected calcium was low at 1.94 mmol/L. She had some seizures when she was much younger, which were attributed to hypoglycaemia.

Investigations

An MRI scan of the brain was reviewed by a neuroradiologist and reported as showing signal abnormality in the left superior middle temporal gyri and left parietal opercular region (Figure 53.1A).

Management

She was treated with lamotrigine and responded well. On one occasion, when she was in hospital, she missed her medication and another epileptic seizure occurred. Subsequently, however, she became seizure-free and was allowed to drive as permitted by the UK Driver and Vehicle Licensing Agency (DVLA).

Presentation 2

History

Three months after starting lamotrigine, she underwent a cautery procedure on her tear ducts for dry eyes. Four days post-operatively, she developed acute left orbital pain, requiring opioid analgesia for symptomatic relief. Two days later, she developed diplopia on left lateral gaze. On examination, eye abduction was reduced in both eyes (70% abduction in the left eye but no abduction in the right eye), with reduced elevation of the left eye. Corneal sensation was intact as were the remaining cranial nerves. The ophthalmoplegia progressed to affect all extra-ocular muscles. Her left visual acuity had dropped to 6/18, right visual acuity 6/6^{-2}. An Ishihara plate reading was 15/17 from the right eye and 13/17 from the left eye.

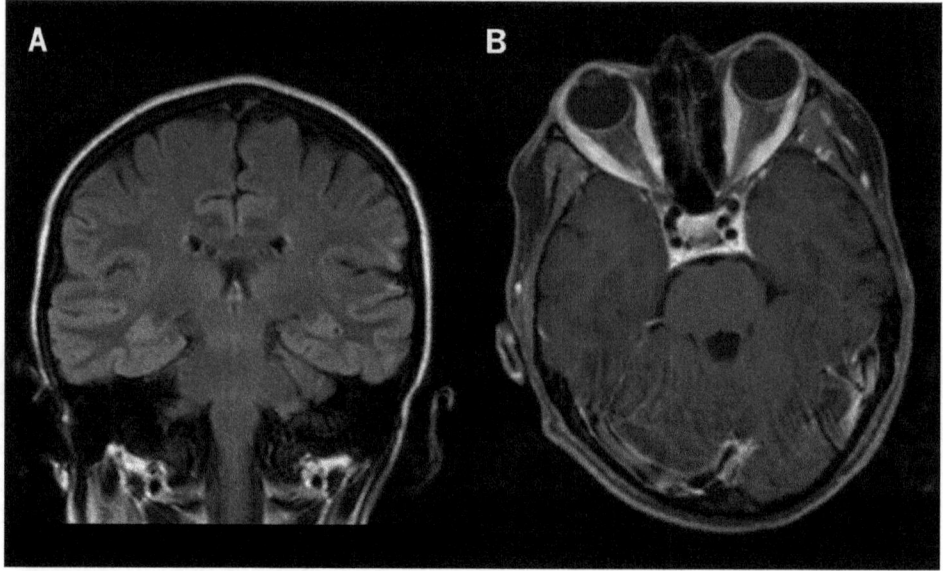

Figure 53.1 (A) A coronal T2 FLAIR MRI scan of the brain showing signal abnormality in the left superior middle temporal gyri and left parietal opercular region. (B) An MRI scan of her orbits with contrast and T1 fat suppression showing symmetrical enhancement of all extra-ocular muscles bilaterally.

Investigations

An MRI scan of her orbits with contrast and fat suppression revealed symmetrical enhancement of all extra-ocular muscles bilaterally (Figure 53.1B). This affected both the muscle belly and tendinous insertions onto the eyes.

Management

She was treated with intravenous methylprednisolone 500 mg/day for five days and then had an oral prednisolone taper. Over the next four months, the pain eased and then her left eye vision (6/12) and eye movements also improved. A prism was fitted to help with ongoing double vision.

Presentation 3

Seven years later, new events occurred. These were different from the previous epileptic seizures. The patient would abruptly stop talking with her mouth open and hold her breath. Head shaking occurred. The events lasted 20–40 seconds and were terminated with a gasp or deep breath. She was able to follow commands and had no loss of awareness. Video-EEG captured one such event; there was no EEG change before or after the event. Muscle artefact occurred during the event. The events stopped after an explanation of the diagnosis and she regained approval to drive as permitted to do so by the DVLA.

Past Medical History

The patient was diagnosed with autoimmune polyendocrine syndrome type 1 aged 3 years and diabetes mellitus aged 13 years. She had epileptic seizures then attributed to hypoglycaemia.

At the time of her first neurological assessment, she also had documented hypoparathyroidism, pancreatic exocrine failure, adrenal insufficiency, chronic renal impairment, vitiligo, pernicious anaemia, keratitis, recurrent candida infections including oesophageal candidiasis, primary ovarian failure, anaemia, iron overload, left renal calculus and gastroparesis. She had a left hip replacement aged 30 years. She did not smoke cigarettes and rarely drank alcohol.

Medications

She had an extensive list of medication including alfacalcidol, hydrocortisone, fludrocortisone, pancrelipase, clobazam, lamotrigine, hormone-replacement therapy, insulin preparations, hydroxocobalamin, prochlorperazine, esomeprazole, gaviscon and the iron chelator, deferasirox.

Investigations

In the *AIRE-1* gene she was homozygous for 13 base pair deletion in exon 8 (c.964del13).

Diagnoses: 1. Focal Onset Epilepsy with Secondary Generalisation

2. Orbital Myositis

3. Dissociative Attacks

Outcome

Multiple hospital admissions with increasing pathologies and complications occurred in her 40s. She became increasingly frail and died at the age of 45 years from sepsis secondary to community-acquired pneumonia.

Comment

Autoimmune Polyendocrine (Also Called Polyglandular) Syndromes

The autoimmune polyendocrine syndromes were first recognised by Martin Schmidt in 1926. The syndromes develop from impaired function of multiple endocrine glands due to a lack of immune tolerance [1]. Autoimmune polyendocrine syndrome type 1 is a rare autosomal recessive disease due to mutations in the autoimmune regulator gene (*AIRE-1*) on chromosome 21q22.3. In autoimmune polyendocrine syndrome type 1, at least two of three cardinal features emerge in childhood – mucocutaneous candidiasis, hypoparathyroidism and primary adrenal insufficiency (Addison's disease). All three features were present in our patient. Multiple other autoimmune diseases can emerge. Red cell aplasia meant that our patient was transfusion-dependent for some years and developed iron overload.

The 13 base pair deletion in exon 8 (c.964del13) of the *AIRE-1* gene appears to be a founder mutation in the British Isles [2]. This mutation causes a frameshift in the autoimmune regulator gene or *AIRE-1* [2].

Malfunctioning of the *AIRE-1* gene (expressed in the medulla of the thymus and in a rare population of peripheral dendritic cells) results in a lack of self-tolerance in which autoreactive T-cells escape deletion; this event seems to initiate autoimmune disease at a later stage [1]. The aire protein enhances regulatory T-cells known as Tregs in the thymus, which can suppress autoreactive cells. More than 100 *AIRE-1* mutations are known but the so-called Finnish major *AIRE* mutation (p.R257X) is prevalent in Finland, Russia and Eastern Europe, where autoimmune polyendocrine syndrome type 1 is more prevalent (about 1 in 25,000 in Finland).

Autoimmune polyendocrine syndrome type 2 is more common and milder than autoimmune polyendocrine syndrome type 1. It is polygenic with complex heritability and is characterised clinically by two of three features of type 1 diabetes mellitus, autoimmune thyroid disease and primary adrenal failure or Addison's disease [1].

Neurological Manifestations of Autoimmune Polyendocrine Syndrome

Autoimmune neurological disease has rarely been recognised in autoimmune polyendocrine syndrome type 1. Berger et al [3] reported Miller Fisher syndrome (also called anti-GQ1b syndrome) in a patient with autoimmune polyendocrine syndrome type 1. Another patient with autoimmune polyendocrine syndrome type 1 and Tolosa Hunt syndrome has also been described [3].

Autoimmune central nervous system demyelination, Guillain–Barré syndrome/Miller Fisher syndrome, autoimmune cerebellar ataxia, extra-pyramidal disorder secondary to basal ganglia calcification (unilateral choreathetosis and hemiballism) and myopathy have all been described in patients with autoimmune polyendocrine syndrome type 1 [3]. The endocrine and metabolic effects can have neurological consequences (e.g. B12 deficiency, hypothyroidism, vitamin E deficiency and coeliac disease).

Our patient also highlights how risk factors can interact or summate to trigger seizures. The brain insult may have been due to a head injury. Structural brain lesions are a risk factor for epileptic seizures as is hypocalcaemia. The development of dissociative seizures may have been associated with the psychological burden of increasing illnesses, which can occur particularly in patients with autoimmune polyendocrine syndrome type 1.

The co-ordination of medical services for complex patients with rare conditions remains a huge challenge, but as testified in the Perspective, patients and their families need a 'captain of the ship' to navigate a fragmented health service.

References

1. Husebye ES, Anderson MS, Kampe O. Autoimmune polyendocrine syndromes. *N Engl J Med.* 2018;378:1132–41.

2. Pearce SHS, Cheetham T, Imrie H et al. A common and recurrent 13-bp deletion in the autoimmune regulator gene in British kindreds with autoimmune polyendocrinopathy type 1. *Am J Hum Genet.* 1998;63(6):1675–84.

3. Berger JR, Weaver A, Greenlee J. Neurologic consequences of autoimmune polyglandular syndrome type 1. *Neurology.* 2008;70(23):2248–51..

Learning Points

*   Autoimmune polyendocrine syndrome type 1 is an autosomal recessive condition due to mutations in the *AIRE* gene.
*   Autoimmune polyendocrine syndrome type 1 has three distinct features – primary adrenal failure, hypoparathyroidism and mucocutaneous candidiasis.
*   Neurological illness can occur in patients with autoimmune polyendocrine syndrome.
*   Dissociative attacks can occur in patients with multiple neurological pathologies. It is not unusual for epileptic and dissociative seizures to occur in the same patient.
*   Co-ordinating medical care for rare and multisystem disease is a challenge for a fragmented health service.

Perspective from Patient's Mother

1   **What was the impact of the condition on your daughter?**

    a. Physical (e.g. practical support)
    B was diagnosed at three years of age with autoimmune polyglandular syndrome type 1. Her older sister had also been diagnosed with same condition when she was three years old.

    When B was three years old her care and management was my responsibility. The impact in early days was one of admissions to hospital to confirm the diagnosis. A new facet of the condition for her life was one of hospital admissions, which she took in her stride. In between hospital admissions she was positive and had a normal childhood.

b. Psychological (e.g. mood, emotional well-being)

B was diagnosed with diabetes mellitus when she was 13 years old. This was a changing moment. Her diabetes was very brittle and a low blood sugar always resulted in a seizure in spite of how fast we reversed the hypo with glucose. B and I had a lot of sleepless nights.

B was referred to a neurologist for seizures in adulthood and was commenced on anti-epileptic medication. This treatment controlled her seizures. Psychologically this had a very positive effect on B, who was by nature a very extrovert and bubbly person.

c. Social (e.g. meeting with friends)

B was an ultra-social person involved in musicals, Feis (festivals of music and dance), choirs, went to Ulster University in Portstewart and completed a degree in Theatre Studies. Her cup was always half full, never half empty.

2. **What could she not do because of the condition?**

   This condition is one of destruction of all endocrine glands. She developed orbital myositis resulting in double vision. B could not drive until it was eventually corrected by wearing glasses with a prism. Her car was her independence and she did not appreciate being told not to drive

   Nurse B always wanted to do nursing and I, being a nurse, didn't encourage her. She was six weeks from completing her nursing degree course with her final hospital placement when she was diagnosed with red cell aplasia. This necessitated blood transfusion every two weeks. The university held her place for two years but her condition worsened and she was unable to complete her training; she was heartbroken.

3. **Was there any other change for your daughter due to her medical conditions?**

   B was working in stage management in Edinburgh, where her younger sister lived who also had autoimmune polyglandular syndrome, and was studying speech and language therapy. B at this time was having a lot of pain in her hip and she had a hip replacement in Edinburgh when she was 30 years old. She very quickly mobilised and came home to recover. She then made the decision she was going to apply to Magee University to do her nursing degree.

4. **What was the most difficult aspect of the condition for your family and daughter?**

   Autoimmune polyglandular syndrome is extremely rare condition caused by a recessive gene. The medical profession was not very knowledgeable about it. All three of my girls had it so I was the victim of my own success, and their entire management was left to me; this was a very lonely place at times. GP answer to any query was to send them into hospital and my aim was to keep them out of hospital, so I had to make a lot of decisions on my own.

   Hospital admissions were a disaster. B had 15 consultants but there was no correspondence between them and each one was only interested in his/her piece of jigsaw regardless of what I knew was going to have an adverse effect on another part. This was very frustrating for me and B, who could see the big picture.

5. **Was any aspect of the condition good or useful? What was that?**

   This chronic condition has many challenges because it's forever changing for the worse and we were always having to cope with another new diagnosis. It encouraged my daughters to be positive and knowledgeable about their condition and not to tolerate arrogance from medical professionals who unfortunately were sometimes unprofessional and bluffing their way.
   All three girls were very successful in their careers but the condition took their lives prematurely.

6. **What do you hope for the future for people with this condition?**

   I hope that on admission to hospital there would be a named consultant who could provide direct access to ward and liaise with other consultants involved in the care of that individual.

   Medical profession to be more knowledgeable and to listen to the patient and their family about ongoing care.

Not a Minor Problem

History

A 59-year-old man was driving to work at 08:20 hrs when he noticed that he had difficulty manoeuvring the gearstick of his car with his left hand. When he arrived at work, he was unsteady walking towards a colleague. An ambulance was called and he arrived in his local hospital emergency department at 09:15 hrs. A thrombolysis call was activated.

Past medical history included headaches. At one stage, he had been taking amlodipine for hypertension. His only current medication was omeprazole. He was an ex-smoker (previous 20 pack year history) and drank no more than 10 units of alcohol per week. He had no history of diabetes mellitus. His father had had strokes in his 60s. He was married with two children.

Examination

In the emergency department, he was alert and orientated. He was hypertensive at 190/108 mmHg. His pulse was 82 beats per minute and regular. His temperature was 37°C. He had mild left finger-nose and left heel-shin ataxia. He had a mild left lower leg sensory deficit. His National Institute of Health Stroke Scale (NIHSS) score was 3 (2 for ataxia in two limbs and 1 for sensory deficit).

Investigations

An ECG showed sinus rhythm and a heart rate of 76 beats per minute. An emergency CT brain showed no hyperdense vessel, no haemorrhage and no loss of the grey-white matter differentiation. An MRI scan of the brain showed multiple foci of restricted diffusion and hyperintense FLAIR signal in the right cortical and subcortical parietal lobe (Figures 54.1A and 54.1B). A CT angiogram showed a 75% right carotid stenosis (Figures 54.1C and 54.1D).

Management and Outcome

He was not treated with intravenous thrombolysis as it was felt he had a mild event. He was given dual antiplatelet therapy (aspirin 300 mg and clopidogrel 300 mg stat) with a plan to reduce both to 75 mg thereafter and to stop aspirin on day 21.

On the day of his assessment, he was referred to a vascular surgery team. Six days later, he had a right carotid endarterectomy without complication.

Fifteen months later, he still had lethargy and had some concentration difficulties but had been well enough to go back to work.

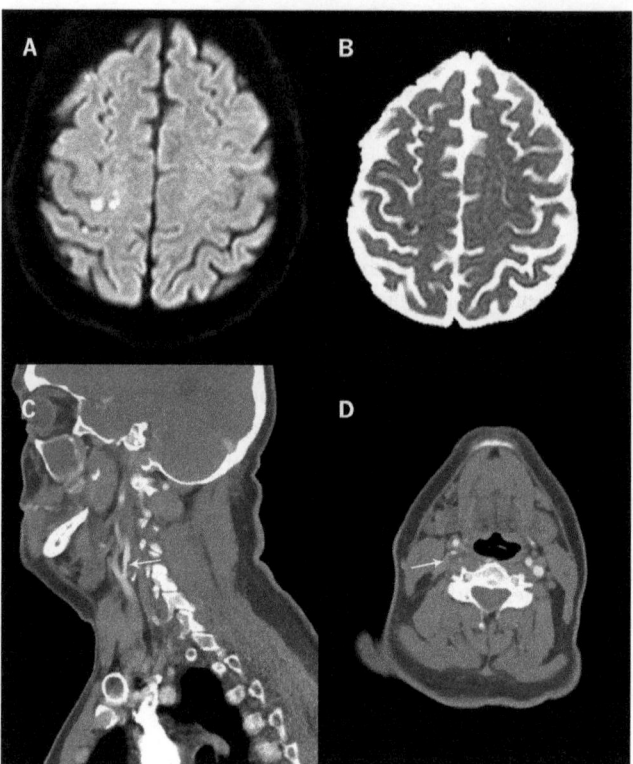

Figure 54.1 An axial MRI scan of the brain with (A) diffusion and (B) apparent diffusion coefficient map demonstrating areas of restricted diffusion in the right hemisphere. (C) A parasagittal and (D) axial CT angiogram showing right internal carotid artery markedly narrowed near its origin

Diagnosis: Right Hemisphere Diffusion-Restricted Infarctions – Minor Stroke

Comment

Transient Ischaemic Attack/Stroke Definition

A transient ischaemic attack or TIA is a sudden clinical deficit of presumed vascular origin lasting less than 24 hours due to focal brain, spinal cord or retinal ischaemia. Most patients have symptoms for seconds to minutes and have complete resolution of symptoms within one hour. Transient ischaemic attack is of clinical importance because up to 25% of ischaemic stroke patients have a preceding TIA, frequently within two days of the stroke. With appropriate treatment, the risk of stroke within 90 days is estimated to drop from 15% to 5%. The frontloading of the risk of stroke following TIA highlights the need for urgent diagnosis and treatment.

The clinical diagnosis of TIA relies on a history of symptoms. The neurological deficit usually lasts less than one hour and frequently no more than a few minutes. A so-called definite TIA includes symptoms such as dysphasia or dysarthria, homonymous hemianopia or monocular blindness, a sensory deficit in face and one limb or in two limbs, a motor deficit in one limb and the face or in two limbs [1]. A patient with more than one symptom in the possible category (unsteady gait, diplopia, vertigo or dizziness and dysphagia) suggests definite TIA [1]. Isolated amnesia, confusion and transient loss of consciousness are not usually thought of as TIAs. Clinicians may differ on a clinical diagnosis of TIA, but such discrepancies are less frequent among stroke experts [2]. It is for this reason that recording a history of TIA should be supplemented with details of the neurological deficit and duration (e.g. TIA – left arm and left leg numbness and weakness for six minutes).

An ischaemic event not visible on appropriate (diffusion-weighted MRI) and timely (within ten days) brain imaging has become the revised 'tissue-based' definition of TIA [1]. The American Heart Association and the American Stroke Association therefore now define TIA as a brief episode of neurological dysfunction with a vascular cause, with clinical symptoms typically lasting less than one hour, and without evidence of infarction on imaging.

The WHO definition of a stroke is a syndrome of 'rapidly developed clinical signs of focal (or global) disturbance of cerebral function, lasting more than 24 hours or leading to death, with no apparent cause other than of vascular origin' [3]. Restricted diffusion on MR imaging even in the presence of transient symptoms constitutes a 'tissue-based' diagnosis of stroke. Up to a third of patients imaged with TIA symptoms have evidence of infarcted brain tissue. Arterial spin labelling MRI may improve the yield of perfusion-weighted imaging for detecting acute ischaemic lesions. Restricted diffusion on an MRI brain scan fulfills the American Heart Association and American Stroke Association definition of stroke or central nervous system (CNS) infarction (i.e. pathological, imaging or other objective evidence of infarction). This has implications for stroke epidemiology, particularly as many parts of the world do not have access to MR imaging.

Some of the most comprehensive epidemiology of TIA has emerged from the Oxford Vascular study, which showed an incident rate of TIA half the incident rate of ischaemic stroke. Modern analyses suggest the risk of stroke after a TIA ranges from 3.9% to 7.4% at 90 days.

TIA Mimics

Table 54.1 itemises conditions diagnosed in one general hospital TIA clinic. These conditions mimic TIA presentations and are frequent diagnoses at clinics or ambulatory settings for patients with suspected TIA. Migraine with aura, migraine aura and epilepsy are the most frequent alternative explanations for transient neurological symptoms. The differential diagnosis of TIA usually consists of conditions managed by a neurologist. To avoid onward patient referrals, neurologists working in acute stroke clinics and 'TIA clinics' can ensure timely diagnosis and follow-up for a wide range of TIA mimics without fragmenting health care.

Clinico-anatomical Correlation

The history is crucial to make a diagnosis of TIA. Language abnormalities can be a lateralising clue. Double vision can be a clue for a posterior circulatory event. A paramedian thalamic lesion can cause diplopia from a vertical upgaze palsy. The thalamus with its vascular supply from the posterior circulation and multiple nuclei can have many different sensorimotor and behavioural stroke presentations.

Following a TIA, a clinical examination in a patient is often normal. Some clinical signs can suggest persisting cerebral or brainstem dysfunction in patients with minor strokes. An extensor plantar response (Babinski sign) is a sensitive indicator of corticospinal involvement in the brain or spine. More recently, an upgoing thumb sign or Hachinski sign has been documented as a sensitive and reliable indicator of brain involvement in patients with TIA or minor stroke. The upgoing thumb sign is elicited with eyes closed and hands raised to the level of the shoulders when an elevated thumb is associated with contralateral brain involvement). It is important to note that an upgoing thumb sign has also been documented in stroke mimics.

Table 54.1 TIA mimics identified in Altnagelvin hospital

TIA mimic
Migraine (migraine with aura and migraine aura)
Epilepsy (small vessel disease and brain tumour)
Peripheral vertigo
Transient global amnesia
Hypoglycaemia
Presyncope and postural hypotension
Multiple sclerosis (transient dystonic posturing)
Cervical spondylosis (and myelopathy)
Peripheral nerve injury (e.g. radial nerve palsy)
Myasthenia gravis
Cerebral amyloid angiopathy-transient focal neurological events
Subdural haemorrhage
(Convexity) subarachnoid haemorrhage
Reversible cerebral vasoconstriction syndrome

Risk stratification

A risk stratification scheme had been used since the early 2000s in an attempt to stratify risk of stroke following a TIA. Although validated, the $ABCD^2$ score (A for age, B for blood pressure, C for clinical speech or limb involvement, D^1 for duration and D^2 for the presence of diabetes mellitus) did not always identify high-risk carotid stenosis-TIA patients. It is now recognised that all patients with a suspected TIA should be assessed immediately to identify risk factors (extracranial carotid stenosis, intracranial artery stenosis or atrial fibrillation) that elevate their risk of stroke irrespective of the $ABCD^2$ score.

Investigations

Once a clinical diagnosis of TIA has been made, investigations should seek to exclude mimics and identify risk factors, which will direct management. Patients with a recent diagnosis of TIA require an ECG, CT angiogram or MR angiogram or Doppler of carotid and vertebral arteries. If an embolic source is suspected, prolonged heart monitoring is advised for suspected embolic aetiology. A bubble transthoracic echocardiograph or trans-oesophageal echocardiograph can help identify and characterise a patent foramen ovale or atrial thrombus. Acute ischaemic stroke in young patients may be cryptogenic even after extensive investigations.

Evidence-Based Management of TIA and Ischaemic Stroke

Timely intervention in patients with a diagnosis of TIA is required to reduce the risk of subsequent stroke. Dual antiplatelet or anticoagulant (for atrial fibrillation) therapy, targeted statin therapy and carotid endarterectomy (for symptomatic carotid stenosis TIA) can all decrease the risk of subsequent vascular complications including stroke [1]. The evidence base for prompt treatment of suspected TIA has been enhanced with the recognition that dual antiplatelet therapy (aspirin and clopidogrel or aspirin and ticagrelor) and targeted statin therapy all enhance outcome (Table 54.2). Anticoagulation has been well established as therapy for stroke due to atrial fibrillation. However, a non-lacunar infarct without proximal arterial stenosis or cardioembolic sources (i.e. absence of atrial fibrillation despite prolonged cardiac recording) classifies the stroke as an embolic stroke of undetermined source (ESUS). Anticoagulation in patients with ESUS has been shown to be no better than antiplatelet therapy, but ongoing research seeks to identify a group of ESUS patients who may benefit from anticoagulation.

A patent foramen ovale is found in 25% of the population. The recurrent risk of stroke in patients with otherwise cryptogenic stroke (patent foramen ovale-associated stroke) can be reduced with closure of the patent foramen ovale plus antiplatelet therapy. A moderate to large shunt and the presence of an atrial septal aneurysm may implicate a patent foramen ovale in ischaemic stroke aetiology. In one study, the number needed to treat to prevent one stroke in five years was 25. Patent foramen ovale closure results in a more than a ten-fold increase in atrial fibrillation during those five years to 1 in 15.

Thrombolysis for Minor Stroke

A minor stroke is usually defined as an NIHSS of ≤ 5. Guidelines suggest that intravenous thrombolysis is usually reserved for patients with disabling deficits. As thrombolysis rates have increased, patients with milder strokes have been treated with intravenous thrombolysis. Trial data have shown benefit from intravenous thrombolysis among patients with an NIHSS of ≤ 5, albeit less benefit than that observed in patients with more severe strokes.

Table 54.2 Management strategies for TIA/minor stroke

Intervention	Comment
TIA/minor stroke	
Antiplatelet therapy	Well established
Dual antiplatelet therapy	Immediate loading and then dual therapy for 21 days, or with intracranial arterial stenosis for 3 months
Anticoagulation (for atrial fibrillation)	Direct oral anticoagulant therapy
Carotid endarterectomy	Most risk reduction achieved with surgery within two weeks
Statin therapy	Low-density lipoprotein <1.8 mmol/L
Blood pressure	<140/80 mmHg target or <130/80 mmHg for patients with lacunar stroke or diabetes mellitus
Smoking	Rapid and considerable stroke risk reduction. Light smokers (<20 cigarettes/day) can reduce stroke risk to that of never smokers within five years
Exercise	Reduces stroke risk factors such as cholesterol, body mass index and blood pressure
Other lifestyle interventions such as reduced alcohol intake and weight reduction	
Screen for sleep apnoea	Emerging evidence of continuous positive airway pressure but poorly tolerated
Patent foramen ovale closure	Moderate to large shunt, atrial septal defect (risk of paradoxical embolism and patent foramen ovale-associated stroke causal likelihood determinants) and otherwise cryptogenic stroke

However, the PRISMS trial in patients with an NIHSS of 0–5 did not show any benefit from alteplase over aspirin in increasing the likelihood of a favourable functional outcome. An Austrian stroke registry study found that thrombolysis for very mild symptoms (an NIHSS of 0–1) did not increase the likelihood of an excellent outcome compared to conservative management, and moreover treated patients were more likely to suffer early neurological deterioration. Like many aspects of acute stroke management, advanced imaging looking for large vessel occlusion may help estimate the risk-benefit ratio of thrombolysis treatment for an individual patient with an acute but minor ischaemic stroke [4].

Driving Issue

The UK Driver and Vehicle Licensing Agency advises no driving for four weeks after a TIA or minor stroke. Driving after a stroke can resume if residual deficit does not impair driving.

References

1. Amarenco P. Transient ischemic attack. *N Engl J Med.* 2020;382(20):1933–41.
2. Lee S, Aw K, McVerry F, McCarron M. Systematic review and meta-analysis of diagnostic agreement in suspected TIA. *Neurol Clin Pract.* 2020;11(1).
3. Aho K, Harmsen P, Hatano S et al. Cerebrovascular disease in the community: results of a WHO collaborative study. *Bull World Health Organ.* 1980;58(1):113–30.
4. Ferrari J, Reynolds A, Knoflach M, Sykora M. Acute ischemic stroke with mild symptoms – to thrombolyse or not to thrombolyse? *Front Neurol.* 2021;12:1–8.

Learning Points

- Transient ischaemic attack is a clinical diagnosis based on a history of a sudden clinical deficit of presumed vascular origin lasting less than 24 hours, but usually seconds to minutes, due to focal brain, spinal cord or retinal ischaemia.
- About a third of patients with a TIA have a focal area of restricted diffusion on an MRI scan of the brain performed within 10 days of the TIA.
- Documentation of TIA should include symptoms, duration and if available, a negative MRI brain diffusion finding.
- Early interventions in patients with TIA or minor stroke (antithrombotic treatment including dual antiplatelet therapy) decrease the risk of subsequent stroke.
- A range of other secondary prevention strategies (smoking cessation, blood pressure control, statin therapy, carotid endarterectomy, avoiding excess alcohol and probably exercise) is often recommended to reduce longer-term stroke risk in patients with TIA or minor stroke.

Patient's Perspective

1. **What was the impact of the condition on you?**

   a. Physical (e.g. practical support, work, activities of daily living)
   Loss of power in left arm and slightly blurry vision from left eye

   b. Psychological (e.g. mood, emotional well-being)
   Very down and emotional with severe mood swings for a few months.

   c. Social (e.g. meeting friends, home)
   For a good few months, I didn't want to see people or meet anyone only my family and grandchildren.

2. **What can you not do because of the condition?**
   I can do most things but my left arm gets weak and has a slight loss of power.

3. **Has there been any other change for you due to the condition?**
   My fatigue has slightly improved but I still get tired very quickly.

4. **What is/was the most difficult aspect of the condition for you?**
   I have found it very hard reading, writing, spelling, texting as I lose my place and can't concentrate as well.

5. **Was any aspect of the experience good or useful? What was that?**
   I found out after my stroke that I had a few other underlying health problems, which have now been sorted, e.g. blood pressure, headache and cholesterol issues.

6. **What do you hope for in the future for people with this condition?**
   I hope that people go to their GP, as I didn't take heed of the signs. My wife and daughter were always saying about my fatigue, headache, moods, redness of face and neck and temper as it was not normal for a man of 59 years to be like that. I didn't talk much and bottled everything inside.

History

A 22-year-old male driver who worked as an electrician presented with a generalised seizure. He had felt dizzy just before he lost consciousness and was observed to have limb- and body-shaking for less than a minute. He took 45 minutes to fully recover. He had not bitten his tongue and had not been incontinent.

Medical history included a fractured right distal radius in a go-carting accident when he was 10 years old. He smoked three or four cigarettes per day and drank no alcohol. He had two children.

Examination

General and neurological examinations were normal.

Investigation

An MRI scan of the brain with contrast was performed (Figure 55.1). A diagnostic procedure was performed.

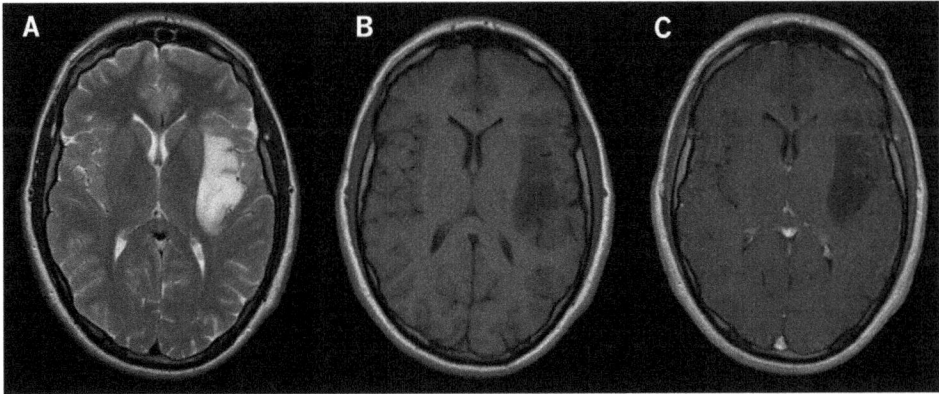

Figure 55.1 (A) An axial T2 MRI scan of the brain at the level of the basal ganglia showing high signal in the left perinsular region. (B) An axial T1 MRI brain scan at the same level shows low signal, which (C) does not enhance with contrast

Diagnosis: Focal-Onset Seizure Secondary to Probable Low-Grade Glioma

Management and Outcome

He was started on levetiracetam and advised not to drive. Other safety precautions were explained, including advice to avoid baths. He underwent a two-staged debulking of the left insular tumour via a left frontotemporal craniotomy. Both procedures were completed within a month. No neurological deficit occurred.

Four months later, he described a fullness in his left ear, then very quickly experienced a transient sensory disturbance down his right arm and right leg. Two such events occurred on the same day. The dose of levetiracetam was slowly increased from 500 mg bd to 1,000 mg bd.

Tumour histology revealed a grade 2 astrocytoma (isocitrate dehydrogenase or *IDH* mutant).

Pathology Description

Diffuse astrocytoma

IDH (nicotinamide adenine dinucleotide phosphate or NADP) mutant

Methylated-DNA-protein-cysteine methyltransferase (MGMT) promoter: no methylation

Chromosome 1p/19q: retained

Chromosome 7p and epidermal growth factor receptor (*EGFR*): no gain and no amplification

Telomerase reverse transcriptase (*TERT*) promoter: technically unsuccessful

Chromosome 10q: retained

Histone H3F3A: no mutation

BRAF (V600E): no mutation

The 2021 WHO classification of tumours recommends a layered report structure

Integrated diagnosis: diffuse astrocytoma, *IDH* mutant

Histopathological classification: astrocytoma

Central nervous system (CNS) WHO grade: 2

Molecular information: *IDH* mutant

The patient developed sudden mood swings on levetiracetam. Lamotrigine was added but he developed a rash on this drug. Sodium valproate was added without complication and levetiracetam was withdrawn. He did well and had no seizures for over a year. He was informed of the epilepsy and grade 2 glioma implications for driving. The UK Driver and Vehicle Licensing Agency guidance involves a driving ban until one year seizure-free *and* an individual with grade 1 or 2 glioma cannot drive until one year from completion of primary treatment. A further seizure ensued with speech arrest and tonic-clonic seizure activity. Valproate was increased to 1,500 mg per day. Imaging surveillance revealed stable appearances.

Focal seizures recurred (dizziness, dysphasia and tingling in his right leg). Lacosamide was added to valproate. Four months later, more seizures occurred. Valproate was increased to 2,000 mg per day and lacosamide increased to 200 mg bd.

Three years after his surgery, imaging surveillance demonstrated tumour growth. Because of ongoing seizures, a third anti-epileptic drug, brivaracetam was added. Further surgical debulking was performed (under general anaesthesia as it was not tolerated awake), which caused significant expressive and receptive dysphasia. Pathology again confirmed WHO grade 2 *IDH1* mutant astrocytoma. Neuro-oncology suggested radiotherapy (54 Gray in 30 fractions) and then adjuvant procarbazine, lomustine and vincristine (PCV) chemotherapy. At last review he had been 10 months seizure-free.

Comment

Glioma Epidemiology and Treatment Advances

The age-adjusted incidence of gliomas is 4.2–5.2 per 100,000 per year. European populations are more affected with gliomas than Asian populations. Survival relates to histological malignancy grading: pilocytic astrocytoma (grade 1) has the best survival while the poorest survival occurs in glioblastoma multiforme (grade 4), which comprises the largest proportion of gliomas with an age-adjusted incidence of 3.16–3.21 per 100,000 per year. Histological grading is now usually quoted in Arabic numerals to reduce error and ensure a uniform approach. Anaplastic astrocytoma and glioblastoma multiforme increase in incidence with age. The Stupp protocol published in 2005 was a landmark study demonstrating for the first time a treatment benefit for the most lethal glioma, gliobastoma multiforme: temozolomide and post-operative radiotherapy increased median survival from 12.1 to 14.6 months.

Another advance in neuro-oncology came in 2012 for low-grade gliomas. Early surgical resection of low-grade gliomas was shown to be associated with improved overall survival compared to a biopsy and watchful waiting. This was the rationale for our patient's initial surgical treatment interventions.

Glioma 2021 WHO Classification

Tumour classification historically relied on histological morphology plus grading based on mitoses, vascular endothelial proliferation and necrosis. Molecular sub-typing was incorporated into the 2016 WHO brain tumour pathology classification. The 2021 WHO classification builds on the use of molecular analyses, particularly using the *IDH1/2* mutant status and the chromosome 1p/19q co-deletion status [1]. Histopathology and molecular analysis are now required to determine tumour grade.

The 2021 WHO classification of tumours of the CNS aims to provide more effective communication of diagnostic and prognostic information. To do so, further advances in molecular diagnostics have been included in the classification while retaining the importance of histology and immunohistochemistry.

Molecular Markers

IDH1 (IDH (NADP) cytoplasmic) or *IDH2* (IDH (NADP) mitochondrial) have been shown to be associated with some types of glioma; collectively, these are known as *IDH* mutations. The 2021 WHO classification for adult diffuse gliomas necessitates this marker because there are markedly varying survivals from tumours of similar histopathology but different *IDH* status.

Methylated-DNA-protein-cysteine methyltransferase repairs the DNA damage caused by temozolomide, reducing its efficacy. The presence of epigentic silencing of MGMT by promoter methylation has been shown to improve survival. Such information and therapeutic responses dependent on molecular information has continued to contribute to the classification of diffuse gliomas.

For adult brain tumours, there are a few changes in the 2021 WHO brain tumour classification. Previously, glioblastomas were diagnosed based on the histological findings of microvascular proliferation and/or necrosis and included *IDH*-mutant and *IDH* wild-type tumours. For adults, the 2021 WHO classification of glioblastoma comprises only *IDH* wild-type tumours.

Astrocytoma *IDH*-wild type in adults without histologic features of glioblastoma but possessing one or more of three genetic parameters (*TERT* promoter mutation, *EGFR* gene amplification, or combined gain of entire chromosome 7 and loss of entire chromosome 10) is now classified as glioblastoma.

Astrocytomas *IDH*-mutant are graded as 2, 3 or 4 according to molecular findings in the WHO 2021 classification. Grade 2 tumours are somewhat inert compared to the elevated mitotic rate of grade 3 tumours, greater cellular crowding and nuclear atypia. Grade 3 astrocytomas may also have multinucleated tumour cells and abnormal mitoses. The presence of *CDKN2A/B* homozygous deletion confers a worse prognosis and has a WHO grade 4 even in the absence of microvascular proliferation or necrosis.

In summary, pathologists produce a layered report providing an integrated diagnosis made up of the histopathological classification, the CNS WHO grade in Arabic numerals and the molecular information.

Risk Factors for Gliomas

There are very few non-genetic risk factors identified in the development of adult diffuse gliomas. Ionising radiation and monogenetic disorders account for a very small number of glioma cases. Intriguingly, a history of allergy such as eczema, hay fever and asthma has been associated with a decreased glioma risk. Pre-disposing genetic conditions include Li Fraumeni syndrome, neurofibromatosis type 1 (astrocytoma and optic nerve glioma), neurofibromatosis type 2 (ependymoma), Lynch syndrome (glioma including glioblastoma), Noonan syndrome (usually dysembryoplastic neuroepthelial tumour) and tuberouse sclerosis (subependymal giant cell astrocytoma).

Treatment of Focal Seizures and Status Epilepticus

Seizures occur in 40–60% of patients with brain tumours. Recurrence or worsening of seizures may signal tumour progression. Surgery, radiotherapy and chemotherapy all contribute to seizure control. The efficacy and tolerability of anti-epileptic drugs in glioma patients has low-quality published evidence because of heterogenous populations – tumour histology, location and concomitant medications – and study design. Levetiracetam has shown the lowest treatment failure rate [2]. Sodium valproate is usually suggested as the second choice for recurring seizures. Thereafter, lacosamide, lamotrigine or zonisamide are additional options. However, a third of brain tumour-related epilepsy patients demonstrate pharmacoresistance, adding to the burden of living with a brain tumour.

Patients can present in status epilepticus. A trial (ESETT published in 2019) using levetiracetam, fosphenytoin or valproate for benzodiazepine-refractory convulsive status epilepticus led to seizure cessation and improved alertness by 60 minutes in about 50% of patients. Just 2% of the patients had a brain tumour implicated in the aetiology of their status epilepticus. About 10% had dissociative seizures. The dosing regime used – levetiracetam 60 mg/kg (maximum of 4,500 mg), fosphenytoin 20 mg phenytoin equivalent/kg (maximum of 1,500 mg phenytoin equivalent) and valproate at 40 mg/kg (maximum of 3,000 mg) – highlights the importance of adequate doses of medications. Refractory status epilepticus is defined as convulsive seizure activity not responding to two or more anti-seizure medications including one non-benzodiazepine drug. Super-refractory status epilepticus is status epilepticus that continues for ≥24 hours despite anaesthetic treatment or recurs on attempted weaning of the anaesthetic regimen.

Non-surgical Treatment of Low-Grade Gliomas
There is an emerging evidence base for treating low-grade gliomas. Patients with biologically favourable high-risk low-grade glioma are thought to derive most benefit (overall survival and progression-free survival) from radiotherapy and adjuvant PCV. The benefit was most marked in patients with tumours harbouring chromosome 1p/19q co-deletion and *IDH1* mutation.

Multidisciplinary Team Management of Glioma
Brain tumour patients benefit from multidisciplinary team management decisions. Neurosurgery, neuro-oncology, neuropathology, neuroradiology and neurology all have a role in optimising management in order to provide more co-ordinated patient care, timely treatment and more evidence-based treatment decisions; this is a national recommendation in the UK for all cancer care [3].

References
1. Whitfield BT, Huse JT. Classification of adult-type diffuse gliomas: impact of the World Health Organization 2021 update. *Brain Pathol*. 2022;32(4):e13062.
2. De Bruin ME, Van Der Meer PB, Dirven L, Taphoorn MJB, Koekkoek JAF. Efficacy of antiepileptic drugs in glioma patients with epilepsy: a systematic review. *Neuro-oncology Pract*. 2021;8(5):501–17.
3. Taylor C, Munro AJ, Glynne-Jones R et al. Multidisciplinary team working in cancer: what is the evidence? *BMJ*. 2010;340(7749):743–5.

Learning Points
- Brain tumours can present with epileptic seizure activity.
- Brain tumour classification has evolved to include not only histology and immunohistochemistry but also molecular diagnostics to improve diagnostic grading and prognostic information.
- Treatments for low-grade glioma and glioblastoma are improving.
- Although of low quality, there is evidence that levetiracetam has been associated with the lowest treatment failure rate in patients with seizures due to brain tumour.

Patient's Perspective
1. **What is the impact of the condition on you?**
   a. Physical (e.g. practical support, work, activities of daily living)
   As I can take seizures at any time, I have to have someone with me at all times. I lost my job as a digger/tractor driver.
   b. Psychological (e,g, mood, emotional well-being)
   My mood is low most of the time – I can get agitated very easily.
   c. Social (e.g. meeting friends, home)
   I don't go far from home. I get anxious if out of my comfort zone.
2. **What can you not do because of the condition?**
   I cannot drive and I cannot work with machinery.

3. **Has there been any other change for you due to the condition?**
    My speech has been affected and my confidence.
4. **What is/was the most difficult aspect of the condition for you?**
    Not knowing when a seizure is going to happen.
5. **Was any aspect of the experience good or useful? What was that?**
    I have found that I am a bit OCD now. I keep things tidy and in order.
6. **What do you hope for in the future for people with this condition?**
    That seizures can be stopped completely and tumours removed.

Perspectives

Neurological disorders are the leading cause of disability and the second leading cause of death worldwide. Population growth and ageing are leading to an increase in the number of people living with neurological disabilities and dying from neurological causes. Such epidemiological change should prompt better research into evidence-based prevention and health care [1]. Making an accurate diagnosis [2] and having an understanding of the patient journey are important components of a neurologist's job.

This book of neurology case reports developed from the diagnoses and the impact of neurological disorders on patients attending a neurology service in a district general hospital (Altnagelvin hospital) in Northern Ireland. The patients prompted the juxtapositioning of the medical history with the experience of living with a neurological disorder. The format allows for a more complete picture of a neurological diagnosis and living with the disorder, either as an acute one-off event with or without resulting disability and/or a chronic disorder with or without an unpredictable outcome for the individual. Some medical journals have employed a similar format but textbooks have not usually adopted the combined patient and doctor case report. Neurology with its many and varied diagnoses offers opportunities for such case histories.

Professor Richard Lehman from Birmingham, UK highlighted the lack of literature in this area in 2017.

> A selection of books about personal experiences of illness can be found in any large bookstore (or online). There may also be a selection of books by physicians describing their experience of practice. Very rarely, and generally only in a few articles in medical journals, have the two sets of experiences been aligned. [3]

Richard Lehman is a professor of the shared understanding of medicine, which is the fusion of evidence-based medicine, shared decision-making and patient-centred medicine.

Patient Perspective of Neurological Disorder

The experience of neurological illness from the perspective of patients, or where required, the relatives or carers, provides an insight into the real life impact of specific neurological diagnoses. While there may be variation even between patients with the same neurological disorder, this format for presenting different neurological disorders highlights common themes among neurological patients. Neurologists should be interested in acknowledging and exploring these consequences of neurological disorders, and helping patients navigate appropriate and timely help.

Patient-Reported Experience of Health Care

The perspectives sought to determine the impact of neurological disorders on individual patients (i.e. the perception of their own disease-related situation). However, the health care experienced by the patient inevitably makes a contribution to any reported experience of ill health. Patient-reported experience measures (PREMs) are used as tools to improve person-centred care. They can increase patient engagement in care and are associated with better outcomes. This has prompted health ministers from different countries in the Organisation for Economic Co-operation and Development (OECD) to promote PREMs, but many PREMs, even for a condition as common as stroke, have inadequate or unknown psychometric properties [4]. Real-time experiences that illustrate patient issues across a variety of neurological disorders may inform future PREMS.

A qualitative analysis of the patient perspective transcripts in this collection of case reports was performed to search for common themes for these patients and their families. In order to explore the relative importance of the themes, quantitative data were collected in order to record the frequency of each theme (a mixed analysis).

All patients or their relatives provided written informed consent or assent to publish the case histories and perspectives. Patients' perspectives were obtained from a series of questions with free text replies/comments. The case report and patient perspective were then combined and a final consent was obtained for each complete case report.

Analyses of Perspectives

A summary of the patient demographics and the classification of the neurological disorders are shown in the Table A.1.

The language of a patient with a medical disorder is very different from that of the medical assessment. Reporting a medical disorder has a different template – employing different words, technologies (imaging, antibodies, pathology features and genetics) – whereas the practical living experience for the individual patient is primarily a composite of the biopsychosocial template. In neurology, the problem is compounded by many uncommon or rare diagnoses and neurophobia (fear of the neurosciences and clinical neurology) among non-neurology medical staff including general practitioners [5, 6].

Seven themes were identified from an analysis of the patient perspective responses (Table A.2).

Table A.1 Demographic details of 55 neurological patients

Variable	Number
Mean age (SD)	47 (18.2) years
Male:female	31:24
Mean follow-up (SD)	6.6 (4.6) years
Neurological disorder category (%)	
• Metabolic	6 (11)
• Nutritional	2 (4)
• Vascular	12 (22)
• Immune	11 (20)
• Infective	5 (9)
• Neurodegenerative	6 (11)
• Neoplastic	6 (11)
• Miscellaneous	7 (15)

Table A.2 Summary of thematic analyses from 55 patient perspectives

Theme	Number (%)
Anxiety	16 (29)
Low mood	25 (45)
Social isolation	36 (65)
Loss of employment	7 (13)
Fatigue/tired/lack of energy	11 (20)
Earlier diagnosis	19 (35)
Research (cure or better treatments)	14 (25)

Anxiety was often present even in patients with transient and/or benign conditions. Uncertainty in diagnosis and prognosis particularly impacted quality of life. Delays in diagnosis seemed to worsen the experience of illness, with some relief occurring when the diagnosis was achieved. Low mood, although not formally assessed, was frequently reported. Patients reported loss of confidence, apathy and loneliness. Social isolation was described by nearly two-thirds of the patients. Stigma was another issue. Patients described reduced or restricted work ability. Many patients expressed the hope for a cure alongside the desire for more research and better treatments.

The findings confirm that timely and accessible psychological support are very important for patients with neurological illness.

Quality of Life in Patients with Neurological Conditions

The Neurological Alliance charity surveys have asked patients about their experience of their neurological condition and their health care service experience (www.neural.org.uk) These have shown that neurological conditions have a substantial negative impact on mental well-being, and have highlighted a lack of signposting of patients to mental well-being supports, a lack of explanation of the condition and the need for physical (books/videos/specialist team support) patient information rather than just a website address. The cases collected in *55 Cases in Neurology* demonstrate that this is a crucial aspect of care for neurological patients.

Interventions to Improve Quality of Life

A number of projects have emerged to help improve the experience of living with a neurological disorder. One such project is What Matters to You (www.whatmatterstoyou.scot).

What Matters to You started in Scotland in 2016 and is now a global phenomenon. It places an emphasis on personalised care by encouraging more meaningful conversations between those who provide health and social care and the people who receive care and support.

Neurologists' awareness of the need for education and patient empowerment with involvement in personalised health plans for chronic neurological conditions has prompted other initiatives. Neurologist Heather Angus-Lappan along with colleagues, patients, carers and digital engineers have created a web-based patient education tool (Confidence College) hosted by NHS England to enable patients to create personalised plans for epilepsy, multiple sclerosis and Parkinson's disease [7].

Research into the quality of life of patients with neurological illness is emerging. Trajectories of Outcome in Neurological Conditions (https://tonic.thewalton.nhs.uk) is one such large national UK research study in this area.

What *55 Cases in Neurology* Add

Personalised medicine aims to focus on the whole person as a unit of analysis [8]. As Rudolf Virchow urged, successful treatment of human suffering may require addressing social determinants of disease as much as the molecular biology of the same disease. The perspectives from the neurological patients in *55 Cases in Neurology* emphasise the need for effective psychological interventions at different stages of a neurological illness. The first part of that journey involves the neurologist adopting strategies in order to make the clinical encounter effective – preparation and focus prior to consultation, listening intently, agreeing on what matters most, connecting with the patient's story, and exploring emotional cues [9].

References

1. Feigin VL, Vos T, Nichols E et al. The global burden of neurological disorders: translating evidence into policy. *Lancet Neurol.* 2020;19(3):255–65.

2. Singh H, Connor DM, Dhaliwal G. Five strategies for clinicians to advance diagnostic excellence. *BMJ.* 2022;376:e068044.

3. Lehman R. Sharing as the future of medicine. *JAMA Intern Med.* 2017;177(9):1237–8.

4. Cornelis C, den Hartog SJ, Bastemeijer CM et al. Patient-reported experience measures in stroke care: a systematic review. *Stroke.* 2021;52(7):2432–5.

5. Loftus AM, Wade C, McCarron MO. Primary care perceptions of neurology and neurology services. *Postgrad Med J.* 2016;92(1088):318–21.

6. McCarron MO, Stevenson M, Loftus AM, McKeown P. Neurophobia among general practice trainees: the evidence, perceived causes and solutions. *Clin Neurol Neurosurg.* 2014;122:124–8.

7. Angus-Leppan H, Caulfield A, Moghim MM et al. Confidence College: an online education tool for neurology patients. *Adv Clin Neurosci Rehabil.* 2022;21(2):6–8.

8. Greene JA, Loscalzo J. Putting the patient back together: social medicine, network medicine, and the limits of reductionism. *N Engl J Med.* 2017;377(25):2493–9.

9. Zulman DM, Haverfield MC, Shaw JG et al. Practices to foster physician presence and connection with patients in the clinical encounter. *JAMA.* 2020;323(1):70–81.

Index

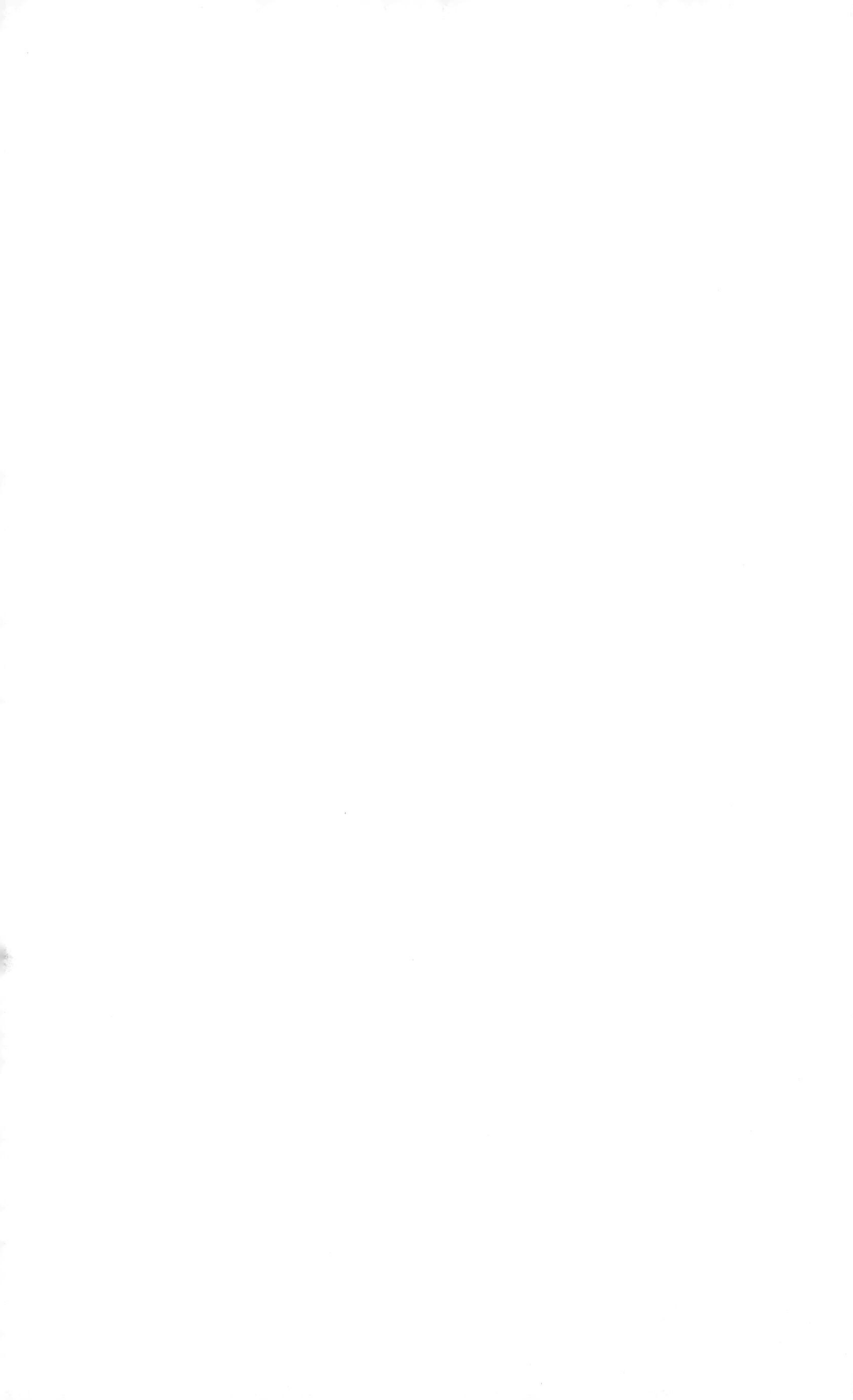

For EU product safety concerns, contact us at Calle de José Abascal, 56–1°, 28003 Madrid, Spain or eugpsr@cambridge.org.

www.ingramcontent.com/pod-product-compliance
Ingram Content Group UK Ltd.
Pitfield, Milton Keynes, MK11 3LW, UK
UKHW050729090126
466816UK00013B/257